AUSCULTATION
OF THE HEART

AUSCULTATION OF THE HEART

A Cardiophonetic Approach

T. Anthony Don Michael, M.D., F.R.C.P., F.A.C.C.

Clinical Professor of Medicine
University of California at Los Angeles
Central Cardiology Medical Clinic
Bakersfield, California

McGraw-Hill
Health Professions Division

New York   St. Louis   San Francisco   Auckland   Bogotá   Caracas   Lisbon
London   Madrid   Mexico City   Milan   Montreal   New Delhi   San Juan
Singapore   Sydney   Tokyo   Toronto

McGraw-Hill

A Division of The McGraw·Hill Companies

AUSCULTATION OF THE HEART: A Cardiophonetic Approach

Copyright © 1998 by *The McGraw-Hill Companies,* Inc. All rights reserved. Printed in the United States of America. Except as permitted under the United States Copyright Act of 1976, no part of this publication may be reproduced or distributed in any form or by any means, or stored in a date base or retrieval system, without prior written permission of the publisher.

1234567890 DOC DOC 9987

ISBN 0-07-018005-9

This book was set in Times Roman by TCSystems, Inc.
The editors were Joseph Hefta and Steven Melvin;
the production supervisor was Richard Ruzycka.

R. R. Donnelley and Sons, Inc., was the printer and binder.

Library of Congress Cataloging-in-Publication Data

Don Michael, T. Anthony
    Auscultation of the heart / T. Anthony Don Michael.
        p.   cm.
    Includes bibliographical references and index.
    ISBN 0-07-018005-9
    1. Auscultation.   2. Heart—Sounds.   3. Heart—Diseases—
Diagnosis.   I. Title.
        [DNLM: 1. Heart Auscultation—methods.   2. Stethoscopes.   WG
141.5.A9 D674a 1997]
    RC683.5A9D66   1997
    616.1′207544—dc21
    DNLM/DLC
    for Library of Congress   97-15124

CONTENTS

Foreword   *vii*

Preface   *xi*

Acknowledgments   *xiii*

Introduction   *xv*

1	Sound and Stethoscopes	1
2	The Basics of Auscultation	17
3	Hemodynamic Basis of Heart Sounds	51
4	Clinical Foundations of Auscultation	73
5	Eliciting Heart Sounds: Timing, Amplitude, and Pitch	113
6	Systolic and Diastolic Murmurs	161
7	Auscultation in Critical Care	219
8	Clinical Antecedents to Auscultation	247
9	Tests Adjunctive to Auscultation	301
10	Auscultation in the Care of Special Populations	315

Appendices

Cardiac Pearls   345
Abbreviations for Cardiac Terminology   353
Heart Sounds: Overview   354
Cardiophonetics   359

Index   *385*

FOREWORD

The art of clinical assessment of cardiac patients is alive, but in need of resuscitation. Current conditions of practice seldom allow the time necessary to conduct an appropriate initial evaluation. Younger practitioners in particular place their trust in laboratory tests rather than in the finer details of clinical history-taking and physical findings on clinical examination. Part of this attitude derives from the actual limitations of clinical assessment, but also in part from an overemphasis in training programs on the use of diagnostic procedures. This trend, which is certainly regrettable, has accelerated in the era of the super-specialist.

Clinical evaluation, on the other hand, is an efficient and inexpensive strategy providing diagnostic direction in all patients and complete diagnosis in many. It is indispensable in the selection of more precise methods of testing. Auscultation does, however, depend on human intention to use it as well as human skill and experience in its application. While auscultation is essential to a thorough cardiac examination, its techniques must be effectively taught and continuously practiced.

In addition to its diagnostic importance, auscultation is a skill that helps to conserve another scarce commodity in contemporary medicine— recognition of the interpersonal dimension of the healing arts. The abbreviation of history-taking to a short-answer questionnaire, and physical examination to a few check marks on a clipboard or computer screen reduces personal contact between doctor and patient—as does a follow-up recital of the latest test results, without even the simple civility of, "How do you feel today?" Are the taking of a detailed medical history, the meticulous physical examination, and the solicitous question obsolete in the practice of medicine today? Are the data obtained by personal attention to the patient of little value or even erroneous, lacking the qualities of specificity, sensitivity, positive-negative predictive accuracy, and the other "scientific" measures of statistical validation?

When my father was new to practice in the early 1920s, he once overheard a patient remark about him, "He's nice, but he needs experience. The old doctor never had to examine me at all!" This meant, of course, that the experienced physician was able to gather all the clinical information he needed and yet the patient was so at ease during the process that he didn't even realize that an examination was taking place. Nowadays, would the patient make the same comment about the young doctor, and instead and be literally correct in his observation?

As we enter the twenty-first century, the health care system in the United States is undergoing changes properly described as unprecedented in their extent and revolutionary in their implications. The coming of "managed care" has compelled physicians and other medical professionals to pay closer attention to efficient allocation of time and other resources. From this we can take a lesson from the field of mechanics, in which efficiency is defined in terms of "work output as a function of energy input." To wit, in health care, using our collective resources wisely serves as a desirable objective as long as this preserves and improves the physical, economic, and psychosocial well-being of patients.

The optimal practice of medicine depends on reaching and implementing sound therapeutic decisions rapidly and efficiently. These actions, in turn, require effective employment of necessary skills. From this perspective, cardiac auscultation is a particularly efficient process, not only in initial evaluation and diagnosis but, perhaps more importantly, in the ongoing management of cardiac patients. Indeed, a careful initial examination and testing by appropriate techniques—including echocardiography—with only occasional follow-up by a cardiologist will be cost-effective yet provide competent care. A conscientious primary care physician skilled in auscultation will recognize the signs of stability, improvement, or deterioration in his or her patients. Must every patient with valve disease have an echo examination? If so, how often? Cannot the relevant questions be posed and answered by clinical methods?

We have seen a steadily increasing tendency to delegate tasks and procedures once reserved to physicians to other members of the health care team. Much to the surprise of doctors in the 1970s, nurses, technicians, and physician assistants proved their expertise in the diagnosis and management of cardiac dysrhythmias in coronary care units. Could these professionals be trained in advanced cardiac auscultation? I, a physician and teacher of many years, see no reason why not—and to the degree that cardiologists and other M.D.s neglect auscultation, it becomes increasingly important that our fellow medical professionals should be so trained.

Cardiac auscultation is a venerable technique of clinical evaluation dating back to the mid-nineteenth century. Although auscultation was used by practitioners into the early part of the twentieth century, this diagnostic art came into its own only in the two decades following World War II. At that time the then-new technique of cardiac catheterization allowed for clinical-physiological correlations, and the definitions of strengths and limitations. Since the mid-1960s, pressure measurements, phonocardiography, and echocardiography have permitted the establishment of more precise relationships. In addition, these techniques allow clinicians to identify the physical characteristics of heart sounds and other intrathoracic auscultatory phenomena, and to relate these findings to other manifestations of disease.

These technological advances, however, have come at the price of relative neglect of auscultation. Until the recent past, stethoscopic virtuosity was the sine qua non of a clinical cardiologist. But times and fashion change. Will the new "high-tech" cardiologist spend the requisite time for a careful auscultatory examination, observing the effects of respiration, the Valsalva maneuver, and the effects of posture? Or will he or she consider it more effective to proceed to a 30-min echocardiographic examination, an angiogram, or an MRI?

In the coming era of limitation, restriction, or redirection of available resources, we must recognize the utility of relevant information obtained with minimal expense. Careful auscultation of cardiac patients is the key to effective care of the patient over the long-term, in that changes in auscultatory findings or clinical symptoms will direct the need for other studies, including echocardiograms, thallium tests, and the like. Although the necessity to return to the stethoscope is clear, young physicians, however, are not learning to auscultate. They deal with the patient according to other methods and criteria, perhaps even relegating cardiac auscultation to determining whether a patient is alive or dead.

It was not always so. I remember the late Dr. Paul Wood's remarkable confidence in the art of auscultation: "When I make the diagnosis, that is the diagnosis." Perhaps a bit of hyperbole had crept into that statement, to be sure, but it was correct with remarkable frequency. Should cardiac auscultation be revived? Yes, emphatically: When properly applied, the stethoscope is a highly effective piece of diagnostic equipment. But the clinical importance of auscultation and its skillful implementation must be expertly taught in training programs in internal medicine and cardiology. The skills so learned will make their practitioners more humane, more efficient, and wiser doctors.

Dr. Don Michael's book presents a new look at this long-established art, using innovative and advanced techniques. His most significant innovation reflects his love of music and his experience as an operatic tenor. The present work introduces a novel phonetic transcription of auscultatory findings that provides a powerful learning tool for students and trainees in the health professions. Computer methodology complements the learning process by reinforcing and refining the learner's clinical experience. In addition, Dr. Don Michael has included a number of anecdotes from his own clinical experience that extend the Campbell-Wood-Leatham era into the present.

To be serviceable in contemporary cardiology, cardiac auscultation requires skills of the highest order developed through appropriate training and then carefully, continuously, and critically applied. It is a worthy skill not only for cardiologists; but for all those who consider themselves a part of the clinical diagnostic team.

H.J.C. Swan, M.D., Ph.D., M.A.C.P.
Professor of Medicine (Emeritus)
University of California at Los Angeles School of Medicine

PREFACE

Does cardiac auscultation still have a role in clinical practice, given the ascendancy of advanced technology? Should auscultation be rehabilitated?

Such questions were the subject of editorial comment in *The New England Journal of Medicine;* the glorious past of auscultation and its uncertain future were commented on by Morton Tavel in *Circulation.* These and other publications have suggested that there is a present imbalance between cost-effective clinical skills and high-cost technology. At last, American medicine seems to be emerging from three decades of apathy regarding the teaching and application of clinical skills. There is a growing realization that bedside evaluation was being neglected, to the detriment of practitioners as well as patients.

A nationwide survey of approved residencies in internal medicine and cardiology in the United States recently called attention to the insufficient emphasis placed on cardiac auscultation: The result is that only a small percentage of students demonstrate reasonable proficiency in this essential clinical skill.

The United States' long-standing fascination with technology, combined with current wide availability of sophisticated equipment, have favored a proliferation of testing procedures that has contributed to a devaluation of the "hands-on" approach to medicine, thus eroding the doctor-patient relationship. It is fortunate that present-day concern with health care expenses has compelled physicians to reexamine their priorities. The need for cost containment directly impacts on the teaching and implementation of clinical skills as we proceed into the 21st century. The new austerity forces practitioners to confront their professional working style, and for the sake of controlling costs, evaluate treatment decisions, and justify expensive testing.

This book is not antithetical to high technology; in fact, the system of cardiophonetics on which it is based uses cutting-edge technology to translate heart sounds into a standardized phonetic lexicon that can be used by students in any language to learn "the language of the heart"—what heart sounds tell us about cardiac function and dysfunction. This knowledge, in turn, when used in conjunction with the basic techniques of using the stethoscope as taught in this book, allows the clinical examiner to make the most effective use of high-technology testing to confirm or expand the preliminary diagnosis that is based on auscultation. In short, *Auscultation of the Heart* is a manual that emphasizes the cultivation and maintenance of the clinical skills that are requisite of health professionals in the present climate of cost-control and managed care.

Good health care and physician-patient relationships involve the interplay of many factors. One must balance cost, time, quality, liability, outcomes, and risk on the one hand against clinical skills in decision-making, diagnosis, and treatment on the other. While this book encourages medical professionals other than physicians to acquire expertise in using the stethoscope, *Auscultation of the Heart* does not advocate the *replacement* of M.D.s but the redirection of their training so as to restore a fully functional partnership with patients. With the rise of managed care, physicians and patients alike stand at the crossroads of competent care and efficient management. The author hopes sincerely that a book that draws on high technology to improve the clinical skills of the next generation of doctors will help to communicate that there are crucial low-tech components, such as the doctor-patient relationship and the effective use of the stethoscope, to high-quality patient care.

ACKNOWLEDGMENTS

As this book undergoes its final pre-publication revisions, I would like to thank a number of people who contributed to its writing in various ways. First, I am indebted to former teachers, Drs. Brigden, Leatham, Oram, Swan, and Wood; and to my colleagues William Parmley, Jim Forrester, Alan Jaffe, and Pravin Shah. In addition, I wish to thank those who critiqued earlier drafts of the book and disk, notably Drs. Roger Chappelka, Mel Cheitlin, Earnest Craig, Michael Crawford, Michael Criley, Proctor Harvey, Victor McKusick, and Dan Mason; with special gratitude to Dr. Jim Shaver, who gave many hours to help with the corrections and clarifications. I also acknowledge the support of Drs. Morton Tavel, Mel Cheitlin, and especially Gordon Ewy; as well as the members of the ACC Committee with whom I served. The publication of the book would not have been possible without the enthusiasm and support of Dr. Sylvan Weinberg, a true friend; the positive reinforcement of my editor, Joseph Hefta; and the hospitality of Maurice Rabot and Dr. Mary Doyle, at whose home much of the manuscript was revised.

In addition, I acknowledge the competence and dedication of my tireless secretary, Inetta Rusciano; Greg Bell, Rose Maestas, Stephanie Bork, Mike Larson, and Lavanne Watson, who helped put the puzzle of this manuscript together. In addition, I acknowledge N. Brannon of the Carden School, who gave me my basic education in phonetics; Sandy Disner, Ph.D., and Peter Ladefoged, Ph.D., of the U.C.L.A Linguistics Department, who provided expert assistance in creating the system of cardiophonetics from heart sounds. Finally, I am grateful to my family, close friends, and staff for bearing with me during the long process of the book's preparation.

THOUGHTS
OF A CLINICAL
CARDIOLOGIST

The clinical art of auscultation comes across as something of an oxymoron! The listening ear is bombarded with a cacophony of noise: Blaring television, the insistent ringing of telephones, the varied sounds of medical equipment, muffled whispers of conversation, the rubbing of the stethoscope against the ribs, the rumble of bowel sounds, singly or collectively, conspire to frustrate the examining ear. "Tuning out" the noise is a constant but worthwhile challenge. Adding to these difficulties is the availability in hospitals of a plethora of stethoscopes, the quality of which seem to vary proportionately to the examiner's skill!

Patients are often fully clothed or examined in an unsuitable position, adding to the tedium of being able to listen to the heart appropriately. It is rare that a patient is examined lying on the left side, the most important position in auscultation.

Despite these difficulties, it is a tribute to human ingenuity that a keen clinical examiner can in most instances set up to perform a complete examination. Only then is the auscultator able to concentrate on the music, which the heart so magically transports to the ears, yielding a symphony of organized information, to reveal its innermost functions.

INTRODUCTION

ORGANIZATION OF THE BOOK

CHAPTER STRUCTURE

INTRODUCTION TO CARDIOPHONETICS

TRADITIONAL METHODS OF TEACHING AUSCULTATION

THE DEVELOPMENT OF CARDIOPHONETICs

THE ELEMENTS OF PHONICS

ADVANTAGES OF CARDIOPHONETICS IN TEACHING AUSCULTATION

LIMITATIONS OF CARDIOPHONETICS

LEARNING CARDIOPHONETICS

As the Latin verb *auscultare* ("to listen") implies, listening is not a skill specific to physicians. Auditory differentiation of heart sounds and murmurs can be learned and practiced by qualified practitioners in all the health professions. This book has been written for all levels of auscultationists: from certified cardiologists and internists to physician's assistants and nurse practitioners to medical and nursing students.

Auscultation of the Heart uses a simplified method for learning and recalling heart sounds. The book is intended to be used with a portable, pocket-sized phonetic *card* and a 3-1/2" floppy *disk,* for personal or laptop computers with speakers or headsets. The latter allows the reader to associate the text with actual auscultated heart sounds. The text and its multimedia accompaniments are designed to achieve the following objectives:

1. To teach the art and science of auscultation using a simplified but accelerated technique of sound reproduction by the use of phonetics; the cardiac conditions are recorded through an acoustic spectrograph to reproduce sounds and are written out phonetically. (See Appendix IV, sound card, computer diskette.)
2. To describe auscultatory findings in a variety of clinical settings.
3. To provide a clinical framework and context for the rational use of auscultation.

The material presented in this book is organized to be read with a referenced summary in the Appendix. That is, the text is intended to be accessible to readers with different levels of previous knowledge of the subject matter. The summary can be used by medical students or other caregivers unfamiliar with the complexities of auscultation; they can then proceed to the appropriate sections in the text for more detailed discussion. More advanced readers can begin with the text itself, with the addition of selected relevant readings from the references at the end of each chapter. It is hoped that all readers will learn the accelerated method of cardiophonics with the combined resources of the text, disk, and card.

ORGANIZATION OF THE BOOK

The text is divided into 10 chapters grouped into three major parts, front matter, and appendices. *Part One* describes the physical, physiological, and clinical essentials of hearing; the art of auscultation; dynamic auscultation and normal auscultatory findings; and the hemodynamics of auscultation. *Part Two* deals with systematic cardiology, heart sounds and murmurs, and the clinical antecedents of auscultation. *Part Three* deals with critical care auscultation, adjunctive tests relevant to clinical findings, and pregnancy and adult/pediatric auscultation. The appendices include diagnostic and treatment algorithms, phonic tables, "Cardiac Pearls," and how-to material.

CHAPTER STRUCTURE

Each chapter is preceded by an outline that can serve either as a guide to the contents or as a synopsis for review. The chapters include sets of clinical vignettes at the end, with questions and answers, which allow students to test their understanding of the material. A list of references at the end of each chapter refers readers to more detailed treatments of topics discussed in the chapter.

INTRODUCTION TO CARDIOPHONETICS

Before there were words in the world, there were sounds. *Cardiophonetics* signifies the use of phonics to express heart sounds; that is, a given heart sound is transcribed by an English phoneme. A *phoneme,* in turn, is the smallest distinctive group or class of phones (individual speech sounds) in a given language. English phonemes include fricatives (e.g., "f" or "v"), sibilants ("s"), glottal stops ("p"), and other similar groups or categories. Cardiophonics uses these building blocks of language to transcribe heart sounds and murmurs. The phonemes are identified by playing the heart sounds into a sound spectrograph and obtaining a *word print.* Word prints have been used by forensic experts for years to identify individual voices. This book, however, is the first attempt to provide a systematic transcription of heart sounds as word prints, each of which designates a specific cardiac condition. For example, the holosystolic murmur of mitral regurgitation, the midsystolic murmur of aortic stenosis, and the diastolic murmur of mitral stenosis have very specific tracings on a sound spectrograph and very different word prints that reproduce the sounds heard through a stethoscope.

To maintain consistency throughout this book, auscultatory findings are transliterated phonetically, in a format referred to as *phonophonics*. This format allows readers to relate the phoneme to phonocardiograms or acoustograms with which they may already be familiar.

Readers who have difficulty with pronouncing the syllables may find the completed phonics on the card for heart sounds and murmurs helpful. The disk can be played on a personal or laptop computer; for best results, it should be used with headphones or reasonably good speakers. The disk provides an animated heart model, as well as visual and auditory phonetic renderings of actual heart sounds and of sounds phonated by the author. The sounds on the disk can be reproduced at different speeds and volumes.

TRADITIONAL METHODS OF TEACHING AUSCULTATION

Teaching the identification of heart sounds relied on audiovisual aids, including CD-ROMs and tape-recorded or videotaped sounds. These media were then coupled with verbal descriptions of cardiac sounds and murmurs. Words such as "rough," "smooth," "blowing," "musical," "train wheel," "sea gull," and the like have been used in these descriptions (Table I-1). The traditional verbal descriptions, however, have two drawbacks. First, they are unspecific and subjective: different students may have very different notions of "rough," "blowing," or "mill wheel" sounds. Second, verbal descriptions are one step further removed from the sounds they represent, in that they are by definition *descriptions* of the sounds rather than *transliterations*. The cardiophonetic syllables, on the other hand, render the sounds themselves into readable phonemes. For example, the so-called "train wheel" rhythm is a quadruple heart rhythm that can be written in cardiophonic form as *luh-dup'-du-dup*. The latter is a clearly readable transliteration of a sound with a pause between the first two syllables, a sound similar to train wheels.

In addition to the lack of precision intrinsic to verbal descriptions, the older methods of teaching auscultation had other limitations. To begin with, they were armchair or library methods that could not be easily transferred to clinical auscultation of actual patients. Students had to associate a plethora of sounds with lengthy descriptions and then rely on rote memorization to master the material. Furthermore, the older methods did not use consistent representations of sounds and hence impaired the student's recall. For example, one text described mitral regurgitation as "a holosystolic murmur and a mid-diastolic murmur," and "a holosystolic murmur and an S_3"—both

Table I-1 Onomatopoeic Sounds and Associated Heart Conditions

Sound Description	Condition
Buzzing, twanging, groaning	Still's murmur
Click	Mitral valve prolapse (MVP)
Cooing diastolic murmur	Retroverted aortic cusp
Crepitus	Pneumomediastinum
Crunch	Pneumomediastinum
Gallop	Triple rhythm
Honk/Whoop	Nonejection click
"Kentucky"	S_3 gallop
Leathery sound	Rub
Mill wheel	Air embolism
Pericardial knock	Constrictive pericarditis
Plop	Myxoma
Rough sound	Stenotic murmurs
Sail sound	Ebstein's anomaly
Sea gull	Mitral or aortic valve disease
Sigh	Aortic regurgitation
Smooth	Regurgitation
Tambour	Loud A_2 in aneurysm
"Tennessee"	S_4 gallop
Train wheel	Quadruple rhythm
Water wheel machinery	Patent ductus arteriosus

variants within the same description. My own experience has convinced me that students will learn to identify holosystolic murmurs much more readily if they hear the same sound repeated without variation and correlated with a phonic representation that can be read at the bedside as well as in the library. The older methods do not provide learners with the "road maps" or analytical tools for analyzing auscultatory data.

THE DEVELOPMENT OF CARDIOPHONETICS

Cardiophonetics can be said to begin with Duroziez, who made the first attempt to represent cardiac sounds in language (in his case, French). He transcribed the murmur of mitral stenosis as *fout'-ta-ta'-rou.* Although present-day spectrographic analysis indicates a different form for the mitral stenosis murmur, Duroziez was nonetheless a pioneer in phonetic translation of heart sounds.

After Duroziez, Victor McCusick made further refinements in the method of cardiophonetics. In the mid-1950s, Dr. McCusick demonstrated that auscultated events could be correlated with acoustic spectrograms. This development was contemporaneous with Leatham's use of the phonocardiogram to characterize the timing of heart sounds and murmurs. The two techniques should not be confused. How does spectrocardiophonics differ from phonocardiography? Dr. Leatham's phonocardiograms only record what could be auscultated; they reproduce the timing and pitch of heart sounds but do not create sounds. McCusick's demonstration of the correlation between specific conditions and spectrograms, however, pre-dated the translation of spectrograms into "word prints." This newer development has made possible the present system of spectrographic phonetics and our own modification, cardiophonetics (heart sound words).

The authors own research group at University of California at Los Angeles collaborated with the Department of Phonics to obtain sound spectrograms of digitally recorded heart sounds. These spectrograms provided us with visual representation of the *timing* of the sound (the X axis), its *frequency* in Hz (the Y axis), its *loudness* in dB (the Z axis), its *shape,* and its *form.* Using modern methods of interpretation, the research group subjected these spectrograms to analysis. They obtained word prints that were specific to each heart sound and reproduced the sound in the phonemes of American English. In some advanced versions of the process, these derivations are performed by computer.

The role of the spectrogram can be illustrated with reference to *spoonerisms.* Spoonerisms, named for the Victorian clergyman, W.A. Spooner of New College, Oxford, are slips of the tongue in which word sounds (usually consonants) are transposed to create different words which change the meaning of the original sentence. Figure I-1 illustrates the process whereby "down train" becomes "town drain." Playing these words into an acoustic spectrogram reproduces the alternating consonants. In a similar manner, playing heart sounds into this instrument allows the tracings to be translated into words. These words are pronounced according to their letters, accents, and phonemes. The principles are universally applicable.

THE ELEMENTS OF PHONICS

Cardiophonetics (heart sounds as words) derive from basic phonetics. The phonemes of American English, represented by letters (e.g., /L/, /T/, and /P/) are built up into syllables (e.g., *lap* or *top*). These syllables in turn are elaborated into words (e.g., *laptop*). The presence of overtones of formants in the spectrograph usually indicates the presence of vowels. The influence of formants was shown in McCusick's work in his characterizations of musical murmurs (e.g., the "sea gull" murmur). Sudden stops can be seen in the spectrographic patterns in such words as *shut,* and are examples of glottal stops. Consonants or fricatives sometimes appear in the spectrograms without vowels, as in our representation of an early systolic murmur as *rrr.* A knowledge of the elements of phonics allows the student to learn the pronunciation of the various heart sounds and murmurs in internationally accepted characters and terminology, as well as the use of pitch marks to indicate changes in pitch, amplitude, and timing. The accent is represented

SPOONERISM

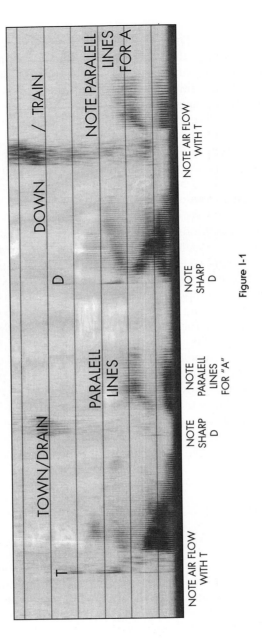

Figure I-1

by a slash (*I*), and the slash is placed *after* the accented syllable. For example, *Lup/Dup*. These are basic principles of instruction in language pronunciation, and they can be applied to heart sounds as well. The letters capitalized are sounded out loud in volume, e.g., Lup at the cardiac apex representing S_1 and dup, in lower case, is soft.

ADVANTAGES OF CARDIOPHONETICS IN TEACHING AUSCULTATION

There are several advantages in using this instructional method:

1. *Phonics is an accepted method of language instruction.* Teaching by means of phonics represents the most effective methodology for rapid mastery of reading or of a foreign language.
2. *Many medical students will already be familiar with phonics.* The teaching of phonics in primary schools is widespread; adult students who were not so instructed can easily pick up on the concept.
3. *Cardiophonetics allows auscultation to be learned as a "language" with a small but precise "vocabulary."* Specific conditions (e.g., holosystolic murmurs) have representative spectrograms and phonic transliterations. These word prints are specific to each condition. All heart sounds or murmurs can be represented by only 13 different word prints. These 13 word prints allow practitioners to write out or sound out heart sounds correctly.
4. *Cardiophonetics can be used in international communications or publications.* Heart sounds can be displayed in cardiophonetics with international or American English phonic symbols.
5. *Cardiophonetics accelerates the student's learning process.* Medical and nursing students rapidly acquire the ability to recall specific sounds and murmurs. This method of learning 13 sounds and building a cardiac "vocabulary" with them is an effective substitution for sound correlations that were originally left to be derived from bedside auscultation a process that take several decades to master. In addition, Table I-2 lists the steps in sequential identification of heart sounds to facilitate the student's learning.
6. *Cardiophonetics allows clinicians to improve the accuracy of their identifications of heart sounds in actual patient examinations.* The syllables and words used in cardiophonetics can be phonated onto a computer disk, and the actual heart sounds from which they are derived can be

Table I-2 Tips for Identifying Heart Sounds

1. Identify S_2 first; then identify S_1. Hence:
2. Identify systole (S_1–S_2) and diastole (S_2–S_1).
3. Listen for the timing: early, mid, or late.
4. Listen for the sound and match the sound to the phonics.

recorded. This disk can then be brought to the patient's bedside; the recorded heart sounds can be altered with respect to rate and loudness to match the unknown. A sound menu allows access to the "best fit" sound.

In addition, a portable pocket-sized cardiophonetics card with visual representations of the phonemes has been produced for clinicians as an aide-mèmoire.

LIMITATIONS OF CARDIOPHONETICS

At present, the primary limitation of our new method is its restricted ability to represent with precision all the possible variations of a given heart sound. Thus, cardiophonetics remains a method for the basic teaching of heart sounds, and offers little or no value as a tool for the diagnosis or treatment of the heart.

Given this limitation, however, the current pressures on apprentice clinicians to master the art of auscultation as rapidly as possible are similar to the pressures on persons who need to learn a new language within a few weeks. Thus, we have had to present our material in such a way that students with average or poor auditory or visual capacities are not unduly disadvantaged. It would be inaccurate or arrogant for our group to claim that, for example, all murmurs indicative of mitral regurgitation are exactly represented by the phonic *Shhhhh*. Variations will clearly occur, and students should be warned to expect them. We have, however, used multiple examples of each heart sound to derive the phonetic transliterations, and we believe that they represent the majority of cases in each category. This holds true for the phonics on the pocket card as well as those on the disk.

LEARNING CARDIOPHONETICS

The optimal way to teach sound is to reproduce sound. In other words, identification of sounds is best taught by having students hear the actual sounds. The sound to be mastered should be reproducible with current recording technology, accurately rendered phonetically, and easily recalled. How can a student use cardiophonetics to accelerate the learning process? My experience as a teacher suggests that the method can be applied in three ways:

1. The student can use cardiophonetics to analyze heart sounds during actual bedside auscultation. He or she can reduce the sounds to their basic phonemes by correlating them with the material on the disk and the card and memorizing the phonetically created sounds. Ideally, the

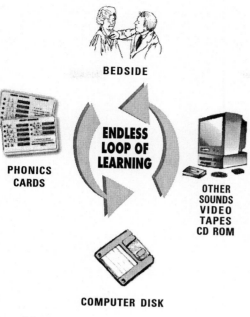

BEDSIDE

PHONICS CARDS

ENDLESS LOOP OF LEARNING

OTHER SOUNDS VIDEO TAPES CD ROM

COMPUTER DISK

Figure I-2

student will match the patient's heart sounds by making changes in the rate and volume on the computer disk in order to reinforce this learning.

2. As Fig. I-2 indicates, the beginner can learn both the visual and the auditory phonemes and correlate these with bedside findings. This process will create a continuous circuit loop for aiding recall.

3. The student can try his or her hand at analyzing the sound descriptions provided by other authors into their component word prints or acoustic signatures in order to build up a vocabulary of sounds analogous to a vocabulary in a new language. This process would be similar to a student's use of grammar to analyze new sentences in a new language, as distinct from rote memorization of sentence paradigms.

Using these tools, the author hopes to lay a firm foundation for a new generation of clinicians who for the rest of their careers will benefit their patients through growing expertise in the art of auscultation.

AUSCULTATION
OF THE HEART

1

SOUND AND STETHOSCOPES

HISTORICAL BACKGROUND

SOUND AND ITS RECOGNITION

PHYSICS OF SOUND

PHYSIOLOGY OF HEARING

PSYCHOACOUSTICS

SELECTIVE HEARING

SOUND ABSORPTION-ACOUSTIC OBLITERATION

TRAINING EFFECT OF SOUND
Tuning Out, Tuning In

STANDARD STETHOSCOPES
Dimensions
Earpieces
The Examining End
Tubes

SPECIALITY STETHOSCOPES
Obstetric and Pediatric
Esophageal

ELECTRONIC STETHOSCOPES
The Stethos
3M
Headphone
Bang & Olafsen
Acoustic Spectrography
Comparison of Stethoscopes

THE DIFFICULT AUSCULTATION

BIBLIOGRAPHY

The doctor being very sore
A stethoscope they did devise
That had a hammer to clear the bore
With a knob to kill the "flies."
(Oliver Wendell Holmes)

HISTORICAL BACKGROUND

Auscultation of the chest using the unaided ear began in the late seventeenth century, but proved unsatisfactory in general, and on the part of female patients, was for the most part unaccepted. Then, in Paris in 1816, Rene Laennec invented the stethoscope (Fig. 1-1). Tradition has it that he learned its princi-

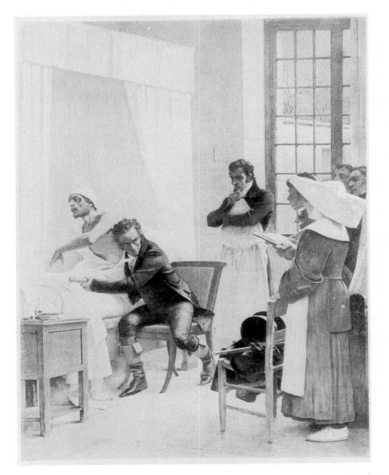

Figure 1-1 Taken from a postcard showing René Hyacinth Laennec using his ear to auscultate the heart prior to his invention of a quire of paper held in his left hand, the forerunner of the stethoscope. Performed at the Necker Hospital in Paris.

ple by watching children tapping messages on one end of a plank, while others listened at the other end. This observation gave Laennec the idea to roll a quire of paper into a cylinder and apply one end of it to the region of a patient's heart and the other end to his ear. As he had hoped, Laennec could hear heart sounds. Encouraged by the results of this simple experiment, Laennec went on to invent a series of rigid, wooden, monaural stethoscopes that are still used in some parts of Europe (Fig. 1-2). The American physician George Camman invented the binaural stethoscope in 1865 (Fig. 1-3).

SOUND AND ITS RECOGNITION

The human threshold of auditory acuity extends from approximately 20 to 20,000 cycles/s, with a range for the average adult of 50 to 14,000 cycles/s (Fig. 1-4). Children may detect frequencies up to 18,000 cycles/s, but with age comes a loss of audibility to the higher frequencies. The ear discriminates frequencies between 8 to 1024 (HRTZ) in recognizing the range for heart sounds. The middiastolic murmur of mitral stenosis is in the low-frequency range, as are the low-pitched, diastolic, third and fourth heart sounds, designated S_3 and S_4. Typical ejection systolic murmurs of aortic stenosis are heard in the intermediate range or frequencies between 600 and approximately 800 cycles/s, while immediate diastolic murmurs due to

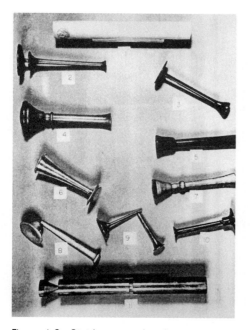

Figure 1-2 Rigid monaural stethoscopes, one replica of Laënnec's "quire of paper," and other multiple varieties.

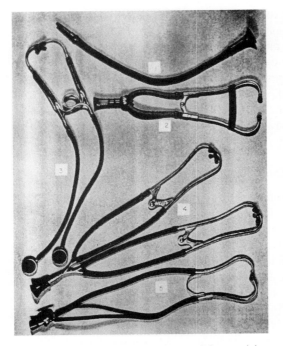

Figure 1-3 Flexible stethoscopes, mostly binaural. Item number 2 was invented by George P. Camman, New York, 1855. These two figures are published by the courtesy of Dr. Victor A. McKusick.

aortic or pulmonary regurgitation are typically high-pitched, in the range of more than 1000 cycles/s. In general, clicks and snaps are of a higher pitch than the first and second heart sounds, S_1 and S_2, and S_2 is higher-pitched than S_1 (Fig. 1-5).

PHYSICS OF SOUND

Sound is a form of pressure. Sound waves are produced by oscillation or vibration in a medium; in the case of the heart, the movement of blood or valves causes the oscillations. Sound waves spread, similar to a ripple, throughout the oscillating medium, which itself does not move. The sound wave travels centrifugally, away from the center, and can react to its environment in five ways. If the sound wave encounters an obstacle:

1. with its identical frequency, the sound wave resonates;
2. and is absorbed, the sound wave is blocked;
3. and changes direction, the sound wave refracts;
4. and bends around it, the sound wave diffracts;
5. that causes oscillations in all directions, the sound wave dissipates.

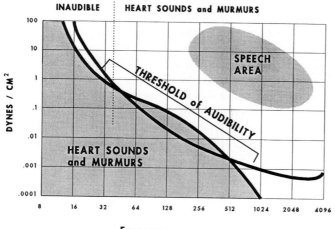

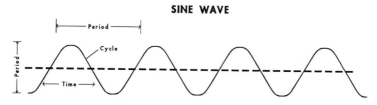

Figure 1-4 Shows the threshold of audibility and the range of hertz that pertain to heart sounds and murmurs. Reprinted with the courtesy of Churchill Davidson.

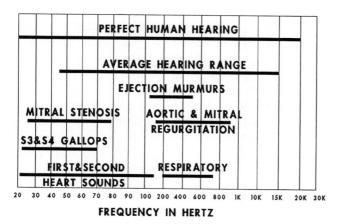

Figure 1-5 Below sine wave showing the propagation of sound. Reprinted from the same source. The correlation of frequency in hertz with auscultated heart sounds and respiratory sounds.

PHYSIOLOGY OF HEARING

A sound wave that ventures into the ear enters through the external auditory meatus and travels downward and forward, causing vibrations of the ear-drum. These vibrations then spread to the organ of Corti, a spiral structure that has nerves to pick up low-amplitude vibrations at its base and high-amplitude vibrations at its top. The sound waves induce perilymphatic and endolymphatic movement within the cochlea. These vibrations, in turn, are picked up by nerve fibers and are transmitted as signals through the cochlear nerve into the brain, to be carried to the superior gyrus of the temporal lobe.

PSYCHOACOUSTICS

Auditory signals that enter the temporal lobe correlate via synapses with other parts of the brain that similarly have received signals from the eyes, nose, and taste buds. All of these signals are experienced as the sensations of sight, smell, and taste, which are interrelated with higher levels of intel-lection, and which associate with each other as well.

SELECTIVE HEARING

Approximately 1 s after they enter the ear, soundwaves are perceived by the brain as sound. The ear can absorb sound, and this ability assists the brain in its filtering function, when a person wishes to focus on sounds selec-tively.

SOUND ABSORPTION-ACOUSTIC OBLITERATION-DAMPING

When a loud sound is followed by a soft sound, the latter is difficult to hear (Cardiac Pearl 2). Also, a low-pitched sound will physically block (obliterate) a high-pitched sound.

   A good clinical illustration of the first principle is seen in the murmur of aortic or pulmonary stenosis, which leads to a softer sound caused by closure of the aortic or pulmonary valve. This makes the soft sound difficult to hear. Similarly, one has difficulty in hearing the soft murmurs of aortic regurgitation that follow a loud midsystolic murmur of aortic stenosis. A classic example of sound obliteration is the acoustic artifact produced by a crescendo-diminuendo ejection systolic murmur, for example, in aortic stenosis, in which no diminuendo is normally heard. The diminuendo por-tion of which is damped out; hence phonetically $\overline{RRR}'$ Dup↓ not $\overline{RRR}'$ Dup.

TRAINING EFFECT OF SOUND

Sound waves have a training effect; a particular sound or kind of sound is better perceived as one listens to it repeatedly. Very complex sound patterns, for example, a musical phrase or a song, can be stored in the brain for later recall. Similarly, sound patterns that are characteristic of certain cardiovascular events can be learned by physicians and other health professionals, and used to diagnose specific heart conditions in patients.

This process is similar to that of learning a new language; before we recognize words, we recognize sounds that are organized as phonetics. When applied to analyzing heart sounds, the process is known as auscultation. We hear as phonetic units (for example, *lup* or *lap*) the basic sound patterns produced by the heart. *Auscultation of the Heart* focuses on the use of the stethoscope in perceiving the various sounds that are representative of a healthy or dysfunctional human heart and vascular system.

Tuning Out, Tuning In

In the same way that smoke can obscure visual perception, extraneous sounds can interfere with auscultation. An examiner must learn not only to *tune out* interfering sound, but also to *tune in* to the salient heart sound pattern that he or she has committed to memory. Matching the pattern that is audible through the stethoscope with the pattern that has been committed to memory allows one to make an accurate diagnosis. An experienced examiner who suspects a particular dysfunction can listen for a specific sound or murmur to either support or cast doubt on his or her preliminary diagnosis. Laboratory comparison of sound recognition and spectrogram findings reveal a *tuning effect* that allows a trained listener to discern clearly what normally would be barely perceptible to the untrained ear.

STANDARD STETHOSCOPES

In the art of auscultation, the best complement to a trained ear is a good stethoscope (*stethos* = chest + *scope* = to view). Hence, choosing the proper stethoscope in terms of both quality and comfort to the examiner is of utmost importance. Of the current products on the market, the author has found the Tycos and the Littman Allen stethoscopes to be superior to the Rappaport Sprague, Hewlett-Packard, and Heiner stethoscopes (Table 1-1).

Dimensions

A modern stethoscope is approximately 10 in. in length. Although a shorter version may be better from an acoustic standpoint, 10 in. offers a more comfortable distance for the patient, thus striking a compromise between auditory effectiveness and professional decorum. While the look of the stethoscope may be important esthetically to the examiner, one should

Table 1-1   Recommended Attributes for Stethoscopes

Component	Description
Bell	Metal
	Small circumference
	No rubbering independently
	Adjustable from diaphragm
Diaphragm	Two-sized (adult, pediatric)
Earpieces	Adjustable independently
	Allows each ear seal to be altered
	Plastic
Tubes	Two tubes from frame to endpiece
	Thick tubing (3/16-in. diameter)
Entire instrument	Easy to carry

be more concerned with the performance of the instrument than with its appearance.

The average commercial stethoscope has an internal diameter of 3/16 in., as do the Tycos and Littman stethoscopes. Leatham and Rappaport Sprague have rubber tubing which is 1/8 in. in diameter (Fig. 1-6). In general, high frequencies are picked up by wide tubing and low frequencies by narrow tubing. Also, the thicker the tubing, the more insulation there is against extraneous noise.

Earpieces

Earpieces connect in most stethoscopes to a bell and a diaphragm. Earpieces are attached to a frame but must be readily movable on hinges created by a joint, a feature that commends the Tycos. Earpieces may be either plastic or rubber. It is important that earpieces fit snugly into the ears and are not obstructed by bends in the examiner's external auditory meatus. The examiner may frequently have to adjust the stethoscope to maintain the earpieces at an angle that is both comfortable and snug. Not all stethoscopes allow individual adjustment of each earpiece; this feature, however, is vital for a proper seal with the external auditory meatus. This emphasizes the need for close-fitting, individually adjustable earpieces to help tune out extraneous noise and tune in to salient sounds.

The Examining End, or Sensor

The Bell   The stethoscope's bell typically forms a seal that should be preserved by applying the bell lightly over a sealable area of the patient's skin. Hence, avoid a nonsealing interspace. The bell is applied to the chest wall with the patient in the left supine position to capture *low frequency* vibrations. This patient position is indicated in listening for S_3, S_4, and the diastolic murmur of mitral stenosis.

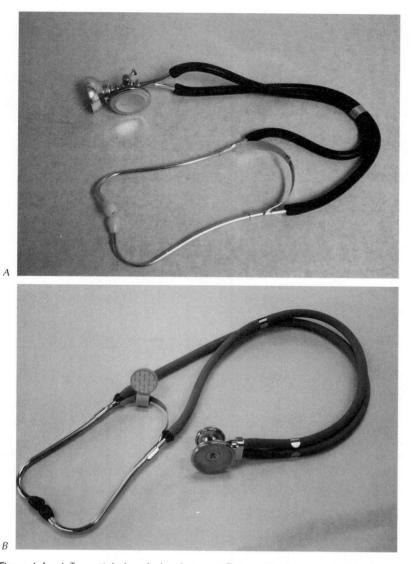

Figure 1-6 *A.* Tycos triple-headed stethoscope. The small bell, corrugated diaphragm, and the flat diaphragm. The earpieces are movable but somewhat heavy. *B.* Rappaport Sprague showing a narrow diaphragm which functions as a bell, a wide diaphragm which picks up high frequencies.

A large bell can make auscultation impossible in a pediatric patient or in a patient with cachexia with prominent ribs and narrow intercostal spaces; in such patients, the bell "rides" the ribs and disallows a good seal with the skin. A smaller bell is good for apical localization in adults as well as children. The metal bell of the Tycos stethoscope is this instrument's

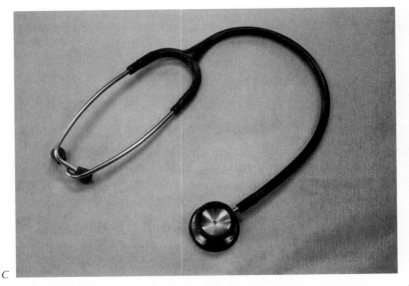

C

Figure 1-6 (Continued) C. Littman stethoscope showing a simple, portable device, which, however, has a rubber ring around a large bell and nonadjustable earpieces.

strongest feature. The Allen bell is quite good, but its enclosed chamber is too wide (Table 1-2).

Too heavy a pressure applied to the chest can muffle the murmur or sound so that it is acoustically "squashed." Also, sound interference can be caused by the stethoscope itself. For example, a diaphragm can produce an interfering sound as it rubs along the ribs, a problem that the Leatham stethoscope circumvents by the use of an inner bell. This inner bell can be awkward, however, because it needs to be pushed out with each use.

The Diaphragm High-pitched, blowing murmurs such as the immediate diastolic murmurs of *atrial regurgitation, pulmonary regurgitation,* or *mitral regurgitation,* described as a "sigh" by Duroziez, are best heard with the diaphragm. The diaphragm may be made of corrugated or flat plastic or of metal. Corrugations enable the examiner to pick up different frequencies by varying the pressure on the chest wall, rendering the capability to pick up low- to high-frequency vibrations. Metal diaphragms are stiffer and pick up higher frequencies. Small bells and corrugated diaphragms are useful in chest deformities. In general, the Heiner and Allen diaphragms are recommended; the Littman and Tycos diaphragms are also good. The Heiner metal portion of the diaphragm has a groove which makes it "finger friendly."

Table 1-2   Comparative Features of Modern Stethoscopes

Component	Instrument			
	Tycos	Littman	Allen	Heiner
Bell	Excellent Small Nonrubber Seals with patient's skin to form chamber	Has rubber ring; too large for reliable seal	Wide bell Plastic No rubber ring; hence, good seal	Small ring does not allow seal in some cases
Diaphragm	Excellent Adjustable diaphragm Useful in some cases	Excellent	Easy to use	Excellent Large Good conduction with metal
Earpieces	Excellent Offer good seal	Not independent of frame Difficult to make seal	Excellent adjustment capabilities	Difficult to adjust Stiff frame connection
End piece	Heavy Somewhat cumbersome	Easy to hold	Cumbersome	Finger-friendly Easy to place on chest

Combination Examining Ends   Some manufacturers, including Littman and Heiner, have produced instruments with a hybrid examining end that in theory offers a combination of low- and high-frequency auscultation. Such instruments do not offer adequate low-frequency sensitivity, however; as previously noted, a bell that creates an airtight seal with the skin is required to auscultate effectively for low-frequency heart sounds.

Tubes

Two tubes are better than one in listening for a murmur of mitral regurgitation, which is high-pitched. By contrast, a single tube, a wooden tube, or a large bell can accentuate the low-pitched S_3 and S_4 and *middiastolic murmurs* in mitral stenosis.

SPECIALITY STETHOSCOPES

Obstetric and Pediatric

Obstetric stethoscopes, the emblem of the obstetrician, are steel funnels to which the ear is applied to listen for fetal heart sounds. Pediatric stethoscopes are small, delicate versions of adult stethoscopes. Electronic versions can aid in detecting fetal cardiac abnormalities (Fig. 1-7).

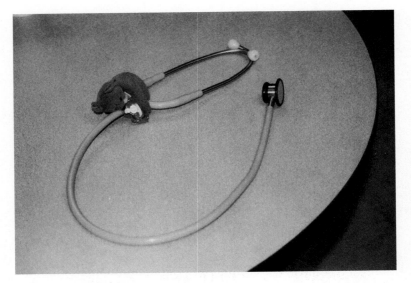

Figure 1-7   Pediatric stethoscope.

Esophageal

Esophageal stethoscopes, once used exclusively by anesthesiologists, have found wider use among medical practitioners. Because these devices allow the examiner to listen from the core of the body, they provide good fidelity and maximize the amount of auscultatory information that can be gathered. Esophageal stethoscopy is recommended for a patient who is undergoing surgery or has had cardiac arrest. Although esophageal stethoscopes can be used in settings in which ambient sound prevents effective chest auscultation with an external stethoscope, due to their limited areas of placement and access, however, these devices are best used in the operating room (Fig. 1-8).

ELECTRONIC STETHOSCOPES

Recently introduced experimental electronic stethoscopes enable heart sounds to be recorded and played back at different rates without pitch change. This feature provides an excellent teaching tool, although pitch variations limit the ability of some newer electronic devices to record sounds and murmurs at slower speeds. Although electronic stethoscopes have proved disappointing in general in the clinical setting, the Klippert nipple stethoscope has proven to be an excellent all-around device. Electronic stethoscopes may be especially helpful to examiners with high-frequency

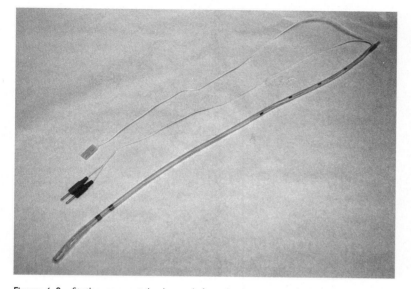

Figure 1-8 Stethoscope at the lower left end, two pacing electrodes used for atrial pacing in the detection of wall motion abnormalities. The stethoscope is useful in detecting "core" heart sounds and breath sounds.

hearing loss (Cardiac Pearl 1). Analogous to the phonocardiogram, electronic stethoscopes pick up whatever can be heard by a standard stethoscope, but they enhance background sound as well, which can cause confusion in the examiner.

The Stethos

The Stethos is an electronic stethoscope produced by Thera Technologies, Inc., in Canada (Fig. 1-9). This stand-alone instrument is intended to replace conventional stethoscopes. Its main features are sound amplification, frequency discrimination, and the capacity to reduce ambient noise. The Stethos can interface with a computer system to simultaneously record phono- and electrocardiograms for teaching purposes and to correlate such data with auscultated events. Background sound interference can reduce the effectiveness of the instrument, however, and its diaphragm is not easy to use. The system's high cost also may discourage its widespread use. The stethoscope with playback tends to be confusing because playback at slower speeds causes a change in pitch from the original sound.

3M

The 3M stethoscope, still in development, is a user-friendly device without playback capabilities. This instrument offers frequency selection and a good heart signal-to-noise ratio.

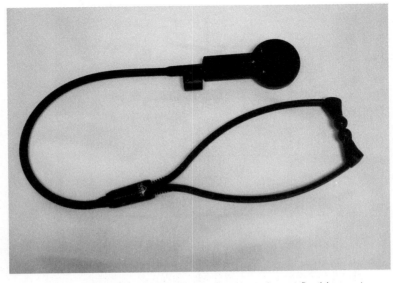

Figure 1-9 The Thera electronic stethoscope showing the nonflexible earpieces and somewhat bulky diaphragm.

Headphone (Fig. 1-9)

The headphone stethoscope, another device still in development, uses headphones with sound-blocking systems for auscultation in noisy critical-care environments (Fig. 1-10). The headphones are designed to be easily attached to a standard stethoscope. This device features recording capabilities and has excellent playback at a fixed rate.

Bang & Olafsen

Bang & Olafsen's experimental device uses accelerometry to reproduce heart sounds electronically. This instrument shows excellent potential for the clinical setting.

Acoustic Spectrography

The acoustic spectrograph (K Elemetrics, used courtesy of the U.C.L.A. Department of Linguistics) that recorded the heart sounds documented in this book provides signal-to-noise ratios as well as a record of ambient noise. These functions were useful in evaluating sounds recorded from patients. Acoustic spectrographs are used in most speech laboratories in the United States.

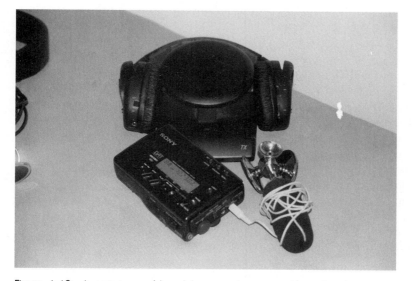

Figure 1-10 A prototype of headphone stethoscope with a digital tape recorder and adaptor to the stethoscope endpiece containing a microphone.

Comparison of Stethoscopes

Comparing stethoscopes, an admittedly subjective task, is important nonetheless because the difficulty of auscultation is compounded by poor stethoscope design; some manufacturers do surprisingly little to relate their instrument's design to the actual practice of auscultation.

The too-frequent emphasis on the appearance or "trendiness" of an instrument over its actual function is emblematic of how the art of auscultation has fallen into neglect. For example, European wooden instruments, the "ugly ducklings" among stethoscopes, are best at picking up low-pitched murmurs, whereas modern stethoscopes with nonadjustable earpieces have no place in serious auscultation.

The author favors the bell of the Tycos, while the plastic diaphragms of the Allen, Littman, 3M, Rappaport Sprague, Tycos, and Heiner stethoscopes are excellent. Bell-diaphragm combinations are not recommended. As for electronic stethoscopes, the need to push frequency selection buttons can be cumbersome. Whereas steel diaphragms can squash sounds, corrugated diaphragms tend to enhance sounds. The Tycos, Allen, Klippert, and the Littman with separate bell and diaphragm are acceptable instruments, although the latter does not have adjustable earpieces. Instruments that have two tubes from the earpieces to the frame, and yet have only one tube from the frame to the endpiece, are not strictly two-tube, binaural instruments, and thus are not recommended.

THE DIFFICULT AUSCULTATION

The practitioner must become accustomed to auscultation in a variety of environments, including the intensive care unit, operating room, emergency department, inpatient rooms, and often-crowded clinics. Each of these settings produces its own kind of noise pollution (Cardiac Pearl 4). For example, the intensive care unit has a variety of instruments—respirators, intra-aortic balloon pumps, suction machines, and the like—that can interfere with auscultation. Outpatient and emergency departments have a great deal of extraneous noise created by staff, patients, and children and others who may accompany patients. Often, clinics provide little privacy for patients, let alone insulation from noise. In inpatient hospital rooms, visitor noise and rustling bed clothes are among the potential causes of interference.

Most important in maximizing the examiner's effectiveness are a well-trained ear and the use of a good stethoscope. Esophageal and electronic stethoscopes are of particular benefit, as are stethoscopes equipped with nipple endpieces that can fit over small intercostal spaces. Headphone stethoscopes also help to block noise. There are other factors, however, in addition to noise interference, that present specific challenges to effective auscultation. Several of these challenges include:

- Kyphoscoliosis. This condition may move the heart to an abnormal location; hence, the examiner may have to "hunt" for the heart.
- Pectus excavatum and carinatum (caved/pigeon chest). This condition may make it difficult to achieve contact with the stethoscope. Use of a tilted corrugated variable-pressure diaphragm often helps.
- Blown chest with soft sounds. Listen from below the xiphoid with the bell tilting up.
- Thin interspaces. Use a small bell to auscultate.
- Large breasts or prostheses. Turn the patient to the right side. Listen at the right sternal border.
- No cardiac impulse. Turn the patient to the left side and listen at the apex.

BIBLIOGRAPHY

Ertel PY, et al: Stethoscope acoustics: Transmission and filtration patterns. *Circulation* 1996; 34:889–899.

Groom D: Comparative efficiency of stethoscopes. *Am Heart J* 1967; 68:220.

Groom D, Chapman W: Anatomic variations of the auditory canal pertaining to the fit of the stethoscope earpieces. *Circulation* 1959; 19:606.

Hampton CS, Chaloner A: Which stethoscope? *Br Med J* 1967; 4:388.

Howell WL, Aldridge CF: The effect of stethoscope-applied pressure in auscultation. *Circulation* 1965; 32:430.

Johnston FD: An acoustical study of the stethoscope. *Arch Intern Med* 1940; 65:328.

Kindig JR, et al: Acoustical performance of the stethoscope. *Am Heart J* 1982; 1104:269.

Olive JP, Greenwood-Coleman J: Acoustics of American English speech. In: *A Dynamic Approach*. New York, Springer Verlag, 1993: 3.11–3.18.

2

THE BASICS OF AUSCULTATION

THE NORMAL HEART
  First Heart Sound (S₁)
  Second Heart Sound (S₂)

AREAS OF AUSCULTATION
  Apex
  Pulmonary Area (PA)
  Aortic Area (AA)

SPECIAL CONSIDERATIONS
  Pregnancy
  Athletes
  Age-Related Changes
  Innocent Systolic Murmurs

ROUTINE AUSCULTATION
  Basic Technique and Locations
  Techniques of Dynamic Auscultation

POSITIONS OF EXAMINATION
  Position 1: 45 Degrees Supine
  Position 2: Left Lateral Supine
  Position 3: Supine with or without Legs Elevated
  Position 4: Sitting Up
  Position 5: Standing
  Position 6: Squatting
  Position 7: Knee-Chest and Knee-Elbow
  Physiology of Auscultatory Positions
  Other Considerations in Auscultation

VASCULAR AUSCULTATION

DYNAMIC AUSCULTATION
  Sustained Fist Clenching or Hand Grip
  Isotonic Exercise

Carotid Sinus Pressure and Atrial Pacing
Drugs
Maneuvers
Other Effects That Enhance Auscultation

The highly publicized phenomenon of sudden death from cardiac disease among some well-known athletes, the increasing numbers of people living into their ninth decade, and new discoveries about physiologic events such as pregnancy have both deepened our understanding about auscultation of the normal heart, and strengthened the ability of clinical practitioners to recognize abnormal heart sounds using auscultation.

THE NORMAL HEART

Auscultation is carried out using the stethoscope end that is appropriate and locating it at the correct position on the chest wall, while the patient is placed in the appropriate position. Abbreviated terminology and cardiophonetics are illustrated in Table 2-2.

First Heart Sound (S₁)

The first heart sound (S_1) in auscultatory phonetics is designated Lup, and is caused by closure of the mitral and tricuspid valves and ventricle systole. This sound is best heard at the apex of the heart where it is phonetically designated Lup. Closure of the mitral valve (M_1) is louder than tricuspid closure (T_1). T_1 is heard normally only at the left sternal edge; hence M_1T_1 are heard together as THRup ↓, as written in uppercase letters (Fig. 2-

Table 2-1   Auscultation of the Normal Heart with Cardiophonetics

Heart sound	Comment	Cardiophonetic
S₁	Normal	LŬP
S₂	Split on inspiration, up to age 40	THRŭp
S₃	Heard at apex, up to age 40 and in pregnancy	LŬP/Dŭ-dŭp
S₄	Audible but low-pitched, in patients over age 65	Lŭh-Lŭp/Dŭp
Ejection sound	Pregnancy	Lŭ-TUK/DUP
Midsystolic murmur	Athletes with bradycardia	Lŭ-RRR/DUP ↗ ↘
Continuous murmur	Heard over breast, jugular veins, and uterus	RRRR
Fetal heart	In pregnant women (after 20 weeks' gestation)	TUK-TUK-TUK

NOTE: Capital L (Lup) indicates that it is loud, while the lower case l (lup) indicates a soft sound. For example, Lup/Dup indicates a pause before the accented syllable Lup while Du-dup indicates tied-in syllables; thus, Lup/Du-dup is Lup (loud, accented), "/" indicates a pause and the syllables Du-dup are loud and soft, respectively.

Table 2-2   Standard Cardiology Abbreviations

Abbr.	Meaning	Abbr.	Meaning
A_2	Aortic valve closure	MSM	Midsystolic murmur
A_2P_2	Aortic pulmonary valve closure	MVP	Mitral valve prolapse
AA	Aortic area	N	Normal
AR	Aortic regurgitation	NEC	Nonejection click
AS	Aortic stenosis	OS	Opening snap
ASD	Atrial septal defect	P_2	Pulmonary valve closure
BP	Blood pressure	PA	Pulmonary area
CO	Cardiac output	PAC	Premature atrial contraction
CoA	Coarctation of the aorta	PDA	Patent ductus arteriosus
ES	Ejection sound	PS	Pulmonary stenosis
HOCM	Hypertrophic obstructive	PVC	Premature ventricular contraction
	cardiomyopathy	RA	Right atrium
HSM	Holosystolic murmur	RBBB	Right bundle branch block
ICS	Intercostal space	RV	Right ventricle
IVD	Isovolemic diastole	S_1	First heart sound
IVS	Isovolemic systole	S_2	Second heart sound
JVD	Jugular venous distention	S_3	Third heart sound
LA	Left atrium	S_4	Fourth heart sound
LBBB	Left bundle branch block	SV	Stroke volume
LLSB	Left lower sternal border	SVR	Systemic vascular resistance
LSM	Late systolic murmur	T_1	Tricuspid valve closure
LV	Left ventricle	TGA	Transposition of the great
M_1	Mitral valve closure		arteries
MDM	Middiastolic murmur	TOF	Tetralogy of Fallot
MR	Mitral regurgitation	VR	Venous return
MS	Mitral stenosis	VSD	Ventricular septal defect

$1D$). The LUP of mitral valve closure is heard best at the apex and is much softer at the base (lup). This sound with ventricular systole makes up S_1 at the apex (Fig. 2-1A).

Second Heart Sound (S_2)

At the apex S_1 is loud and S_2 is soft. Hence, the closure of the mitral valve and tricuspid valve $M_1T_1(S_1)$, designated LŬP, is followed by the second heart sound (S_2), designated dŭp. S_2 is actually made up of two components, A_2 and P_2, which is sharp, high-pitched, and softer than A_2. A_2 is heard in the left second intercostal space, hence DRŭp (Fig. 2-1B) in the pulmonic area and in the aortic area a single second sound is heard (DUP) (Fig. 2-1C).

AREAS OF AUSCULTATION

Apex

The classic auscultatory phonetics of S_1 (LUP) is followed by S_2 (dup), hence—Lŭp/dŭp, Lŭp/dŭp, Lŭp/dŭp—signify normal first and second

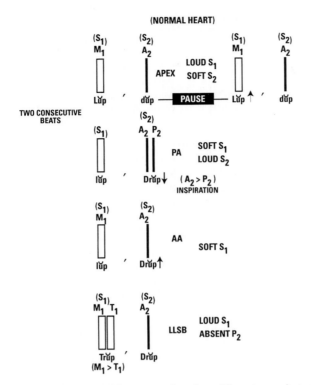

Figure 2-1 Normal heart sounds at four different auscultatory locations.

sounds in sequence. Note that Dŭp-Lŭp interval corresponds with diastole and is longer than the Lup/dup interval, corresponding with systole. At normal heart rates (60 to 80 beats per minute) a third sound (S_3) may be heard at the apex up to age 40, hence LUP/du-dup.

Pulmonary Area (PA)

Auscultation is carried out with a stethoscope diaphragm over the second left intercostal space in the pulmonary area. S_1 is soft, S_2 loud, and on inspiration, physiologically S_2 may divide into two components. After S_1 is heard as lup (note the lower case letter l, indicating a soft sound), S_2 is heard as a louder Dup sound, as denoted by its upper-case D, or Drup (A_2-P_2) written with an upper-case "D." This depends on the phase of respiration; S_2 is split in inspiration (Fig. 2-1*B*). In older patients, splitting on inspiration may not be evident (Fig. 2-1*D*). The louder DR designates A_2 preceding the softer up, designated P_2.

Aortic Area (AA)

A_2, the first component of S_2, is louder than P_2, the second component. The sounds heard are a soft S_1 and loud A_2, designated lup-Dup (Fig. 2-1D) since S_1 is soft in the aortic area.

In a normal adult up to the age of 40, an S_3 may be heard in the left lateral position. This is a low-pitched sound—Lŭp/dŭ-dŭp (S_4, S_1, S_2) at the apex. Although the S_3 heard up to age 40 is usually normal, in a patient with a diseased heart, S_3 indicates significant elevation of left atrial pressure, heart failure, or a noncompliant ventricle. S_3 in children and young adults is higher-pitched; hence LŬP/dŭ DŬP. DUP ↑ increases in pitch in the normal heart in contrast to dup ↓, which is soft and low-pitched in heart failure.

An S_4—Lŭ-Lŭp/dŭp (S_4, S_1, S_2)—is not normally heard. A very soft S_4, in the absence of a double apical impulse coincidental with S_4 and S_1, may be heard in older persons and may indicate presbycardia. Decreased ventricular compliance is implicated as the cause. It has been shown that in physically conditioned elderly persons an S_4 is rarely heard. In these patients only a single apical impulse is felt. This corresponds with the findings on the Doppler atrial tracing of a prominent a wave in elderly patients; it is not seen in conditioned elderly patients (Chanderatna et al).

In athletes who are in training, a soft S_3 (LUP/du-dup) and S_4 (luh-Lup/dup) may be heard; they do not necessarily signify underlying pathology.

SPECIAL CONSIDERATIONS

Pregnancy

While S_3 is commonly heard in pregnancy, it is normal. Pregnant women often have systolic murmurs. These arise from the right ventricular outflow tract, are mid-systolic, grade III, and are associated with an ejection sound. S_2 may be widely split, but the split moves and is narrow on expiration.

Accentuation of S_1 occurs in a triple cadence simulating mitral stenosis in pregnancy. Thus, LŬP/dŭ-dŭp (S_1, S_2, S_3) is heard best in the left lateral supine position with the bell of the stethoscope at the apex. This combination needs to be distinguished from the Lŭp/dŭ-drr of mitral stenosis. This is a common mistake. Systolic murmurs may be heard above the clavicle and over the pulmonary artery, and a prominent jugular venous hum may simulate a patent ductus in pregnant patients. A continuous murmur representing a prominent mammary soufflé may be heard over the breasts in pregnancy and is usually extinguished with stethoscope pressure. It is a normal finding. A continuous murmur over the uterus may be present, as well as fetal heart sounds. Occasionally an ejection sound may be heard as well (Fig. 2-2).

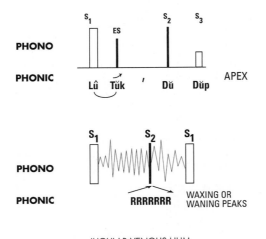

Figure 2-2 Phonophonic representation of ejection sound and mammary souffle in pregnancy.

Athletes

Athletes often have resting bradycardia, and may have systolic murmurs at the left sternal border unassociated with clicks. S_2 is physiologically split. A soft S_4 and an S_3 may be heard. Pulse pressure is wide in athletes, but usually does not exceed 50 mmHg. Bradycardia is associated with a loud S_1—LŬP/dŭp at the apex due to increased contractility.

Age-Related Changes

As patients age, the ventricle becomes less compliant and an S_4 may be present. Midsystolic ejection murmurs may be heard over the left ventricular outflow tract and in the neck. S_2 is usually single, and is considered normal in this population. A physiologically split S_2 (A_2P_2), however, points to the need to exclude mitral regurgitation, a ventricular septal defect, or right bundle branch block; or, if the split is fixed (A_2-P_2), atrial septal defect. If the split is paradoxical (P_2-A_2), left bundle branch block, aortic stenosis, and hypertension may be implicated. Cardiophonetically, the latter split is heard on expiration drUP corresponding with a soft P_2 and a loud A_2, signifying reversed splitting of S_2 in contrast with DRup (loud A_2 preceding soft A_2). Hence, it is possible to distinguish physiological splitting of S_2 from reversed splitting, both cardiophonetically as well as by the effects of respiration if A_2 and P_2 are of normal amplitude.

Midsystolic murmurs in elderly patients are commonly heard. These are soft to moderate and unassociated with a thrill. In these patients, pulse pressures are elevated but seldom more than 60 mmHg. During exercise, diastole is attenuated. Hence, the gap between dŭp and lŭp is shortened and under exceptional conditions is shorter than systole. This phenomenon causes "tic-tac rhythm" and is often present in patients in shock. It sounds like TUK-TUK-TUK-TUK, incorrectly called "tic-tac." Similarly, in brady-cardia, stroke volume is increased and S_1 may be accentuated, due to prolonged diastolic filling time, with resultant augmented stroke volume (Lup).

At birth, patent ductus arteriosus yields a systolic (only) murmur. This murmur is cardiophonetically SHH-DUP, is physiological and disappears over the first few days of life.

Innocent Systolic Murmurs

Salient features of innocent systolic murmurs include a buzzing, groaning, or croaking character called Still's murmur. Innocent systolic murmurs may present as blowing midsystolic murmurs that are heard best at the left sternal edge, and are ejection in type. They are thought to arise from the right ventricular outflow tract. Innocent murmurs are not associated with a thrill (i.e., grades I to III). "These murmurs keep innocent company," specifically meaning that they are not associated with ejection sounds or clicks. Murmurs arising from the right ventricular outflow tract and supra-clavicular murmurs are examples of innocent systolic murmurs. The latter disappear when the patient's shoulders are braced. Chest deformities are a common cause of innocent murmurs as in the straight back syndrome and may be caused by mechanical compression of the cardiac outflow tracts. Innocent murmurs are not associated with clicks or other murmurs.

ROUTINE AUSCULTATION

In preparation for auscultatory examination, be sure to close the doors to the examining room, and check to see that the room temperature is comfortable for the unclothed patient. Ask the patient to undress to the waist and put on an examination gown. If the patient is uncomfortable with disrobing, explain kindly but firmly that listening to the heart cannot be accomplished through clothing. Allow the patient a private area for chang-ing clothes and time to disrobe.

Basic Technique and Locations

Figure 2-3 indicates the positions on the chest for stethoscope placement during the examination. The stethoscope is inched from the cardiac apex to the left lower sternal edge, the midsternal edge, the pulmonary area, the aortic area, the right and left sternal borders, and below the xiphoid.

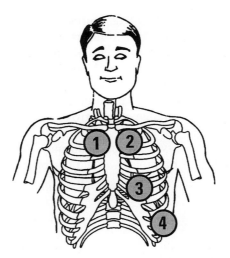

Figure 2-3 Positions on chest for stethoscope placement during auscultation. Reading clockwise: (1) aortic area; (2) pulmonary area; (3) tricuspid area (lower left sternal border); (4) mitral area (apex).

Radiating murmurs are detected from axillary to the scapular line in mitral regurgitation; right clavicle and above in aortic stenosis; and axillary in rubella syndrome.

Techniques of Dynamic Auscultation

A number of techniques may be used during stethoscope examination to augment auscultation and accentuate murmurs that may not be ordinarily heard. These techniques include:

1. Placing the patient in various positions for examination using the correct stethoscope end.
2. Having the patient sustain a clenched fist (an isometric exercise) during part of the examination.
3. Accentuating heart sounds with the assistance of drugs (e.g., amyl nitrite and pressor or conducting a cold pressor test).
4. Instructing the patient to perform the following maneuvers:
   a. Carvallo
   b. Valsalva (straining)
   c. Müller.
5. Applying carotid sinus pressure.
6. Auscultating during the pause that follows premature ventricular contractions (PVCs) (Brockenborough-Braunwald-Morrow test).
7. Selecting the correct site and correct stethoscope end piece for that site.

The cold pressor test involves immersing the patient's hands in ice, which increases peripheral systemic vascular resistance (afterload) for a longer period of time than the clenched-fist technique. While the cold pressor test achieves the same result as clenched fist, its effects are more difficult to reverse because of the test's characteristic rapid increase in afterload and increased contractility of the noncompliant ventricle.

POSITIONS OF EXAMINATION
Position 1: 45 Degrees Supine

Preparation The patient is asked to lie supine on the examining table with the head of the table tilted upward at a 45-degree angle (Fig. 2-4). This allows the physician to establish eye contact with the patient and gather valuable clinical information from the patient's appearance. These external signs include the patient's general demeanor; signs of dyspnea or relief in sitting up; pulsations of the carotid arteries and jugular veins; and the presence of pulsations over the precordium above the clavicle and subxiphoid area. You should also check for xanthomata, tophi, the diagonal ear crease, periodic apnea, and stridor.

Use your hands to warm the stethoscope. A few moments spent warming the hands and stethoscope are well worth the effort; it is extremely unpleasant to the patient to have a cold stethoscope or icy hands applied to the chest. In addition, applying cold hands or implements to the patient may elicit rapid breathing or nervous conversation, which interferes with effective auscultation. In general, it is best to discourage nonessential conversation during stethoscope examination.

Finally, remove other potential physical impediments to an effective examination by stethoscope. For instance, if the patient has pharyngeal secretions, perform suction if possible prior to auscultation. After such preparations, the examiner is ready to begin the examination.

Auscultation Sequence Listening to the heart begins at the mitral area or apex, with the examiner placing one finger on the carotid pulse to time

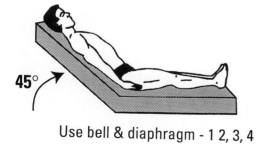

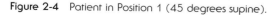
Use bell & diaphragm - 1 2, 3, 4

Figure 2-4   Patient in Position 1 (45 degrees supine).

S_1 (Fig. 2-5). Proceed, inching the stethoscope into the left lower intercostal space, up along the left border of the sternum to the second intercostal space (pulmonary area) and across to the second right intercostal space (aortic area). Listen to both carotid arteries with the patient holding his or her breath for a few seconds during auscultation. Listen for the sharpness and loudness of S_2 in the second intercostal space; these qualities provide the sound landmarks that distinguish S_2 from S_1. Lup sounds like "a ball thrown into a mitt" (Criley); Dup, a sharp sound, is like "a stone falling into a pond."

Next, note the heart rate, inspect the neck veins, and palpate the thyroid. Check the venous meniscus in the neck during breathing; it will normally fall during inspiration. Look for the presence of Kussmaul's sign, in which the opposite (venous distention during inspiration) will occur. Also, venous pressure is observed to rise in patients with heart failure when pressure is exerted on the abdomen. This test is performed as described by Ewy, by pressing on the patient's abdomen with the closed fist.

Position 2: Left Lateral Supine

The head of the examining table is dropped to approximately 15 degrees' elevation and the patient instructed to turn on the left side (Fig. 2-6). This position moves the heart against the chest wall and may allow the character

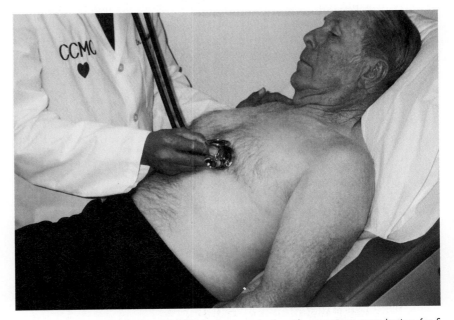

Figure 2-5 Patient in Position 1 (45 degrees supine), with examiner auscultating for S_1 while taking carotid pulse.

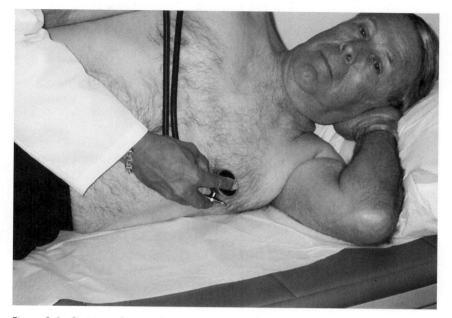

Figure 2-6 Patient in Position 2 (Left lateral supine).

of the apical impulse to be felt, and sometimes seen, as well. Examination is customarily performed with the practitioner standing behind the patient, on the patient's right side, and reaching over the shoulder to auscultate the chest. Depending, however, on the patient's size and the examiner's height, the practitioner may reverse this position and stand in front of the patient, on the patient's left side.

While lying in the left supine position, the patient is instructed to breathe in, breathe out, and hold his or her breath for a few seconds. With the patient holding the breath, the physician can then palpate at the apex for thrills and for impulses. When the bell of the stethoscope is very lightly applied to the apex, the physician can usually hear mitral valve closure, ventricular systole, and closure of the aortic valve (designated LUP/dup); and in patients up to age 40 (LUP/Du-dup) (S_1 S_2 S_3) as well.

Heart sounds that may be heard in this position include a summation gallop or quadruple rhythm; the diastolic murmurs and thrill of mitral stenosis can be both heard and palpated. Also audible from this position are the holosystolic murmurs due to mitral regurgitation which may radiate to the axilla ($\overrightarrow{\text{SHHH}}$ or $\overrightarrow{\text{SHHH}}$), late systolic murmurs of mitral regurgitation, and the opening snap of the mitral valve. Use the bell to listen for low-pitched acoustic events such as middiastolic murmurs (MDM), and S_3-S_4; use the diaphragm to listen for high-pitched sounds such as holosystolic murmurs. For intermediate frequencies, the corrugated diaphragm is sometimes useful in certain cases of aortic regurgitation; increasing the frequency of pickup from low to high by pressure on the diaphragm helps in listening for the Austin Flint and Cecil Cole murmurs (Chap. 5).

Position 3: Supine with or without Legs Elevated

For this position, have the patient turn over onto his or her back and lie supine with the head elevated about 10 to 15 degrees (Figs. 2-7 and 2-8). Position 3 is the ideal position to palpate the right ventricular (RV) and pulmonary and aortic areas, and to feel for thrills. Abdominal bruits are listened for, and pulsation and tenderness are noted. The bell of the stethoscope is used in auscultation for deeper penetration.

Neck veins will become evident in position 3 if the patient's venous pressure is low (Cardiac Pearl 49). If patients are in heart failure, they will not tolerate this position and will develop shortness of breath. In this event, you may need to elevate the patient's head between 30 and 40 degrees from the horizontal. Auscultation also may be carried out with the legs supported and elevated to 15 degrees. Leg elevation increases venous return, augments S_3 and S_4 sounds, and delays nonejection clicks (Fig. 2-8). Return the legs to a horizontal position and listen for the murmurs of pulmonary branch stenosis in the axilla. Listen for continuous murmurs at the pulmonary area for patent ductus arteriosus; at the left lower sternal border for aortopulmonary windows; and at the apex for coronary arteriovenous fistulae.

Percussion   It is useful to percuss the liver, parallel to the upper border, then at right angles to the right cardiac border. Next, percuss for the left heart border, moving tangentially from left to right and from the lower areas cephalad. By using this pattern of percussion, the examiner can detect possible right atrial enlargement and cardiomegaly.

Palpation   Following percussion, palpate the abdomen for enlargement or pulsation of the liver using the closed-fist method abdominal thrust

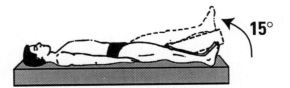

Use bell & diaphragm - 1 2, 3, 4 (normal breathing)
Supine and legs elevated

Figure 2-7   Patient in Position 3 (Supine with legs elevated).

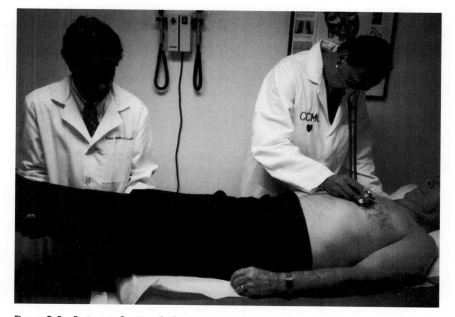

Figure 2-8   Patient in Position 3 (Supine with legs elevated), to increase venous return. An assistant is holding the patient's legs at the proper angle (15 degrees).

as described by Ewy, while observing the venous pressure as previously described. Be sure to note whether the upper border of the liver is in the normal location. Check the epigastric and subcostal areas for the expanding pulsations of an abdominal aneurysm, or for right ventricular pulsations. Examine the patient's groin and loin areas for renal artery bruits, using the bell of the stethoscope.

Inspection   Inspect the patient's abdomen for an everted umbilicus, distension, and upper truncal obesity. Also perform percussion of the abdomen; dullness in the flanks on either or both sides indicates fluid accumulation in dependent areas. Then listen for bowel sounds. In male patients, inspect for a lower right testis, which may be a sign of dextrocardia. Palpate the femoral pulses and listen for murmurs over the femoral and iliac pulses. Palpate and inspect all four extremities and their pulses, and check for brachiofemoral lag.

Position 3 (supine) is excellent for listening below the xiphoid for an RV, S_3, an S_4, or for tricuspid regurgitation. Listening is facilitated by tilting the stethoscope caudad to the heart on held inspiration. Listening below the xiphoid is also useful in the presence of emphysema in detecting right ventricular impulses and sounds. Look for accessory nipples from the breast to the inguinal line.

Position 4: Sitting Up

Have the patient sit up on the horizontal part of the examining table or bed with legs hanging down over the edge (Fig. 2-9). Instruct the patient to lean forward slightly, chin up, with hands behind the back to support the patient (Fig. 2-10). If the patient cannot fold his or her arms behind the back, ask him or her to raise the arms above the head as an alternative technique (Fig. 2-9B). Both these methods displace the aorta and pulmonary artery toward the examiner's stethoscope. Twisting the trunk may bring out an occult rub of pericarditis. Palpation for a thrill, for pulsations, and for subsequent auscultation is carried out at the base of the heart, in the second left intercostal space. Inspiratory splitting of S_2 is elicited in this position and is usually heard in younger patients. Inspiratory splitting in an older patient in the absence of right bundle branch block suggests an atrial septal defect, ventricular septal defect, or mitral regurgitation, as normally S_2 is heard as a single sound in these patients (DÚP).

Position 4 (sitting up) is ideal for listening to the continuous murmur of patent ductus arteriosus, ejection midsystolic murmurs of pulmonary and aortic stenosis, and ejection sounds and clicks at the base; while Still's murmur and an innocent midsystolic buzzing murmur can be heard at the right or left sternal edge (Fig. 2-11) below the nipple line.

In position 4 (sitting up), the nonejection click of mitral valve prolapse falls close to S_1 and may be partially obscured due to proximity to S_1. Nonejection clicks are an indication to perform rapid sequential auscultation, in the supine, upright, and standing positions. This technique will cause the heart to become smaller in sequence and the mitral click to be heard closer to S_1. It is position-induced heart size change that alters the

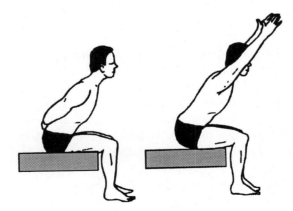

Use diaphragm - 3, 4 (normal breathing)

Figure 2-9 Patient in Position 4 (Sitting up). (A) and (B) illustrate the positions of the patient's arms for displacing the aorta and pulmonary artery toward the examiner's stethoscope.

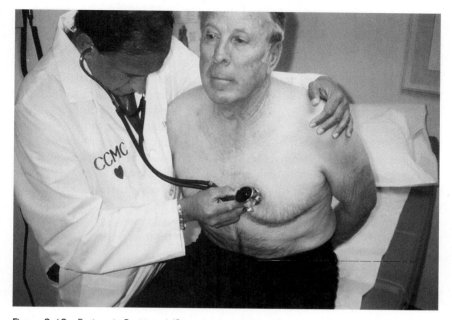

Figure 2-10   Patient in Position 4 (Sitting up) with hands behind back, chin up, and leaning forward. The examiner is performing auscultation with the patient in full expiration.

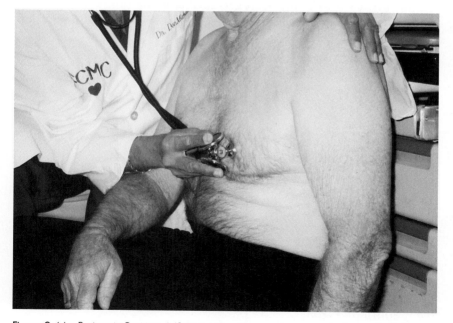

Figure 2-11   Patient in Position 4 (Sitting up), with examiner auscultating at the left sternal edge with the diaphragm of the stethoscope.

timing of the NEC with respect to S_1, enabling it to be distinguished from an ES or S_4. It is important to note that inspiration, which selectively increases right heart size, delays the click caused by tricuspid prolapse after S_1. The musical Gallavardin murmur of aortic stenosis may be heard at the left lower sternal edge or apex. Position 4 (sitting up) also is ideal for listening for aortic regurgitation, pulmonary regurgitation, and for pericardial friction rubs. To do this, the practitioner uses the diaphragm with firm pressure on the chest wall or the corrugated diaphragm with progressive pressure to coapt the stethoscope end and/or pick up higher sounds.

The sitting-up position is ideal to interrogate S_2 and elicit splitting (A_2P_2). Held respiration is mandatory to examine bruits in the neck, the back of the chest, and the loin area and axilla. Deep breathing elicits rales at the base and axilla of each lung; rales can be readily auscultated in this position. A soft early diastolic murmur in the right second and third intercostal spaces in a patient with diastolic hypertension usually indicates an aneurysm of the ascending aorta.

Position 5: Standing

This is an excellent position for distinguishing ejection from nonejection clicks and from S_4 (Figs. 2-12 and 2-13). S_4 tends to disappear; and the ejection and nonejection clicks grow louder when the patient sits or stands. Furthermore, the timing of S_1 to ES is relatively fixed, although the timing of S_1 to NEC narrows as the heart gets smaller in this position. Pulmonary ejection sounds in pulmonary stenosis soften or disappear on inspiration.

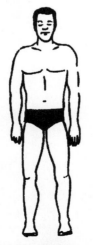

Use diaphragm - 2, 3

Figure 2-12 Patient in Position 5 (Standing).

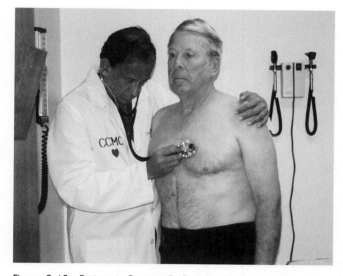

Figure 2-13 Patient in Position 5 (Standing), with examiner using the diaphragm of the stethoscope.

The sitting-up or standing positions decrease venous return. Thus, inspiration, by increasing the volume of blood drawn into the right side of the heart, may allow detection of physiologic splitting of S_2 into A_2 and P_2. Use both positions 4 and 5 to examine the lungs and the thorax for deformities, rales, and bronchi and to look for sacral edema (Fig. 2-13). If venous pressure is high, stand a short distance behind the patient's head to check for lateral displacement of the ears and sternomastoids, caused by pulsating internal jugular veins, the "rocking ear sign."

Position 5 (standing) augments the murmur of hypertrophic obstructive cardiomyopathy (HOCM). Prompt movement into position 6 (squatting) from position 5 will diminish this murmur and suggest the diagnosis. By having a patient in position 5 (standing) lean forward with their hands hanging down, the examiner can elicit Suzman's sign (pulsation of the axillary intercostal arteries in coarctation of the aorta and Fallot's tetralogy). A continuous murmur may be heard in the axilla in this position.

Position 6: Squatting

As squatting is awkward for many patients, this position (Fig. 2-14) can be made more convenient if there is a low stool available or if the examining table has a step built in at the bottom to allow for squatting. Ensure sufficient space for squatting safely. Support the patient as he or she moves into the squatting position, to ensure against injury. After this portion of the examination is completed, assist the patient in returning to the standing

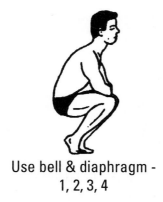

Use bell & diaphragm -
1, 2, 3, 4

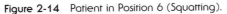

Figure 2-14   *Patient in Position 6 (Squatting).*

position (Fig. 2-12). The examiner can squat with the patient if possible, and come up with him or her, supporting the patient.

In position 6, venous return is increased due to squeezing action on the calf veins; an increase in systemic vascular resistance (SVR) also occurs because of partial clamping of the femoral arteries. Position 6 may augment filling sounds; they are detected by using the variable-frequency concertina diaphragm or bell and are further augmented by the clenched fist maneuver. By increasing heart size, the squatting position makes the nonejection click of mitral valve prolapse occur late. Also, cyanosis is reduced and the systolic murmur of tetralogy of Fallot increases as more blood is ejected into the pulmonary artery. The reduction of right-to-left shunting and increased pulmonary flow in the squatting position often relieves dyspnea in younger patients.

Position 6 (squatting) cannot be assumed by many older patients, and may be impossible in patients with orthopedic injuries. Thus, however useful, position 6 is not often used.

Position 7: Knee-Chest and Knee-Elbow

In the knee-chest position, the patient lies prone with face and chest elevated. It is another awkward position that is rarely employed. When the patient must be asked to assume this position, examination is kept brief for the sake of his or her comfort. Occasionally the patient is asked to get on his or her elbows and knees on the examining table [knee-elbow position (Fig. 2-15)]. The knee-chest position is preferred for detection of minimal aortic regurgitation and pericardial friction rubs, while abdominal fluid in small quantity can be detected by percussion over the inverted abdomen in the knee-elbow position. Position 7 facilitates elicitation of: (1) murmurs of aortic regurgitation, and (2) pericardial friction rubs. This position allows

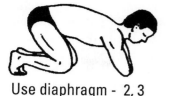

Use diaphragm - 2, 3

Figure 2-15 Patient in Position 7 (Knee-elbow variation).

the heart in an emphysematous patient to drop into the location of the stethoscope. By turning the supine patient onto his face and elevating his head, the discomfort of this awkward position is reduced.

Physiology of Auscultatory Positions

Table 2-3 summarizes the changes in venous return, blood pressure, and heart rate in the five most commonly used auscultatory positions.

Other Considerations in Auscultation (Cardiac Pearl 12)

In patients with chronic obstructive pulmonary disease (COPD), heart sounds and murmurs may be heard best in the subxiphoid area (Cardiac Pearl 67). The stethoscope may need to be tilted caudad in held inspiration, similar to an echo probe during a subcostal study, with the patient supine at a 45-degree angle. In dextrocardia (so-called situs solidus), the heart sounds and murmurs are heard on the right side, with P_2 louder than A_2. The clinician must distinguish whether there is isolated dextrocardia, isolated levocardia, or mirror-image dextrocardia.

Altered positions of auscultation also allow the examiner to adapt to orthopedic considerations in the patient's chest. Thus, the presence of pronounced abnormalities of the sternum, such as the pigeon chest (pectus carinatum), funnel chest (pectus excavatum), marked scoliosis or kyphosis with thoracic asymmetry, mastectomy, infiltration of the chest wall by tu-

Table 2-3 Physiological Changes Associated with the Most Commonly Used Auscultatory Positions

Position	VR	BP	HR
Supine	↑	N	N
Supine, legs elevated	↑	N	N
Sitting	↓	↑	↑
Standing	↓ ↓	↑	↑
Squatting	↑	↑	N

mor, crepitus over the chest wall in pneumomediastinum, and the presence of anasarca with peau d'orange (orange-peel skin), will require different positions in which auscultation can best be carried out. In the presence of breast prosthesis or in patients with large breasts, turning the patient to the right may allow auscultation to be carried out without stethoscope-prosthesis rattle (Cardiac Pearl 86). In pectus excavatum, tilting the stethoscope to the left on the sternum and using a non-rigid concertina diaphragm may be helpful. In certain cases aortic regurgitation can be heard if the patient is asked to lean in a standing position against the wall. Having the patient twist the trunk during auscultation may disclose a friction rub.

VASCULAR AUSCULTATION

Vascular auscultation should be carried out over the carotid arteries, subclavian arteries, abdominal aorta, and arteries of the flanks and groin (Fig. 2-16). Examination should continue over the femoral and iliac arteries, overlying arteriovenous fistulae, enlarged thyroid glands for continuous murmurs, and over the uterus for continuous murmurs, systolic murmurs, and fetal heart sounds. Auscultate over the head in patients with suspected aneurysms.

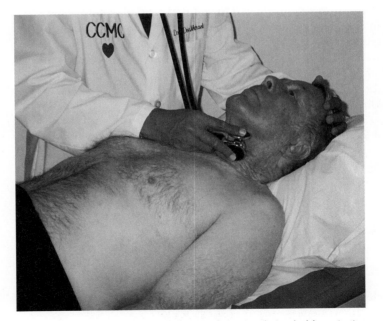

Figure 2-16 Auscultation over the carotid arteries during held respiration.

DYNAMIC AUSCULTATION

Table 2-4 summarizes the physiological changes related to the various maneuvers used in dynamic auscultation.

Sustained Fist Clenching or Hand Grip (Fig. 2-17)

This technique, which is helpful in evoking and enhancing a variety of heart sounds, should be used with caution in a patient with symptoms of heart failure. In addition to enhancing S_3 and S_4, the procedure can increase mitral regurgitation, and even cause the heart to fail. Hence, it should not be used under any circumstances for more than a brief period of time. The sounds to listen for with sustained clenched fist include: S_3; S_4; nonejection clicks; and the aortic second sound (A_2). Accentuation of diastolic murmurs occurs in mitral stenosis, aortic regurgitation, and mitral regurgitation. A clenched fist will also accentuate the click and murmur of mitral valve prolapse, ventricular septal defect, and importantly, decrease the murmur of hypertrophic obstructive cardiomyopathy.

Isotonic Exercise

Isotonic exercise (e.g., treadmill exercise) is useful in bringing out the murmurs of mitral stenosis, which are also evoked by a few rapid breaths. Exercise reduces diastolic filling time and markedly increases diastolic flow and gradient across the mitral valve; hence, it produces a loud, long murmur.

Conversely, vasodilatation caused by exercise may cause reduction in regurgitant murmurs. Murmurs of the heart that are stenotic, including those of aortic and pulmonary stenosis, increase with exercise and atrial pacing. Murmurs that are associated with aortic regurgitation and mitral regurgitation do not change or soften.

Carotid Sinus Pressure and Atrial Pacing

Carotid sinus pressure applied with the fingers was first used by Levine to relieve angina. Application of pressure to the carotid sinus or gentle massage over the area may be used to observe the disappearance of S_3, S_4, and the late systolic apical murmur that may be concomitants of angina.

The use of a pacing electrode in the esophagus to increase the atrial rate evokes changes similar to those seen with treadmill testing.

Drugs

Amyl nitrite, a short-acting inhalant that is used to treat angina, can also be administered as a test to accentuate or decrease certain murmurs in

Table 2-4 Physiology of Dynamic Auscultation Indicating Changes[a]

Function	Supine, left side	Sitting	Squatting	Clenched fist	Carvallo maneuver	Valsalva phase 2	Valsalva phase 4
SVR	N	↑	↑	↑	N	↑	↓
VR	↓	↓	↑	O	↑	↓	↑
HT size	↑	N	↑	N	↑	↓	↑
SV	↑	N	↑	↑	↑	↓	↑
HR	N	N	N	↑	O	↑	↓

Function	Amyl nitrite	Pressors; carotid sinus pressure	Post-ectopic pause	Treadmill exercise	Beta-blockers	Cold pressors	Standing
SVR	↓	↑	N	↓	↑	↑	↑
VR	↓	N	↑	↑	N	N	↓
HT size	N	↑	N	↑	↑	N	↓
SV	↓	N	↑	N	↓	N	↓
HR	↑	↓	N	↑	↓	↓	↑

[a] Illustrates physiological changes caused by changing patient's position and dynamic auscultation with drugs and maneuvers.

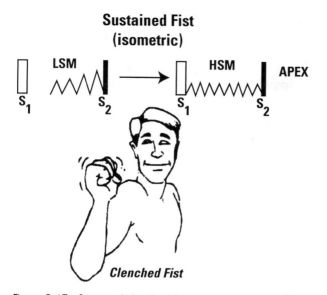

Figure 2-17 Sustained clenched fist maneuver. NOTE: S₁, first sound; S₂, second sound; SM, systolic murmur; LSM, late systolic murmur; HSM, holosystolic murmur.

characteristic ways (Table 2-5). This test is carried out with the patient lying completely supine. The examiner breaks the drug ampoule and instructs the patient to sniff three to five times (Fig. 2-18).

Amyl nitrite accentuates the murmur of hypertrophic obstructive cardiomyopathy by decreasing heart size. Because the drug also causes a fall in venous return to the heart and decreases systemic vascular resistance, amyl nitrite decreases the murmur of mitral regurgitation (Cardiac Pearl 3), functionally increasing the gradient. With the heart size reduced, the click of mitral valve prolapse falls earlier. Amyl nitrite causes the murmurs of mitral stenosis, pulmonary stenosis, and tricuspid stenosis to increase, as it does innocent murmurs. Murmurs of aortic and mitral regurgitation and the diastolic component of patent ductus arteriosus decrease in intensity.

In cyanotic congenital heart disease associated with the tetralogy of Fallot, amyl nitrite decreases venous return and also causes a reduction in systemic vascular resistance, resulting in an increase in right-to-left shunting across the unrestricted ventricular septal defect (VSD). This phenomenon is not uniformly seen, however. A fall in blood pressure in tetralogy of Fallot may cause increased right-to-left shunting, offsetting the effect of squatting.

Amyl nitrite may have no effect on the systolic murmur in tetralogy of Fallot in the presence of severe pulmonary stenosis with an unrestricted ventricular septal defect. In the presence of a large VSD with a systemic resistance higher than pulmonary resistance—so-called pink Fallot with predominant pulmonary stenosis—the right-sided murmur may increase.

Amyl Nitrite Inhalation

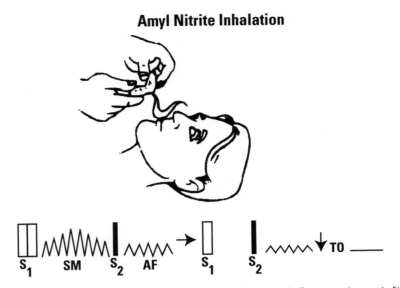

Figure 2-18 Amyl nitrite inhalation. NOTE: S_1, first sound; S_2, second sound; SM, systolic murmur; AF, Austin Flint middiastolic murmur.

Whereas, if pulmonary resistance exceeds systemic resistance in the presence of an unrestricted VSD—blue Fallot—the murmur may decrease as a result of increased right-to-left shunting and decreased pulmonary flow (Chap. 5).

Pressors decrease the murmur of hypertrophic obstructive cardiomyopathy; amyl nitrite increases it. Amyl nitrite is useful in diagnosing patients with aortic regurgitation, because it causes the diastolic murmur to be delayed or softened, and the Austin Flint late diastolic murmur to disappear. This change contrasts with the murmur of mitral stenosis, which gets louder. The drug extinguishes S_4 and the late systolic murmurs heard during an episode of angina. Pressors such as methoxamine (Vasoxyl) and angiotensin increase systemic vascular resistance (SVR), enhancing S_3, S_4, atrial regurgitation (AR), and mitral regurgitation (MR) murmurs.

Maneuvers (Table 2-5)

Carvallo Maneuver First described by Rivera Carvallo, this maneuver consists of holding deep inspiration for 3 to 5 s (Fig. 2-19). This breath-holding increases venous return to the right side of the heart and accentuates right-sided events such as right ventricular third and fourth sounds and tricuspid regurgitation. The pulmonary ejection sound, or click, in pulmonary valvular stenosis becomes softer because of preopening of the pulmonary valve on inspiration. This preopening is caused by an increase in right

Table 2-5 Positions for Auscultation with Related Maneuvers and Physiological Changes.

Position	Auscultatory action(s)	Maneuver(s)	Physiology			
			VR	SVR	CO	BP
1 (45° Supine)	Observe patient's facial expression and general appearance Check for xanthomata, tophi, crease sign, arcus, periodic apnea, stridor Check for JVD Take pulses in upper extremities Take BP in both arms Listen for bruits Identify S_1 by S_2	None				
2 (Left Lateral)	Feel apex and LV Listen with bell gently at apex, full expiration, for thrills Note S_3, S_4, MDM Listen for M_1 A_2 ± S_3	Clenched fist		N		
3 (Supine, Legs Elevated)	Observe neck and neck veins Palpate RV, PA, AO Percuss right border, left border Auscultate at second ICS; listen for bruits Observe (in males) scrotum and testes for possible situs inversus Percuss liver	Amyl nitrite Valsalva Carotid sinus NTG SL		N		
4 (Sitting)	Palpate liver, spleen, kidneys Listen to PA and AA Listen for A_2P_2 on inspiration Note whether A_2 is louder than P_2 Listen for ES, NEC, systolic ejection murmurs Listen to lungs	Carvallo Full expiration Valsalva				
5 (Standing)	Check for sacral edema and leg swelling Listen for ejection sounds	Valsalva				
6 (Squatting)	Listen for NEC and early systolic bruit Listen for delay in nonejection click Listen for increased S_3 and S_4 Listen for increased HOCM bruits	None				
7 (Knee-Chest)	Listen for pericardial rub Listen for AR murmur	None				

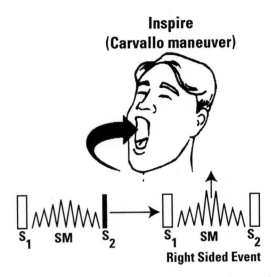

Figure 2-19 Carvallo maneuver (inspiration). NOTE: S_1, first sound; S_2, second sound; SM, systolic murmur.

ventricular end diastolic pressure. Do not forget to have the patient resume normal breathing after the completion of the Carvallo maneuver.

Valsalva Maneuver   Described below is a useful bedside test that employs the Valsalva maneuver; it has four phases. Phases (2) and (4) are the major phases in causing hemodynamic changes (Table 2-4). Straining is done against a closed glottis.

1. Initial straining. This phase causes a transient increase in blood pressure caused by the sudden increase in intracardiac pressure.
2. Sustained straining. Venous return decreases with a falling of the right ventricular and subsequently left ventricular stroke volume. This fall initiates a basoreceptor-mediated tachycardia with reflex increase in heart rate.
3. Release. A transient decrease in blood pressure occurs secondary to the fall in intrathoracic pressure.
4. Postrelease, or "overshoot." An increase in right-sided filling is followed by an increase in left-sided filling. Increased stroke volume and blood pressure volume cause a basoreceptor-mediated bradycardia.

The Valsalva maneuver itself is produced by pushing the patient's abdomen against an unyielding fist [with the patient lying supine (Fig. 2-20)]. It can also be performed by asking the patient to bear down with an obstructing finger in the mouth—sometimes called the "whistle blower" position (Fig. 2-21).

Supine Position

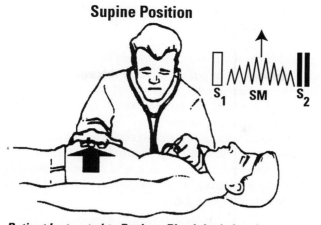

Patient Instructed to Push on Physician's hand

Figure 2-20 Valsalva maneuver, patient exerting abdominal pressure against examiner's hand. NOTE: S₁, first sound; S₂, second sound; SM, systolic murmur.

The Valsalva maneuver is the opposite of the Müller maneuver described below. The Valsalva maneuver is useful in detecting murmurs or hypertrophic obstructive cardiomyopathy. The murmur grows louder due to the reduced filling of the left heart that occurs late in phase 2. The click and murmur of mitral valve prolapse tend to occur earlier. The Valsalva maneuver decreases right-sided murmurs during phase 1, and left-sided murmurs during the late part of this phase. Initially, right heart sounds are accentuated in phase 4 after release; then left-sided sounds are heard. This enables a distinction to be made between left- and right-sided murmurs.

Valvasa "Whistle-blower" position

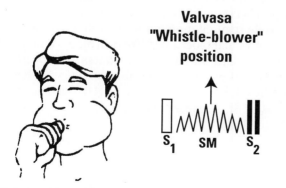

Exhaling Into Closed Fist

Figure 2-21 Valsalva maneuver, "whistle blower" position. NOTE: S₁, first sound; S₂, second sound; SM, systolic murmur.

A two-component pericardial rub becomes three components with the Valsalva maneuver (Cardiac Pearl 20).

Müller Maneuver   In the Müller maneuver, the patient breathes in against a closed glottis. Hence the abdomen is pulled in while the glottis is closed, as opposed to pushing the abdomen out when the glottis is closed. As described in the diagnosis of HOCM, the patient would be instructed to push the abdomen out without sucking in air.

The Müller maneuver causes venous return and right ventricular stroke volume to increase. It also causes increases in ventricular afterload and right-sided murmurs. The Müller maneuver is less useful and more difficult to perform than the Carvallo maneuver. It is not commonly used but is mentioned here for completeness (Table 2-6).

Other Effects That Enhance Auscultation

Postpause   During the pause produced by electrical activity that follows premature ventricular contractions or atrial fibrillation, a well-known physiological enhanced response occurs. The normal pulse, blood pressure, heart sounds, and murmurs are enhanced. After the pause in hypertrophic obstructive cardiomyopathy and aortic stenosis, the heart murmur is increased. In HOCM and aortic stenosis the heart murmur is increased; the pulse pressure and blood pressure after a pause show attenuation, indicating a positive Braunwauld-Brockenborough-Morrow response. The murmur paradoxically is unchanged.

Atrial Pacing   In this technique, the bipolar electrode performing pacing is placed in the esophagus and the atrium to produce contractions. The electrode is stimulated electrically by an outside battery. Placement of the electrode is guided by the esophageal P wave. Atrial pacing is a useful means of obtaining a stress echocardiogram. In general, stenotic murmurs get louder during pacing, while regurgitation murmurs soften. At the time second-degree Type I atrioventricular block (Wenckebach block) is induced by pacing, S_1 displays the standard variation in loudness (Chap. 5). If ischemia is produced, an S_4 and apical systolic murmur may be heard transesophageally. As the PR interval increases, LŬP/DŬP becomes lup' DŬP, signifying the softness of S_1. A pause follows, succeeded by a short PR interval and loud S_1 (LUP/DŬP).

TRUE OR FALSE

1. S_4 over age 65 is always abnormal.
2. S_3 up to age 40 is normal.
3. S_4 in pregnancy is normal.

4. Innocent murmurs keep innocent company.
5. S_1 is loud in sinus bradycardia.
6. Diastolic murmurs may be benign.
7. A valvular click is always abnormal.
8. S_2 is often single in older patients.
9. Amyl nitrite increases the murmur of HOCM.
10. Amyl nitrite causes a predictable effect on murmurs in tetralogy of Fallot.
11. The Müller maneuver is highly useful, offering significant advantages over the Carvallo and Valsalva maneuvers.

CLINICAL VIGNETTES

The following vignettes present actual cases of patients who were affected by diseases and conditions discussed in this chapter. At the end of each case, choose the one answer that best describes the diagnosis indicated by the vignette.

1. A 34-year-old woman presents in the ER with angina and dyspnea that began when she was lying on her left side. A diagnosis of mitral valve prolapse has been made by the referring physician. On turning the patient on her left side during your examination, her complaint is confirmed by both the chest pain and shortness of breath that are elicited in this position. Using auscultation at the apex with the stethoscope bell, a loud S_1, an S_2, and an S_3 followed by a middiastolic murmur (MDM) which simulates mitral stenosis are heard. At the apex, a loud diastolic low-pitched sound occurs approximately 100 ms after A_2 and preceding the MDM. The echocardiogram is uninformative, although mitral valve excursion appears diminished.
The diagnosis is:

A. Mitral stenosis
B. Left atrial myxoma
C. Tricuspid regurgitation

2. A 16-year-old male was referred with a diagnosis of mitral regurgitation. He was in sinus rhythm with frequent premature ventricular contractions (PVCs). When the clinician auscultated at the apex, she heard a harsh grade IV systolic murmur. After administering amyl nitrite to the patient, the murmur increased. The pulse beat after a pause following a PVC diminished markedly. The diagnosis is:

A. Aortic stenosis
B. Mitral regurgitation
C. Hypertrophic obstructive cardiomyopathy.

3. A 54-year-old male presented with shortness of breath and a history of asthma. His heart was enlarged. In the course of examining the patient in the left lateral position, the clinician discovered an S_4. With the patient in this position, the examiner asked him to clench his fist, and the following sequence of events occurred:
    a. An S_3 appeared.
    b. A quadruple rhythm was present.
    c. The patient developed a summation gallop, tachycardia, shortness of breath.
        In response to these signs, the patient was asked to release his clenched fist and to stand up. Signs a–c disappeared, and the patient returned to normal status.
    The diagnosis is:

A. Increased systemic vascular resistance.
B. Transitory heart failure.
C. A. and B.

4. You are a physician working for a health maintenance organization and are obliged to see approximately 30 to 40 patients a day. The head of the HMO's utilization review committee asks you for advice as to whether there is any way for clinicians to cut down on the time involved in auscultation without compromising the effectiveness of the examination.
    The answer is:

A. Yes; use positions 1, 2, and 4, and omit the rest.
B. Yes, use positions 1 and 3 and omit the rest.
C. No, there is no way to do this.

ANSWERS

True or False

1. F; 2. T; 3. F; 4. T; 5. T; 6. F; 7. T; 8. T; 9. T; 10. F; 11. F

Clinical Vignettes

1. *B. Atrial myxoma.* This patient had immediate cardiac catheterization performed with a presumptive diagnosis of left atrial myxoma. The levophase of the pulmonary angiogram revealed a large mass originating from the atrial septum and filling the left atrium, prolapsing through the mitral valve. The auscultatory findings with this patient in the left lateral position gave the diagnosis. Surgical removal of the mass and pathological examination confirmed the diagnosis of a myxoma.

2. *C. Hypertrophic obstructive cardiomyopathy* due to ventricular outflow tract dynamic obstruction. This diagnosis is indicated by an increase in the loudness of the murmur induced by amyl nitrite. If the murmur had disappeared or diminished, mitral regurgitation would have been considered. The S_2 in mitral regurgitation is physiologically split, enabling the examiner to distinguish between aortic stenosis and HOCM. The decreased pulse pressure, which is characteristically induced by the pause after a PVC or atrial fibrillation, is in character with hypertrophic obstructive cardiomyopathy (Brockenborough maneuver).

3. *C. Transitory heart failure* produced by increased systemic vascular resistance. The examiner had the patient clench his fist to increase systemic vascular resistance, or afterload, and thus increase venous return. Whereas the clenched-fist maneuver is safer than the cold pressor test as a useful bedside means of stressing the heart, both maneuvers must be used with caution when the patient is at risk of heart failure.

4. *A. Yes; use positions 1, 2, and 4, and omit the rest.*

The Art of Auscultation

Chatterjee K: Bedside evaluation of the heart physical examination. In Gowers (ed): Cardiology: An Illustrated Text/Reference, vol. 1. Philadelphia, New York, and London, Lippincott, 1993:3.25.

Chizner MA: Art of Auscultation, vol. 1. Cedar Grove, NJ, Laennec, 1995:108–118.

Hurst JW: The initial examination. In Auscultation of the Heart Arteries and Valves. St. Louis: Mosby, 1993:147–183.

Levine SA, Harvey WP: Clinical Auscultation of the Heart, 2nd ed. Philadelphia, Saunders, 1959.

Marriott HJL: Textbook of Bedside Diagnosis. Philadelphia, Lippincott, 1993.

Shaver JA, Salerni R: Auscultation of the heart. In Hurst JW (ed): The Heart, 7th ed. New York, McGraw-Hill, 1990:175–242.

Dynamic Auscultation

Beck W et al: Hemodynamic effects of amyl nitrite and phenylephrine on the normal human circulation and their relation to changes in cardiac murmurs. Am J Cardiol 1961; 8:341.

Cochran PT: Auscultatory clues elicited by physical maneuvers and pharmacologic agents. In Abrams J (ed): Essentials of Cardiac Physical Diagnosis. Philadelphia, Lea & Febiger, 1987:177–183.

Crawford MH, O'Rourke RA: A systematic approach to the bedside differentiation of cardiac murmurs and abnormal sounds. Curr Probl Cardiol 1977; 1:1–42.

Criscitiello MG: Physiologic and pharmacologic aids in cardiac auscultation. In Fowler NO (ed): Cardiac Diagnosis and Treatment, 3rd ed. Hagerstown, MD, Harper & Row, 1930:77–90.

Criscitiello MG, Harvey WP: Clinical recognition of congenital pulmonary valve insufficiency. Am J Cardiol 1967; 20:765.

de Leon AC, Harvey WP: Pharmacological agents and auscultation. Mod Concepts Cardiovasc Dis 1975; 44:23.

Lauson HD, et al: The influence of the respiration on the circulation of man. Am J Cardiol 1946; 1:315.

Lembo NJ, et al: Bedside diagnosis of cardiac murmurs. N Engl J Med 1988; 318:1572–1578.

McCraw DB, et al: Response of heart murmur intensity to isometric (hand grip) exercise. Br Heart J 1972; 34:605–610.

Morrison A: The value of amyl nitrite inhalation in the diagnosis of mitral stenosis. Br Med J 1918; 1:452.

Nellen M, et al: Effect of prompt squatting on the systolic murmur in idiopathic hypertrophic obstructive cardiomyopathy. Br Med J 1967; 3:140–143.

Nutter DO, et al: Isometric exercise and the cardiovascular system. Mod Concepts Cardiovasc Dis 1972; 41:11–15.

Sharpey-Shafer EP: Effects of squatting on the normal and failing circulation. Br Med J 1976; 1:1072.

Thapar MK, et al: Changing murmurs of patent ductus arteriosus. J Pediatr 1978; 92:939.

Vitums VC, et al: Bedside maneuvers to augment the murmur of tricuspid regurgitation. Med Ann DC 1969; 38:533.

Vogelpoel L, et al: The value of squatting in the diagnosis of mild aortic regurgitation. Am Heart J 1969; 77:709.

The Normal Heart

Carceres CA, Perry LW: The Innocent Murmur. Boston, Little, Brown, & Co., 1967:64–115.

Cutforth R, Macdonald CB: Heart sounds and murmurs in pregnancy. Am Heart J 1966; 71:74.

de Leon AC, Jr: "Straight Back" Syndrome. In Leon DF, Shaver JA (eds.) American Heart Association Monograph No. 46, Physiologic Principles of Heart Sounds and Murmurs. New York: American Heart Association, 1975:197–200.

Fowler NO, Marshall WJ: The supraclavicular atrial bruit. Am Heart J 1965; 69:410.

Griffiths RA, Sheldon MG: Clinical significance of systolic murmurs in the elderly. Age Ageing 1975; 4:99.

Groom D, et al: Venous hum in cardiac auscultation. JAMA 1955; 159:639.

Harvey WP: Alterations of the cardiac physical examination in normal pregnancy. Clin Obstet Gynecol 1975; 18:51.

Hurst JW, et al: Precordial murmurs during pregnancy and lactation. N Engl J Med 1958; 259:515.

Jones FL: Frequency, characteristics, and importance of the cervical venous hum in adults. N Engl J Med 1962; 267:658.

Leatham AL: Auscultation of the Heart and Phonocardiography, 2nd ed. Edinburgh, London, and New York: Churchill Livingstone, 1975.

Leatham AL, et al: Auscultatory and phonocardiography in healthy children with systolic murmurs. Br Heart J 1963; 25:451.

Levine SA, Harvey WP: Clinical Auscultation of the Heart, 2nd ed. Philadelphia, Saunders, 1959.

Martin CE, et al: Ejection sounds of right-sided origin. In Leon DF, Shaver JA (eds.) American Heart Association Monograph No. 46, Physiologic Principles of Heart Sounds and Murmurs, New York, American Heart Association, 1975:35.

Segal BL: Innocent murmurs. In Segal BL, et al (eds): The Theory and Practice of Auscultation. Philadelphia, Davis, 1964.

Shaver JA, et al: Ejection sounds of left-sided origin. In Leon DF, Shaver JA (eds.) American Heart Association Monograph No. 46, Physiologic Principles of Heart Sounds and Murmurs, New York, American Heart Association, 1975:35.

Tavel ME: Innocent murmurs. In Leon DF, Shaver JA (eds.) American Heart Association Monograph No. 46, Physiologic Principles of Heart Sounds and Murmurs, New York, American Heart Association, 1975:105–106.

3

HEMODYNAMIC BASIS OF HEART SOUNDS

HEMODYNAMIC DIAGRAMS

DYNAMIC CARDIAC PHASES

HEART SOUNDS
   The First Heart Sound (S_1) (D)
   Ejection Sounds
   Nonejection Clicks
   The Second Sound (S_2)
   The Third Heart Sound (S_3)
   The Fourth Heart Sound (S_4)
   Opening Snaps

HEMODYNAMICS OF ABNORMAL CONDITIONS
   Aortic Regurgitation
   Aortic Stenosis
   Pulsus Paradoxus and Tamponade
   The Echocardiographic Tamponade Sign
   Hypertrophic Cardiomyopathy with Obstruction
   Shunting
   Constrictive Pericarditis

QUESTIONS

The loudness, quality, and its correlation with other attributes of heart sounds reflect the character of the valve or ventricle causing the sound. From this anatomical connection evolved an understanding of the hemodynamics of heart sounds. The sounds are modified by such factors as the degree of fibrosis of the valve; the compliance of the ventricle; the velocity, volume, acceleration, and deceleration of blood flow; vibration of the valve or of the blood column; and the tautness, or resistance to flow, of the valve or chamber.

These factors can be analyzed by recording their electrical properties using electrocardiography, and by using a variety of instruments that measure changes in blood volume and pressure. Together these technologies provide the data for the study of blood flow, or hemodynamics. This chapter presents hemodynamic data from studies of normal as well as pathological heart conditions, and discusses their implications for effective auscultation.

HEMODYNAMIC DIAGRAMS

Numerous attempts have been made to combine electrical events, mechanical events, and sounds on one page. As this is confusing, an alternative, stepwise approach has been adopted. For example, the sequence of events is shown in terms of ECG (*top*) and mechanical events (*bottom*). These diagrams apply to both right and left sides of the heart. Figure 3-1 emphasizes that electrical events precede mechanical events. Thus, (1) the P wave signals atrial systole (depolarization); (2) the AS(1) signifies atrial mechanical systole; (3) the QRS signals ventricular depolarization; (4) (2–4) ventricular systole shows mechanical events following the QRS; (5) the T wave signifies ventricular depolarization; (6) (6 + 7) ventricular diastole follows the QRS; (7) the T_A wave of atrial repolarization is buried in the QRS complex and is not seen.

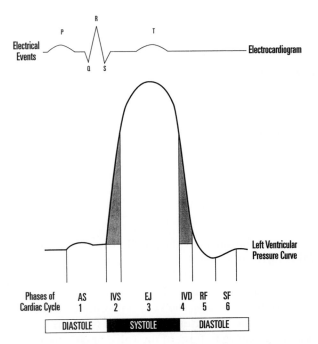

Figure 3-1   Electrocardiogram combined with ventricular pressure curves. 1. AS, atrial systole; 2. IVS, isovolumic systole (note shading); 3. IVD, isovolumic diastole (note shading); 4. EJ, ejection; 5. RF, rapid filling; 6. SF, slow filling.

An important principle illustrated by Fig. 3-1 is that electrical events precede mechanical events. For instance, note that atrial systole in late diastole, a mechanical event, occurs after the p wave, an electrical event that signals depolarization.

Note also that the top line of Fig. 3-1 indicates that the qrs complex occurs before ventricular systole, represented on the lower graph in its two phases: (1) isovolumic systole and (2) ejection (hatched section under curve). Ventricular diastole is electrocardiographically indicated on the upper graph by the t wave. The lower line shows that isovolemic diastole (IVD), rapid filling (RF), and slow filling (SF) are mechanical events. The t_a wave is embedded in the qrs complex on the upper graph and is not seen in this figure. Systole (hatched area) and diastole (open area) are distinguished.

DYNAMIC CARDIAC PHASES

Figure 3-2 illustrates the changes in cardiac structure and size that occur during normal heartbeat. These phases are featured in many of the pressure diagrams that are presented in this chapter.

Phase 1. Atrial systole.

Phase 2. Commencement of ventricular isovolumic systole. The ventricle increases its wall tension with resultant closing of the mitral and tricuspid valves. Aortic and pulmonary valves remain closed while ventricular contraction occurs and the atrioventricular ring is pulled downward, allowing the atria to fill by increasing its volume.

Phase 3. Ejection. The aortic and pulmonary valves open. This opening enables the ventricles to eject blood into the outflow tracts; the aorta and the pulmonary arteries. During this phase, the mitral and tricuspid valves remain closed. The atria continue to fill and expand while the ventricles get smaller as blood is ejected out into the outflow tracts.

Phase 4. Isovolumic diastole. The atria continue to fill as the ventricles begin to relax. Immediately prior to this event, the aortic and pulmonary valves close. Thus, isovolumic diastole is a phase in which the aortic and pulmonary valves are closed; the mitral and tricuspid valves are closed; and the atria fill, with the ventricles beginning to relax. There is no change in ventricular volume.

Phase 5. Rapid phase of ventricular diastole. The mitral and tricuspid valves open, allowing the atria to rapidly fill the right and left ventricles. The aortic and pulmonary valves are closed. The ventricles enlarge; the atria get smaller.

Phase 6. Diastasis. Slow filling of the ventricle occurs during this phase. The atria contract and the ventricle grows larger, but less rapidly than during Phase 5. The aortic and pulmonary valves remain closed.

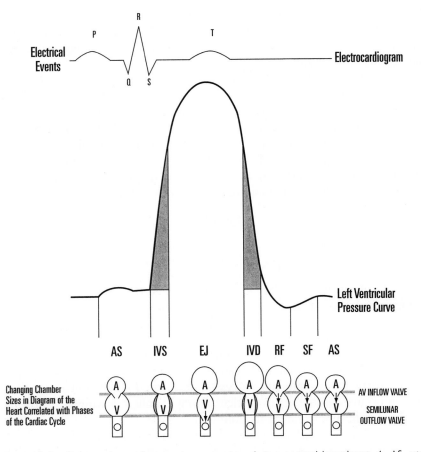

Figure 3-2 Changes in cardiac structure occurring during normal heartbeat. 1. AS, atrial systole; 2. IVS, isovolumic systole (note shading); 3. IVD, isovolumic diastole (note shading); 4. EJ, ejection; 5. RF, rapid filling; 6. SF, slow filling.

Phase 7. Atrial systole. The atria contract, opening the mitral and tricuspid valves with rapid filling of the ventricles, referred to as the "atrial kick." The atrial kick contributes up to about 25 percent of the volume of blood filling the ventricle. During this phase the atria shrink and the ventricles expand.

The upper graph in Fig. 3-3 shows the electrocardiogram as hemodynamic pressure crosses over between the atrium and ventricles. Atrial and ventricular pressures in Fig. 3-3 indicate a sequence of pressure waves. Atrial systole commences on the left side, as shown by the pressure curves in the lower graph. When atrial pressures are exceeded by ventricular pressures, closure of the mitral and tricuspid valves occurs prior to the 'v' wave.

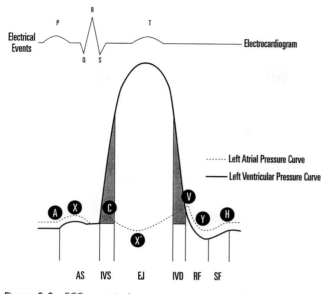

Figure 3-3 ECG, ventricular pressure curves, and atrial pressure tracings. A, atrial systole (emptying); X and X', atrial filling in atrial diastole; C, transmitted pulsation; V, crossover of atrial and ventricular pressures; Y, rapid atrial emptying; H, slow atrial emptying.

In Fig. 3-4, the aortic pressure curve shows crossover pressures between the left ventricle and the aorta. A similar sequence of events occurs on the right side of the heart. The aortic pressure drops in diastole, as shown at the upper left side of the diagram. As ventricular ejection begins, pressures in these chambers exceed aortic and pulmonary pressure, causing the pulmonary and aortic valves to open, in that order. Blood flows into the aorta and coronary artery during the ejection phase. As ventricular ejection slows, ventricular pressure drops. Aortic and pulmonary pressures drop and cross over ventricular pressures, leading to closure of the aortic and pulmonary valves; beginning Phase 4, ventricular isovolemic diastole. Aortic and pulmonary valve closures occur soon after this, during reflux into the outflow tracts (Chandraratna). Thus, the aortic and pulmonary valves open and close in the opposite sequence in early and late systole, i.e., P_{2E} precedes A_{2E} when opening, A_2 precedes P_2 when closing (P_E and A_E represent ejection sounds).

Figure 3-5 superimposes phonocardiographic events on pressure curves and the electrocardiogram. S_4 occurs during atrial systole. M_1 and T_1 (S_1) occur shortly after crossover of pressure between the atria and ventricles. Ejection sounds and opening snaps are not normally heard. When they do occur, it is sequentially after the pulmonary and aortic valves begin to open. A_2 and P_2 (S_2) (aortic and pulmonic valve closure) occur after pressures cross over between the ventricles and outflow tracts. An opening snap (OS)

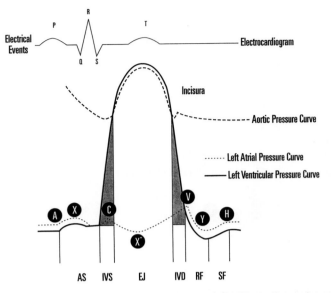

Figure 3-4 Crossover of atrial and ventricular pressures in aortic pressure curves. A, atrial systole (emptying); X and X', atrial filling in atrial diastole; C, transmitted pulsation; V, crossover of atrial and ventricular pressures; Y, rapid atrial emptying; H, slow atrial emptying.

is not normally heard in diastole but occurs after the crossover pressures between the atrium and ventricles. S_3 is heard at the peak of rapid filling, when elongation of the ventricle suddenly ceases.

Figure 3-6 shows ventricular pressure curves of the right ventricle (RV), left ventricle (LV), aorta (AO), and pulmonary artery (PA) on inspiration and expiration. The phonocardiogram of S_2 is represented by the horizontal line at the bottom of the figure, to indicate the physiologic splitting of S_2 on inspiration. Pressure curves are superimposed in order to contrast the lower pressures in the right ventricle and pulmonary artery with the higher pressures in the left ventricle and aorta. Vascular resistance (VR) in the aortic circuit is approximately 7 to 10 times that of the pulmonary circuit.

Figure 3-6 illustrates the physiology behind the so-called splitting of S_2, in which A_2 precedes P_2, and P_2 is displaced to the right, leading to wide splitting of S_2 on inspiration. This displacement of A_2 and P_2 is caused by increased venous return to the right side of the heart and some decrease to the left side of the heart on inspiration. This leads to (1) delay in right ventricular ejection due to increased stroke volume; (2) slowing in pressure fall in the pulmonary artery due to increased compliance in the pulmonary circulation as compared with systemic compliance; and (3) a slight decrease in left ventricular volume induced by inspiration due to increased pulmonary venous compliance in inspiration. All three factors lead to the phenomenon of hangout. In 15 percent of cases, a shortening of left ventricular

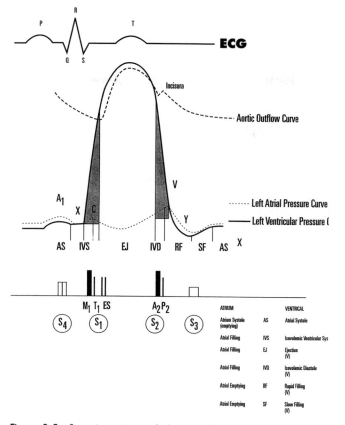

Figure 3-5 Superimposition of phonocardiogram on ECG and pressure curves.

ejection during inspiration leads to early aortic valve closure as compared to pulmonary valve closure has been aptly likened to a tight hinge with quick rebound A_2 and a loose hinge with slow rebound P_2 (Shaver).

Figure 3-7 is a video print sheet that illustrates the pressure curves previously described, as well as their associated echocardiographic events. The echocardiogram of aortic (upper line) and mitral (lower line) valve movement are indicated in this figure. The mitral valve shows two distinct positive displacements, an a wave and an e wave. Aortic valve motion is illustrated above the phonocardiogram above the zero pressure line. Ventricular posterior wall motion appears as the lowermost horizontal component of Fig. 3-7. S_4 is an acceleration phenomenon caused by sudden distention of the ventricle, as shown by sharp outward ventricular movement. This acceleration is visible in tissue Doppler imaging, in which ventricular wall motion is color-coded as a velocity. Ventricular systole is shown to occur prior to or coincidental with crossover pressures, and persists after the mitral and tricuspid valve closure causing S_1. Valve closure and

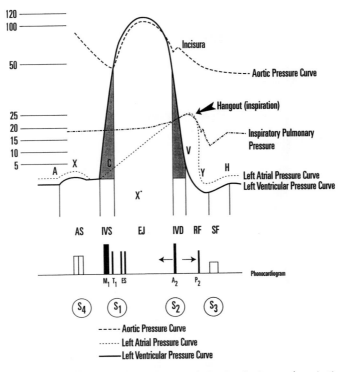

Figure 3-6 Ventricular pressure curves during inspiration and expiration. ----, aortic pressure curve; ·····, left atrial pressure curve; ——, left ventricular pressure curve.

ventricular systole immediately follow the pressure crossover between the atria and ventricles.

An ejection sound is not normally heard. Vascular root sounds occur in relation to the opening of the valves. These sounds usually coincide with full opening of the valve.

In valvular stenosis, however, the ejection sounds correspond with the early phase of valvular opening. Since opening of the semilunar valves may be followed by an ejection sound, and the pulmonary valves open before the aortic valves, pulmonary sounds precede aortic sounds, conversely, in the genesis of S_2, aortic valve closure precedes pulmonary valve closure (Fig. 3-5, phonocardiogram) (A_2P_2) (D).

HEART SOUNDS

The First Heart Sound (S_1) (D)

S_1 is caused by two physiologic events: (1) ventricular systole with contraction of the ventricle, and (2) mitral valve closure. These physiologic events

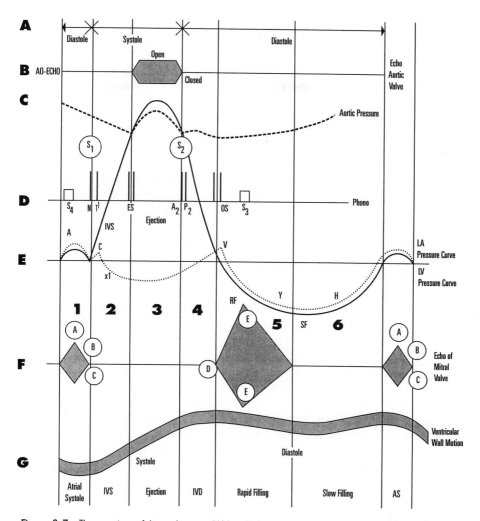

Figure 3-7 The motion of the valves and LV wall during the cardiac cycle. *Echocardiogram*: B, opening and closing of the aortic valve during phase 3; F, opening of the mitral valve providing the atrial kick in late diastole phase 1; DE, opening of the mitral valve, corresponding to the opening snap if heard in (D) phase 5; EF, rapid filling of the ventricle as the mitral valve closes, corresponding with the atrial 'v' wave (E) phase 5; F-A, corresponds with slow filling of the ventricle in diastasis shown on color Doppler ventricular imaging in black (low velocity) phase 6. *Phonocardiogram*: S₁, corresponds with ventricular systole and the A wave ending phase 2; S₂, corresponds with closure of the aortic valve of the echotrace phase 3/4.

have temporal relationships with the sound that is heard by the clinician. Thus, the pressure that causes the sounds constituting S_1 can be attributed to the mechanical effect of ventricular systole as well as to valvular closure, which immediately precedes the sound.

Wexler and associates have demonstrated that as the PR interval is prolonged from 200 to 500 ms, separation of the mitral valve leaflets decreases and the closure sound (S_1) is softened due to reduced valve tension. After 500 ms, however, S_1 normalizes in intensity. As the PR interval shortens to less than 200 ms, the valve leaflets are in the fully open position and are tense; hence, S_1 is louder, due to rapid closure of the valves. Mills and Craige showed that a correlation exists between terminal rates of closure of the anterior leaflet of the mitral valve and the amplitude of S_1 in atrial fibrillation. This finding would support the hypothesis that valvular closure plays a role in the creation of S_1. Administration of inotropes at a constant PR interval, however, has been shown to increase contractility and increase the loudness of S_1, adding support to the role of ventricular systole in S_1. Administration of beta-blockers decreases the loudness of S_1.

Finally, beat-to-beat variations of S_1 occur in conditions with alternating ventricular contractility (e.g., pulsus alternans) and after pauses, which are followed by postextra systolic potentiation. This enhances ventricular systole, thus augmenting the loudness of S_1. This post-pause phenomenon of enhanced ventricular contractility is probably caused by the increased flow of calcium ions into sarcolemma and enhanced actin-myosin sliding, with consequent enhanced contractility at an intracellular level.

Ejection Sounds

Ejection sounds are not heard in normal hearts. Ejection sounds may be valvular or vascular in origin. As noted above, pulmonary ejection sounds usually precede aortic sounds: P_{ES} A_{ES}. Mills and associates have indicated that valvular sounds occur at the opening of the aortic and pulmonary valves. Mills and Craige had attributed the sounds to the opening of the outflow tract valves (aortic and pulmonary). It is of interest that vascular or root sounds in systemic hypertension occur early, but are heard late after valve opening—if the aorta is dilated, or ventricular conduction is delayed as in left bundle branch block, or heart failure. In pulmonary hypertension, these vascular sounds occur earlier, corresponding to the early opening of the valve. Tight pulmonary stenosis may cause a click which may even precede S_1 in mild pulmonary stenosis; the ejection sound occurs later at valvular opening. In moderate pulmonary stenosis, the sound may be fused with S_1 and not heard by the clinician.

Nonejection Clicks

Nonejection clicks are not heard in normal hearts. These clicks, whether single or multiple, are caused by distortions in the mitral or tricuspid valves as they close. Nonejection clicks may be musical in tone, sharp, or rattle-like. They commonly occur in either mitral or tricuspid valve prolapse, in systole or diastole.

Timing   Valve clicks arising from mitral and tricuspid valve closure occur early after S_1 if the heart volume is small, as in the standing position, which reduces heart size and venous return. Clicks occur late when heart volume is increased, as when the patient is lying down; or in deep inspiration, as in clicks originating from the tricuspid valve. In the latter case, the late timing is caused by increased venous return to the right ventricle.

The Second Sound (S_2) (Cardiac Pearl 41)

S_2 is a high-frequency sound comprised of an aortic (A_2) and a pulmonary (P_2) component. Both these components relate to the closure of their associated valves, as demonstrated by Craige. Several studies, however, have shown that there may be a delay between the actual valve closure and the presence of A_2 and P_2. Chandraratne and colleagues provide evidence that S_2 occurs during the reflux of blood towards the semilunar valves. Thus S_2 may be recorded in early diastole (Brutsart; Don Michael).

Timing   In S_2, the A_2 component precedes P_2. A_2 is delayed in left bundle branch block, left ventricular failure, and aortic ectasia. An early A_2 may occur in acute hypertension. P_2 is delayed on inspiration. An early P_2 may be caused by early valve closure in pulmonary hypertension. A late P_2 in the absence of pulmonary hypertension may indicate the presence of a dilated pulmonary artery, right heart failure, or right bundle branch block.

The Third Heart Sound (S_3)

S_3 has been studied extensively. Physiologic third sounds are heard in young children and can continue to be heard in some adults up to the age of approximately 40. S_3 in children is high-pitched, corresponding with rapid tissue Doppler velocities (Don Michael).

This finding in the pediatric population contrasts with the low-pitched S_3 that occurs in a variety of adult heart conditions, such as mitral regurgitation, hypertrophic obstructive cardiomyopathy (HOCM), and left ventricular dysfunction or failure. S_3 also may be associated with tricuspid stenosis and regurgitation, and with right ventricular failure.

Diastolic events are the genesis of S_3. This was demonstrated by Ozawa and Craige with the combined use of a miniature accelerometer and noninvasive techniques (e.g., echocardiography) in laboratory studies of the genesis of S_3 in dogs. These researchers showed that dimensional changes in the short axis of the ventricle played a minor role in causing S_3. In invasive laboratory animal studies, Ozawa and colleagues measured the ventricular dimension in the transverse and long axis during early diastole. Their work indicated that S_3 results from the sudden intrinsic limitation of longitudinal expansion of the ventricle in early diastole. Hence S_3 is caused by arrested elongation of the filling ventricle.

The Fourth Heart Sound (S₄)

S_4 is a diastolic sound preceding ventricular systole. It is caused by atrial systole inducing rapid filling of the ventricle, termed the *atrial kick*. Atrial sounds are heard in heart block, as dissociated 'P' waves give rise to atrial sounds in P/QRS dissociation, seen in complete heart block. These findings support the theory that the motion of the heart, rather than ventricular volume or pressure changes, is responsible for S_4, i.e., it is a kinetic phenomenon.

S_4 is associated with an acceleration/deceleration effect: acceleration causes rapid filling and impaction of the ventricle against the chest wall. This process is combined with the deceleration of the blood caused by ventricular stiffness. Evidence for this effect has been provided by tissue Doppler imaging studies in which both high velocities of ventricular filling and large degrees of displacement (Don Michael) have been shown to coincide with fourth sounds.

Opening Snaps

Opening snaps are not heard in normal hearts. They commonly occur, however, in mitral and tricuspid stenosis. Hemodynamic studies, combined with angiography, have shown that the sudden checking of the mitral valve as it opens leads to deceleration of the blood column. This deceleration sets up cardiohemic vibrations, causing opening snaps. Tensing of the valvular components may also be responsible for the sounds.

HEMODYNAMICS OF ABNORMAL CONDITIONS

Aortic Regurgitation

Figure 3-8 depicts the hemodynamics of aortic regurgitation. The pressure curves shown are simultaneous and represent those of the ventricle and aorta. Change in aortic regurgitation occurs during diastolic flow toward the aortic valve, causing increased filling of the left ventricle after aortic valve closure. This increase in volume causes a steep upslope in both aortic and left ventricular pressure and is followed by a sharp downslope in diastole. The diastolic downslope is caused by reduced systemic vascular resistance (SVR). Because the rapid upslope is responsible for raising the systolic pressure and the downslope for lowering diastolic pressure, this combination leads to bounding pulses, described as pulses with a rapid rise and fall, empty between beats.

Figure 3-9 depicts the difference between the hemodynamics of acute aortic regurgitation and those of normal cardiac physiology. In acute aortic regurgitation, there is a precipitous fall in aortic diastolic pressure; an attenuated left ventricular rapid filling phase, with a premature rapid rise

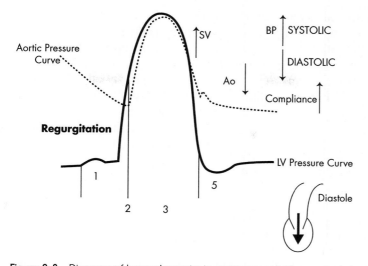

Figure 3-8 Diagram of hemodynamics in aortic regurgitation. NOTE: 4, isovolumic diastole is absent.

in left ventricular pressure, which exceeds left atrial pressure. This phenomenon leads to audible preclosure of the mitral valve in diastole (pseudo-S_3). S_1 is absent. Figure 3-9 illustrates the reversal of pressures in late diastole in the rapid filling phase of the ventricle, exceeding atrial pressures.

The early diastolic murmur and the Austin Flint murmur are caused by the gradient between the left atrial and the left ventricular pressure, which occurs only in middiastole and is absent. Hence no presystolic murmur is present in this condition. An Austin Flint murmur is thus caused

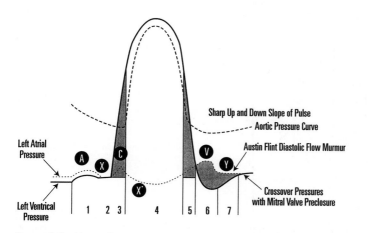

Figure 3-9 Hemodynamics of acute aortic regurgitation and normal cardiac function.

by parallel downward flow between the aorta and the mitral valve into the ventricle, with ventricular pressure opposing the leaflets of the mitral valve and even causing flutter. In aortic regurgitation, this flow in diastole may occur early across the mitral valve, and giving rise to a middiastolic and presystolic murmur. In acute or severe aortic regurgitation, flow across the mitral valve ceases in early diastole and the presystolic murmur is not present. Diastolic mitral regurgitation may, however, be seen on echocardiography. The hatched pressure area in Fig. 3-9 illustrates these changes relative to pressure flow alterations in atria and ventricles.

Aortic Stenosis

Figure 3-10 illustrates the hemodynamics of aortic stenosis, in which ventricular pressure exceeds aortic pressure. These two pressure curves, however, peak at different points, with the aortic pressure curve cresting later than the ventricular. Peak-to-peak gradients are thus inaccurate. The area between the curves is more representative of the mean gradient, best determined by echo Doppler techniques. In aortic stenosis, the left ventricular pressure elevation above the aortic pressure corresponds with the severity of stenosis. In general, aortic pressure curves are slower and less steep, and interrupted by a notch on the upslope, which accounts for the lower pulse pressure. The atrial 'A' wave is prominent in severe aortic stenosis and may cause a fourth sound to be heard.

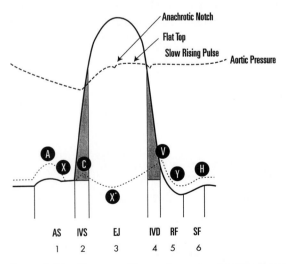

Figure 3-10 Diagram of hemodynamics of aortic stenosis. A, atrial systole (emptying); X and X', atrial filling; C, transmitted pulsation; V, crossover of atrial and ventricular pressures; Y, rapid atrial emptying; H, slow atrial emptying.

Figure 3-11 represents the hemodynamics of acute mitral regurgitation. The rapid increase of atrial pressure, crossing the ventricular pressure curve, attenuates the systolic murmur, replacing it with an early systolic murmur ending before S_2, as depicted by the jagged line on the phonocardiogram at the bottom of the figure. The large left atrial volume is dumped into the left ventricle causing S_3 in the phonocardiogram.

Pulsus Paradoxus and Tamponade

Figure 3-12 illustrates the hemodynamics of pulsus paradoxus. The right ventricular pressure curve is superimposed on the aortic and pulmonary pressure curves. In pulsus paradoxus, on inspiration, negative intrathoracic pressure decreases less than the pleural pressure and the increase in lung capacity. This phenomenon causes filling of the right heart as well as a slight bulging of the intraventricular septum, thus decreasing the volume of the left heart. This process is called reciprocal filling. In pulsus paradoxus, a fall in blood pressure of more than 10 mmHg is seen clinically on inspiration resulting from this phenomenon.

In the presence of increased intrapericardiac pressure due to fluid or an enlarged right ventricle following infarction, inspiration exaggerates the process of right heart filling at the expense of the left heart. It is this resulting fall in left-sided output on inspiration that causes the drop in blood pressure.

The Echocardiographic Tamponade Sign

In severe tamponade, however, intrapericardiac pressure is high. The elevated intrapericardiac pressure and right atrial pressure are identical, and cannot accommodate increased right-sided volume on inspiration. Under

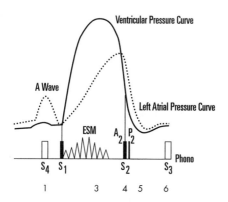

Figure 3-11 Diagram of hemodynamics of acute mitral regurgitation. NOTE: 2, isovolumic systole is absent.

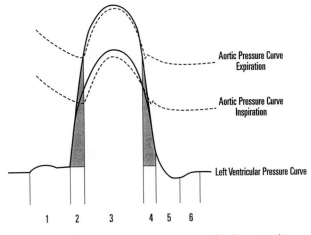

Aortic Pressure Curve
Expiration

Aortic Pressure Curve
Inspiration

Left Ventricular Pressure Curve

1   2   3   4 5   6

Figure 3-12   Diagram of hemodynamics of pulsus paradoxus.

these circumstances, instead of the fall in venous pressure that normally occurs on inspiration, venous pressures are elevated. The result is Kussmaul's sign (increase in jugular venous pressure during inspiration) as inspiration causes right-sided pressures to rise.

Pericardial tamponade may be indicated by the presence of either Kussmaul's sign or pulsus paradoxus (Fig 3-13). Kussmaul's sign, however, occurs late in severe tamponade. Although the 'y' wave of the venous pressure in the right atrium is absent, the x′ descent is prominent in ventricu-

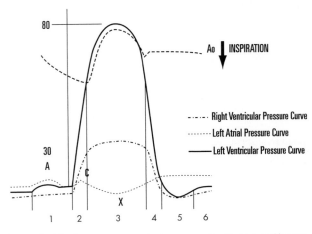

80

Ao   INSPIRATION

----- Right Ventricular Pressure Curve
········· Left Atrial Pressure Curve
——— Left Ventricular Pressure Curve

30
A

C

X

1   2   3   4   5   6

Figure 3-13   Pressure curves in tamponade. Note equilibrium of diastolic pressures in all four chambers. On inspiration the right-sided diastolic pressures and flow reciprocate with left-sided flows as right-sided (atrial) pressure rises systolic systemic BP falls (Kussmaul's sign). Note prominent X descent with no Y.

lar systole. This is caused by the shrinkage in cardiac volume as the left valve ejects blood and by facilitated filling of the atrium within the pericardium. Rarely elevated left ventricular filling pressure may prevent shock from occurring, a fact known to clinicians in treating tamponade.

Hypertrophic Cardiomyopathy with Obstruction

Figure 3-14 juxtaposes aortic and ventricular pressure curves in hypertrophic obstructive cardiomyopathy (HOCM). In HOCM, pressure increases in the left ventricle because of dynamic obstruction, as shown in panel *A* of the figure. In panel *B*, the gradient increases with standing (Fig. 3-14*C*) and with the use of inotropic agents such as amyl nitrite. The left ventricle may be enlarged by: having the patient lie supine and increasing venous return by elevating the legs; rapid intravenous therapy; or having the patient squat, which squeezes more blood through the veins into the heart. Increased pressure in the aorta increases the afterload and decreases the gradient. Standing decreases heart size and increases the gradient. Inotropic drugs increase the gradient and hence lower blood pressure (Fig. 3-14*C*).

Shunting

Left-to-right shunting is caused by atrial septal defects; ventricular septal defects or patent ductus arteriosus; or rupture of a sinus of Valsalva into

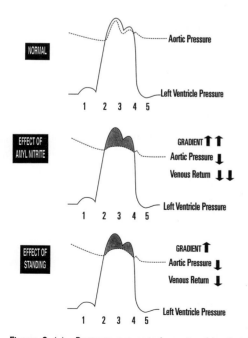

Figure 3-14   Pressure curves in hypertrophic obstructive cardiomyopathy.

the right side of the heart. The capacity of the pulmonary arteries is such that up to three times the normal flow can be accommodated without an increase in pulmonary artery pressure. If such increased flow volume is maintained long-term, however, pulmonary artery pressures increase and right-sided cardiomegaly may occur.

In atrial septal defect, there is characteristic hemodynamic alteration in right ventricular filling and left/right shunt that occurs with inspiration and expiration. Specifically, with inspiration, right ventricular filling increases and the left-to-right shunt decreases. With expiration, right ventricular filling decreases and the left/right shunt increases. As the right heart fills, the negative intrathoracic pressure causes an increase in lung capacity, a decreased impedance in the pulmonary circuit, and a delay in P_2. Hence, A_2 and P_2 are widely split and the split is relatively unaffected by phases of respiration. In pulmonary hypertension, narrow fixed splitting of A_2 P_2 occurs.

Constrictive Pericarditis

Figure 3-15 shows the pressure curves, apexcardiogram, and phonocardiogram in constrictive pericarditis, a condition in which the filling of the

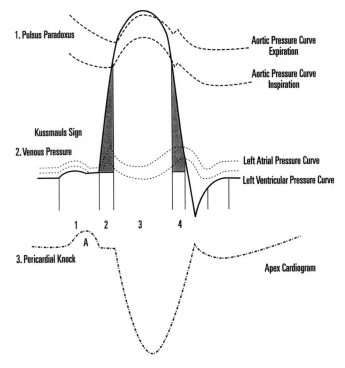

Figure 3-15 Triad of signs in constrictive pericarditis.

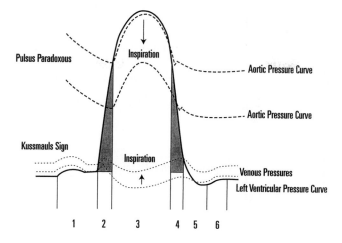

Figure 3-16 Pressure curves in severe tamponade.

ventricle is halted, giving rise to a pericardial knock. This knock is thought to be caused by impaction of the ventricle on a rigid encased pericardium early in diastole. On inspiration, the hemodynamics are very similar to pericardial tamponade. The right ventricle expands on inspiration, but is constrained by the calcified pericardium. The patient may demonstrate pulsus paradoxus. The rigidly encased heart has minimal right-sided filling on inspiration and venous pressure may rise in the jugular veins leading to Kussmaul's sign. The triad of signs, pulsus paradoxus, Kussmaul's sign, and a pericardial knock, are shown in Fig. 3-15. Figure 3-16 shows tamponade in which the right and left heart pressures look similar in diastole with an M configuration. The reading that resembles a square root in constrictive pericarditis is caused by the dip and rise of the ventricular pressure caused by the rigid pericardium.

TRUE OR FALSE

1. An S_3 is caused only by rapid ventricular filling.
2. An S_2 occurs when the aortic and pulmonary valves close.
3. S_3 is caused by deceleration of ventricular elongation.
4. Nonejection clicks depend on position in systole.
5. An S_3 up to 40 and an S_4 over 60 may be normally found.

ANSWERS

1. *F*; 2. *T*; 3. *T*; 4. *T*; 5. *T*

BIBLIOGRAPHY
Heart Sounds Hemodynamics

Mills PG, et al: Echocardiographic and hemodynamic relationships of ejection sounds. Circulation 1977; 56:430–435.

O'Toole JD, et al: The contribution of tricuspid valve closure to the first sound. Circulation 1976; 53:752–758.

Ozawa Y, et al: Origin of the third sound. Circulation 1983; 67:393–404.

S_1

Burgraff GW, Craige E: The first heart sound in complete heart block. Circulation 1974; 50:17.

DiBartolo et al: Hemodynamic correlates of the first heart sound. Am J Physiol 1961; 201:888–892.

Dock W: Mode of production of the first heart sound. Arch Intern Med 1933; 51:737.

Faber JJ: Origin and conduction of the mitral sound in the heart. Circ Res 1964; 14:426.

Heintzen P: The genesis of the normally split first heart sound. Am Heart J 1961; 62:332.

Hultgren HN, Leo TF: The tricuspid component of the first sound in mitral stenosis. Circulation 1958; 18:1012–1016.

Kincaid-Smith P, Barlow J: The atrial sound and the atrial component of the first heart sound. Br Heart J 1959; 21:470.

Lakier JB, et al: Mitral components of the first heart sound. Br Heart J 1972; 24:160.

Leatham A: Splitting of the first and second heart sounds. Lancet 1954; 2:607.

Leech G, et al: Mechanism of influence of PR interval on loudness of the first heart sound. Br Heart J 1980; 43:138–142.

Luisada AA, et al: Mechanisms of production of the first heart sound. Am J Physiol 1952; 168:226.

Sakamoto T, et al: Hemodynamic determinants of the amplitude of the first heart sound. Circ Res 1965; 16:45–57.

Shah PM, et al: Hemodynamic correlates of the various components of the first heart sound. Circ Res 1963; 12:386.

Shah PM, et al: Influence of the timing of atrial systole on mitral valve closure and on the first heart sound in man. Am J Cardiol 1970; 26:231.

Stept ME, et al: Effects of altering PR interval on the amplitude of the first heart sound in the anesthetized dog. Circ Res 1969; 25:255.

Thompson ME, et al: Pathodynamics of the first heart sound. In Leon DF, Shaver JA (eds.) American Heart Association Monograph No. 46, Physiologic Principles of Heart Sounds and Murmurs, New York, American Heart Association, 1975.

Waider W, Craige E: First heart sounds and ejection sounds. Am J Cardiol 1975; 35:346.

S_2

Dickerson RB, Nelson WB: Paradoxical splitting of the second heart sound: An informative clinical notation. Am Heart J 1964; 67:410.

Gray I: Paradoxical splitting of the second heart sound. Br Heart J 1956; 18:21.

Kardilinos A: The second heart sound. Am Heart J 1962; 64:610.

Leachman RD, et al: Narrowed splitting of the second heart sound upon inspiration in patients with giant left atrium. Chest 1971; 60:151.

Leatham A: The second heart sound, key to auscultation of the heart. Acta Cardiol 1964; 19:395.

Luisada AA: The second heart sound in normal and abnormal conditions. Am J Cardiol 1971; 28:150.

MacCannon DM, et al: Direct detection and timing of aortic valve closure. Circ Res 1964; 14:387.

Perloff JK, Harvey WP: Mechanisms of fixed splitting of the second heart sound. Circulation 1958; 18:998.

Shafter HA: Splitting of the second heart sound. Am J Cardiol 1960; 6:1013.

Shaver JA, O'Toole JD: The second heart sound: Newer concepts. Part 1: Normal and wide physiological splitting. Mod Concepts Cardiovasc Dis 1977; 46:7–12.

Shaver JA, O'Toole JD: The second heart sound: Newer concepts. Part 2: Paradoxical splitting and narrow physiological splitting. Mod Concepts Cardiovasc Dis 1977; 46:13–16.

Shaver JA, et al: Second heart sound: The role of altered greater and lesser circulation. In Leon DF, Shaver JA(eds.) American Heart Association Monograph No. 46, Physiologic Principles of Heart Sounds and Murmurs, New York, American Heart Association, 1975.

Stein PD, Sabbah HN: Origin of the second heart sound: Clinical relevance of new observations. Am J Cardiol 1978; 41:108.

Stein PD, Sabbah HN: Second heart sound: Mechanism and clinical utility of auscultatory changes. Am J Noninvas Cardiol 1987; 1:68.

Zuberbuhler JR, Bauersfeld SR: Paradoxical splitting of the second heart sound in the Wolff-Parkinson-White syndrome. Am Heart J 1965; 70:595.

S_3

Braunwald E, Morror AG: Origin of heart sounds as estimated by analysis of the sequence of cardiodynamic work. Circulation 1958; 18:971–974.

Nixon PGF: The genesis of the third heart sound. Am Heart J 1963; 65:712–714.

Ozawa Y, et al: Origin of the third heart sound. II: Studies in human subjects. Circulation 1983; 67:399.

Sakamoto T, et al: Genesis of the third heart sound—Phonoechocardiographic studies. Jpn Heart J 1976; 17:150–162.

Shaver JA, et al: Genesis of the third heart sound. Am J Noninvas Cardiol 1987; 1:39–55.

Sloan AW, et al: Incidence of the physiological third heart sound. Br Med J 1952; 2:853.

Timmis AJ: The third heart sound. Br Med J 1987; 294:326.

S_3 and S_4

Leonard JJ, et al: Modification of ventricular gallop rhythm induced by pooling of blood in the extremities. Br Heart J 1958; 20:502–506.

Leonard JJ, et al: Observations on the mechanism of a trial gallop rhythm. Circ 1958; 20:502–506.

Stapleton JF: Third and fourth heart sounds. In Horwitz LD, Groves BM (eds): Signs and Symptoms in Cardiology. Philadelphia, Lippincott, 1985:214–226.

S_4

Tavel ME: The fourth heart sound: A premature requiem? Circulation 1974; 49:4.

Others

Braunwald E, Morrow AG: Origin of heart sounds as elucidated by analysis of the sequence of cardiodynamic events. Circulation 1958; 18:971.

Fontana ME, et al: Functional anatomy of mitral valve prolapse. In Leon DF, Shaver JA(eds.) American Heart Association Monograph No. 46, Physiologic Principles of Heart Sounds and Murmurs, New York, American Heart Association, 1975.

Grayzel J: Gallop rhythm of the heart: II. Quadruple rhythm and its relation to summation and augmented gallops. Circulation 1959; 20:1053.

Haber E, Leatham A: Splitting of heart sounds from ventricular asynchrony in bundle branch block, ventricular ectopic beats and artificial placing. Br Heart J 1965; 27:691.

Ikram H, et al: Genesis of diastolic sounds in mitral incompetence. Br Heart J 1969; 31:762.

Karnegis JN, Wang Y: Phonocardiogram of idiopathic dilatation of the pulmonary artery. Circulation 1963; 28:747.

Keenan TJ, Schwartz MJ: Tricuspid whoop. Am J Cardiol 1973; 31:642.

Rackley CE, et al: The precordial honk. Am J Cardiol 1966; 17:509.

Reddy PS, et al: The genesis of gallop sounds: Investigation by quantitative phono and apex cardiography. Circulation 1981; 63:922.

Shaver JA, et al: Ejection sounds of left-sided origin. In Leon DF, Shaver JA (eds.) American Heart Association Monograph No. 46, Physiologic Principles of Heart Sounds and Murmurs, New York, American Heart Association, 1975:27.

Tavel ME, et al: Opening snap of the tricuspid valve in atrial septal defect: A phonocardiographic and reflected ultrasound study of sounds in relationship to movements of the tricuspid valve. Am Heart J 1970; 80:550.

Wiggers CJ, Dean AL Jr: The nature and time relations of the fundamental heart sounds. Am J Physiol 1917; 42:476.

Wittaker AV, et al: Sound-pressure correlates of the aortic ejection sound: An intracardiac sound study. Circulation 1969; 39:475.

4

CLINICAL FOUNDATIONS
OF AUSCULTATION

CORONARY SYNDROMES
  Chronic Stable Angina
  Accelerated Angina and Preinfarction Angina (Unstable Angina)
  Silent Ischemia
  Prinzmetal's Angina
  Coronary Spasm
  Acute Myocardial Infarction

VALVULAR HEART DISEASES
  Valvular Sequelae of Rheumatic Fever
  Mitral Stenosis
  Mitral Regurgitation
  Acute Mitral Regurgitation
  Mitral Valve Prolapse
  Calcification of Mitral Ring
  Aortic Stenosis
  Hyperlipidemia Presenting as Aortic Stenosis
  Aortic Regurgitation
  Tricuspid Stenosis
  Tricuspid Regurgitation
  Pulmonary Stenosis
  Pulmonary Regurgitation

MYOCARDITIS AND THE CARDIOMYOPATHIES
  The Cardiomyopathies

CARDIAC ARRHYTHMIAS
  Atrial Fibrillation
  Atrial Flutter and Supraventricular Tachycardia
  Ventricular Tachycardia
  Atrioventricular Conduction Defects

PERICARDIAL DISEASES
  Friction Rubs

> *Atrial Pacing*
> *Effusion*
> *Tamponade*
> *Constrictive*

INFECTIVE ENDOCARDITIS

HYPERTENSION

> *Systemic Hypertension*
> *Pulmonary Hypertension*

CARDIAC FAILURE

> *Left Heart*
> *Right Heart*
> *Congestive*
> *High-Output*
> *Low-Output*

For auscultation to be performed effectively, the clinician must have a working knowledge of conditions and diseases that can affect the heart. Hence, in describing a range of heart dysfunctions and their causes, this chapter lays the groundwork for Chaps. 5 and 6 by describing the clinical context of auscultated events.

CORONARY SYNDROMES

Coronary syndromes refer to modes of presentation of ischemic heart disease. These syndromes usually present with chest pain (Fig. 4-1), but occasionally may be clinically silent. Auscultatory findings in coronary syndromes may be evanescent, an S_4, apical systolic murmur; or may demonstrate filling sound S_3S_4 in heart failure. Pericardial friction rubs and persistent S_4 are seen in myocardial infarction. In addition, friction rubs are seen in:

1. Rupture of the myocardium;
2. Pericarditis associated with anticoagulant therapy;
3. Dressler's syndrome, a postcardiotomy pericarditis that is most likely an autoimmune disorder.

Chronic Stable Angina

Transient findings during an attack of angina often may include: an audible S_4 that may be palpable as a presystolic impulse; late systolic murmur due to papillary muscle dysfunction; an S_3; rarely, splitting of the S_2; and a softened S_1. These physical findings are signs that usually disappear with administration of nitroglycerin or with the application of carotid sinus pressure.

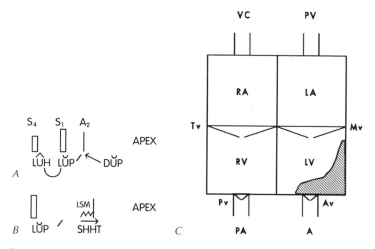

Figure 4-1 Ischemic myocardium. *A.* Phonophonic representation of transient S_4 with ischemia. *B.* Phonophonic representation of late systolic murmur. *C.* Box diagram with ischemic tissue represented by hatched area. Vc, vena cava; PV, pulmonary veins; RA, right atrium; LA, left atrium; RV, right ventricle; LV, left ventricle; PA, pulmonary artery; A, aorta, Tv, tricuspid valve; PV, pulmonary valve; Av, aortic valve; MV, mitral valve.

Accelerated Angina and Preinfarction Angina (Unstable Angina)

Auscultatory findings are similar to those for chronic angina. Murmurs and abnormal filling sounds are transient associated stethoscope findings.

Silent Ischemia

This coronary syndrome may present with a soft S_1 following S_3, and an S_4 followed by ST-T change on the electrocardiogram (ECG). The patient may then also report chest pain; note that the auscultatory signs precede ECG changes and pain. Apical systolic murmurs may be transient findings. The ischemic cascade (Fig. 4-2) is the temporal progression of events caused by ischemia; the order in which these changes appear typically is: (1) the development of auscultatory findings; (2) electrocardiographic changes; (3) chest pain.

Prinzmetal's Angina

Prinzmetal's angina is nocturnal angina often found in women under age 50. It is caused by a reversible obstruction of a coronary artery, i.e., spasm, usually of the right coronary artery, and is associated with ST segment elevation on ECG.

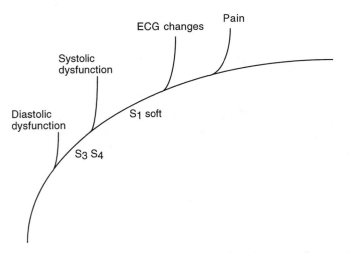

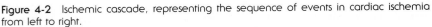

Figure 4-2 Ischemic cascade, representing the sequence of events in cardiac ischemia from left to right.

Auscultatory findings include an S_4 as well as atrioventricular (AV) block with associated variations in the intensity of the S_1. Apical systolic murmurs or papillary muscle dysfunction may be present during attacks. Diastolic murmurs or sounds due to atrial contraction may also be heard. S_1 may be variable during an attack.

Coronary Spasm

Coronary spasm, as opposed to occlusion, is the reversible obstruction of a coronary artery.

Acute Myocardial Infarction

An acute myocardial infarction (MI) may present with pericardial rubs and an S_4 papillary muscle dysfunction with late systolic murmurs or with complications such as a ventricular septal defect (VSD) or mitral valve papillary muscle rupture. Myocardial free wall rupture is a catastrophic complication heralded by a friction rub, and heart failure may be evident by the presence of gallop rhythms (Fig. 4-3).

Myocardial infarction requires careful diagnosis and management because it may be followed by changes in which the damaged area remodels or ruptures, leading to heart failure and cardiogenic shock. [Other changes may occur in which the damaged muscle temporarily loses its function; with arterial occlusion causing stunting of the myocardium and absence of blood flow to areas of muscle (no reflow), caused by blood vessel wall damage. Arrythmias are common.]

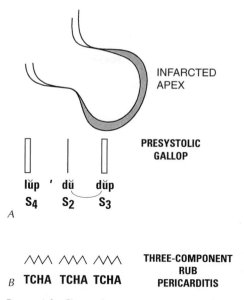

INFARCTED
APEX

PRESYSTOLIC
GALLOP

lŭp ' dŭ   dŭp
S₄   S₂   S₃

A

∿∿ ∿∿ ∿∿   THREE-COMPONENT
                            RUB
B TCHA TCHA TCHA   PERICARDITIS

Figure 4-3 Phonophonic representation of myocardial infarction. A. Presystolic gallop; B. three-component rub pericarditis.

VALVULAR HEART DISEASES

Valvular heart diseases still represent a major category of cardiac dysfunction worldwide, even though rheumatic fever is no longer the single most common cause in developed countries.

Valvular Sequelae of Rheumatic Fever

The incidence of acute rheumatic fever has declined over the past century with the development of antibiotics as well as improved living standards. Rheumatic fever has, however, recently re-emerged in the Western world as a result of immigration from developing countries where it is endemic. Clinicians should, therefore, familiarize themselves with the diagnostic criteria of rheumatic fever (Table 4-1). The disease is often not recognized because it is not suspected.

Patients with the disease typically present with fever and joint pains that they characteristically describe as "fleeting" and "flitting," i.e., transient and migratory. Patients may report a history of sore throat, tonsillitis, scarlet or rheumatic fever, and may develop heart failure. Patients may double over with severe chest pain on extension, swallowing, or turning (Cardiac Pearl 48). Due to pericarditis, 50 percent of patients with rheumatic valvular disease have a previous history of rheumatic fever; 50 percent of patients with rheumatic fever develop heart disease.

Table 4-1   Duckett Jones Criteria for Rheumatic Fever

Major Criteria	Minor Criteria

Carditis, established by any of these signs
  Pericarditis
  Endocarditis
  Cardiomegaly
  Congestive failure
  Mitral or aortic regurgitation murmurs
Erythema marginatum
Sydenham's chorea
Migratory polyarthritis
Subcutaneous nodules
	Previous history of rheumatic fever; or
	  evidence of antecedent beta-
	  hemolytic streptococcal infection
	Polyarthralgia
	Fever
	Rapid ESR
	Reversible prolongation of PR interval

NOTE: The presence of two major criteria, or of one major and one minor criterion, establishes the diagnosis.

Auscultatory findings connected with carditis in rheumatic fever are summarized in Table 4-2. Of note is the soft middiastolic murmur without an associated thrill opening snap or loud S_1 described by Cary Coombs. Electrocardiographic findings include a prolonged PR interval associated with a soft S_1. Sinus tachycardia with advanced heart block may occur. With pericarditis, ST segments are elevated and T-wave inversion occurs. QT_c prolongation may occur.

Mitral Stenosis

Mitral stenosis is obstruction of the inflow to the left ventricle by an abnormally narrowed mitral valve. This narrowing may resemble a buttonhole, funnel, or fish's mouth. The left atrium enlarges due to the obstruction, and clots may form within it. As the valve area is reduced in size, pulmonary venous congestion may result. The left atrium may develop a patch of rheumatic disease (McCallum's patch); Aschoff nodules, collections of cells pathognomonic of rheumatic fever, are a pathological finding that may also be detected if the atrium is biopsied during surgery.

Hemodynamic Changes   The hemodynamic changes resulting from mitral stenosis include the development of pulmonary hypertension, initially pulmonary venous distention, which leads in turn to congestive heart failure (CHF). Biatrial and right ventricular enlargement may occur. The left

Table 4-2   Auscultatory Findings in Rheumatic Fever

Soft S_1 middiastolic murmur (Cary-Coombs)
Apical holosystolic murmur
Early diastolic murmur
Atrial sounds in heart block
Friction rubs
S_3 S_4 tachycardia, gallop rhythm

ventricle and aorta are typically small. Atrial fibrillation and pulmonary hypertension may develop, altering the auscultatory signs of mitral stenosis.

Mitral stenosis is more common in women and may become evident with atrial fibrillation in pregnancy. The heart rate is important because diastolic filling time of the left ventricle is markedly diminished by increased heart rate. In the presence of a fixed obstruction, an increased heart rate causes left atrial hypertension and heart failure. Mitral stenosis may present with hoarseness; the vocal difficulty is caused by Ortner's syndrome, compression of the left recurrent laryngeal nerve between the enlarged pulmonary artery, the aorta, and the ligamentum arteriosum. Chest pain may occur and is related to pulmonary hypertension.

Clinical Features   Patients with mitral stenosis may present with orthopnea, paroxysmal nocturnal dyspnea, fatigue, weakness, and hemoptysis produced by the rupture of bronchial submucosal varices. Heart failure with pulmonary edema may follow. Pulmonary hypertension may result in right-sided heart failure; ventricular enlargement; tricuspid regurgitation; enlargement and pulsation of the liver; and peripheral edema. The symptoms of mitral stenosis may develop over decades; may wax and wane; and without intervention progress to disability or death.

Physical Findings   In advanced cases, the patient may have a cachectic pink-tinged face (mitral facies) with scleral icterus and cyanotic blush over the cheeks. Systemic and pulmonary venous pressures may be elevated. The pulse is of low volume. The cardinal diagnostic impulse is felt by placing the patient on the left side and feeling for a tapping impulse and diastolic thrill with the base of the fingers. The liver may be enlarged and pulsatile, with associated venous systolic (cv) and rapid-filling diastolic (y) venous pulsation. This cv-y pulsation can move the ears laterally. Pedal edema may be present.

Differential Diagnoses   Patients with Libman-Sacks endocarditis may present with the murmur of mitral stenosis and signs of systemic lupus erythematosus. Nodules on the mitral valve and on the ventricular side of the aortic valve may be present.

Ball valve clots may present in patients with the murmur of mitral stenosis.

A middiastolic murmur of mitral stenosis can be heard in association with fixed splitting of the second sound in Lutembacher's syndrome (congenital atrial septal defect and mitral stenosis).

Mitral stenosis may be suggested by aortic regurgitation in which the murmur is heard in middiastole, late diastole, or both, at the left sternal border and disappears with amyl nitrite (Austin Flint murmur). Aortic regurgitation and pulmonary regurgitation may present with middiastolic murmurs that are not Austin Flint murmurs or those to pulmonary hypertension (Graham Steell murmurs). These entities need to be sorted out.

Flow middiastolic murmurs may be present in patients with ventral septal defect and patent ductus arteriosus arising from the mitral valve.

Carey-Coombs murmur: This murmur, which is due to mitral valvulitis, has already been discussed. This is a middiastolic murmur associated with a soft S_1, a long PR interval in acute rheumatic fever, thought to be due to mitral valvulitis. There is no presystolic accentuation and no opening snap.

A left or right atrial mass can produce murmurs similar to that of mitral stenosis, due to inflow tract flow obstruction, e.g., a myxoma thrombus or vegetation (Cardiac Pearl 52).

Increased left-sided flow in ventral septal defect and patent ductus arteriosus may cause diastolic flow murmurs. Middiastolic murmurs are heard in tricuspid inflow tract obstruction, i.e., tricuspid stenosis myxomas, and with increased flow across the tricuspid valve in atrial septal defect. Also due to increased flow in mitral and tricuspid regurgitation, and after valvuloplasty of mitral and tricuspid valves.

Mitral Regurgitation

Mitral regurgitation (MR) is characterized by ejection of blood from the left ventricle into the left atrium (LA), commencing in early systole (Fig. 4-4). The murmurs of mitral regurgitation may become more prominent

MITRAL REGURGITATION

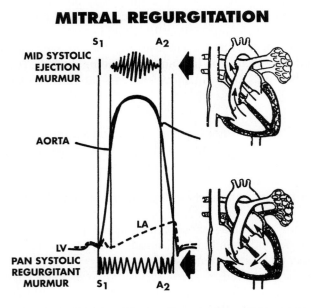

Figure 4-4 Mitral regurgitation. Note the holosystolic murmur of mitral regurgitation and the absence of isovolumic systole with atrial filling in early systole.

with heart failure. For a more detailed discussion, see "Changing Murmurs," Chap. 6.

Pathology   Mitral regurgitation may have several causes: rheumatic disease; mitral valve prolapse, sometimes called *myxomatous degeneration;* endocarditis; and dilatation of the valve ring in dilated cardiomyopathy, in hypertrophic obstructive cardiomyopathy (HOCM), as well as in restrictive cardiomyopathy. Mitral regurgitation may occur in calcification of the mitral valve ring and in diseases of the papillary muscle or chordae tendineae. The condition is a common feature in AV canal defects and ostium primum. Aortic rupture of a chordae or belly of a papillary muscle may cause acute mitral regurgitation. Diastolic mitral insufficiency occurs in AV block and in conditions in which slow filling of the ventricle occurs, associated with severe aortic regurgitation.

Hemodynamics   In mitral regurgitation, the ejection fraction of the left ventricle (LV) is increased and ventricular pressure is transmitted to the left atrium (LA). Both the LV and LA may be enlarged and pulmonary hypertension may be associated with cor pulmonale (right ventricular hypertrophy and eventual failure associated with pulmonary disease). Enlargement of the left atrium may lead to atrial fibrillation and systemic embolism.

Symptoms   Patients with mitral regurgitation may be asymptomatic, or may complain of fatigue, dyspnea, or palpitations. Most patients are female; some have minor chest wall deformities.

Physical Signs   The pulse is small in volume and rises and then falls sharply and is empty between beats (small collapsing pulse). The apical impulse is hyperkinetic. A (pseudo) parasternal heave due to left atrial enlargement displacing the right ventricle anteriorly may be felt in the area between the apex and the left lower sternal border (Cardiac Pearl 16).

Acute Mitral Regurgitation

Mitral regurgitation may occur acutely, due to a ruptured chordae tendineae, papillary muscle belly rupture, endocarditis, or trauma; less commonly, MR occurs because of rupture of a chordae tendineae in a parachute valve. Chronic mitral regurgitation may be due to ventricular dilatation as in dilated cardiomyopathy; fibroelastosis and restrictive cardiomyopathy in association with tricuspid regurgitation; dilatation of the mitral annulus; mitral valve prolapse; papillary muscle dysfunction due to ischemia or infarction; or, less commonly, rheumatic heart disease. See Chap. 6 for a more detailed discussion.

Mitral Valve Prolapse

Mitral valve prolapse (MVP; Fig. 4-5; sometimes called "floppy" or "billow-ing" mitral valve) occurs when the mitral valve slips down from its normal position with or without mitral regurgitation.

Causes   Mitral valve prolapse typically is caused by congenital degenera-tion of the mitral and tricuspid valves secondary to trauma or rheumatic fever. Both the mitral valve and spine develop in the sixth week of intrauter-ine life, and abnormalities in both structures frequently occur during this period.

Clinical Features   Patients with mitral valve prolapse commonly present with anxiety, chest pain (usually atypical), left-sided fatigue, lassitude, palpi-tations, dyspnea, syncope, dizziness, or panic attacks. Mitral valve prolapse is rarely associated with sudden death, embolism, or skeletal disorders. Marfan's syndrome may be present as well as atrial septal defect (ASD). Patients may have associated psychiatric problems (e.g., agoraphobia and panic disorder). Chest pain occasionally closely simulates angina. Dyspnea, or inability to "get one's breath," is atypical. Chest pain may closely simulate angina, with treadmill provocation and st segment depression on exercise.

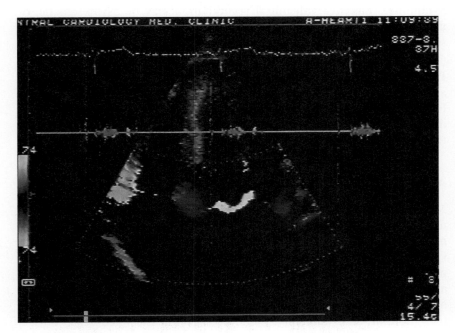

Figure 4-5   Mitral valve prolapse, S_1 and S_2.

In patients with mitral valve prolapse, one may observe a flattening of the spine at the level of T_3 to T_1 in the midline at the back with winged scapulae into which the examiner's hand can sink (Fig. 4-6A, 4-6B). This "oval" may be associated with numerous skeletal abnormalities seen in this condition, including kyphoscoliosis. Such abnormalities may also be associated with a proclivity to major accidental injuries.

Prognosis Most patients have a good prognosis; however, some may develop mitral regurgitation, and rarely, sudden death, systemic embolism, or endocarditis. Mitral regurgitation develops acutely due to chordal rupture.

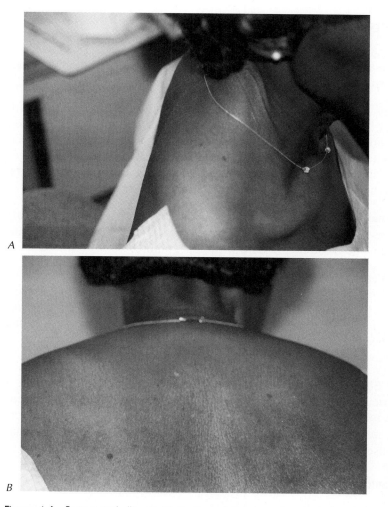

Figure 4-6 Patient with "oval" (flattening of the thoracic spine) characteristic of mitral valve prolapse.

Calcification of Mitral Ring

Idiopathic valve calcification occurs in conditions associated with mitral valve prolapse (e.g., chronic renal disease or hyperparathyroid disorders). Valve calcification also occurs in disorders of calcium metabolism that may be associated with hypertension. Other associated conditions include: aortic stenosis, diabetes, Marfan's and Hurler's syndromes, and hypertrophic obstructive cardiomyopathy. Calcification of the mitral valve ring may lead to an apical systolic murmur due to mitral regurgitation, and less commonly to mitral stenosis. Patients develop embolic episodes and surgery may be required. There is an association with Rytand syndrome (Chap. 5) and coronary artery disease.

Aortic Stenosis

Aortic stenosis (AS, Fig. 4-7) is characterized by abnormal narrowing of the aortic valve orifice. It is the most common valvular lesion in developed countries.

Pathology   Aortic stenosis is usually asymptomatic in adults until the fifth decade or later. In middle-aged patients it is typically caused by calcified bicuspid aortic valves. In older patients Mönckeburg sclerosis of calcified valves is the common cause. Bicuspid aortic valves may be seen in younger patients (ages 8 to 40 years), and unicuspid valves in ages 1 to 8 years. Aortic stenosis may also be caused by rheumatic fever.

Hemodynamics   The concentric left ventricular hypertrophy found in aortic stenosis leads to elevated left ventricular systolic pressures and eventually to elevated diastolic pressure with heart failure.

Clinical Features   Patients with aortic stenosis may be asymptomatic; or may present with the tetrad of angina, syncope, heart failure, and gastrointestinal (GI) bleeding (Heyde's syndrome). Less commonly they may develop hemolysis or dissecting aneurysms (Fig. 4-8). In addition, patients with aortic stenosis are prone to endocarditis. Patients in atrial fibrillation usually have concomitant rheumatic mitral valve disease.

Physical Signs   An anacrotic notch on a small delayed volume pulse, a left ventricular apical impulse, reduced pulse pressure, and neck vein distention due to septal interference with ventricular filling (Bernheim's effect) are seen in aortic stenosis. Occasionally pulsus alternans is seen with anacrotic pulses and alternating loudness of the midsystolic murmur.

Hyperlipidemia Presenting as Aortic Stenosis

Hyperlipidemia (Cardiac Pearl 24) has no direct clinical relevance to auscultation in most cases; however, aortic stenosis-like murmurs have been de-

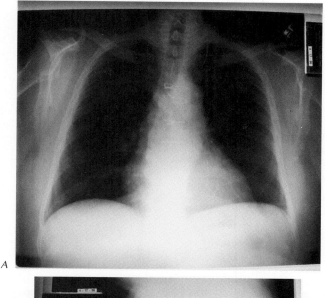

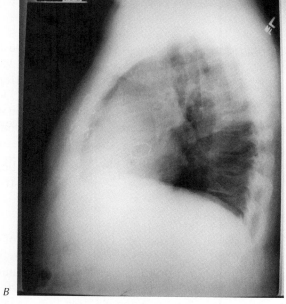

Figure 4-7 Chest x-rays of elderly patient with aortic stenosis, showing dilated ascending aorta and cardiomegaly.

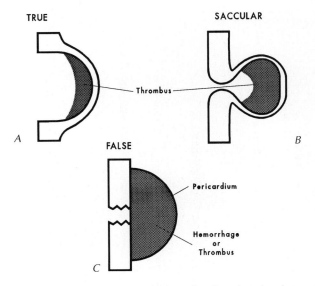

Figure 4-8 Ventricular aneurysm, showing the development of a pseudoaneurysm. *A.* Dilated ventricle. *B.* Rupture. *C.* Walling-off with communication with the cardiac lumen.

scribed in children with Friedrichsen's type II homozygous hypercholesterolemia and are caused by xanthomata in the aorta above the valve (Fogelman). A variety of auscultatory findings due to stenosed arteries may be seen in hyperlipidemia, e.g., an early localized diastolic "Dock murmur in coronary stenosis, continuous murmurs over renal carotid and peripheral arteries and systolic murmurs with pulsation over abdominal aneurysms. The latter are common in young patients with type II heterozygous hypercholesterolemia. Tendon xanthomata (Fig. 4-9) are seen in the hands (Fig. 4-9*A*) and Achilles tendons (Fig. 4-9*B*).

Aortic Regurgitation

Aortic regurgitation (AR; Fig. 4-10), the diastolic filling, or reflux, of the aortic blood into the left ventricle, and diastolic murmur can be caused by a variety of conditions. These include trauma associated with rheumatic heart disease, luetic (syphilitic) aortitis, Marfan's syndrome, and bacterial endocarditis. Aortic regurgitation is seen in Asian children in association with congenital supracristal ventricular septal defects. Aortic nonvalvular regurgitation is seen in patients with acute rupture of the sinus of Valsalva. There is runoff from the aortic valve back into the left ventricle. Aortic valve regurgitation is common in patients with connective tissue disorders, including polychondritis, Marfan's syndrome, and Ehlers-Danlos syndrome. It is also encountered in patients with type I dissecting aneurysms. Minimal aortic regurgitation murmurs are common in the presence of dissection and

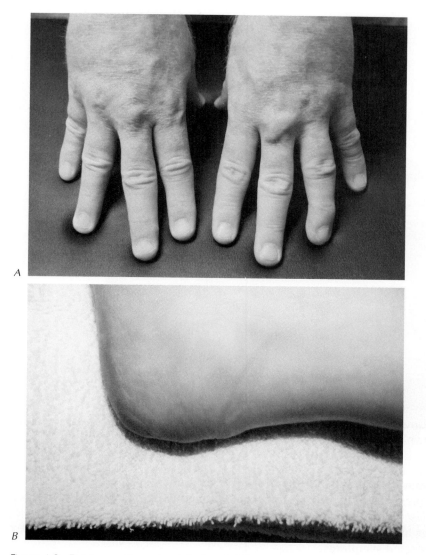

A

B

Figure 4-9 Tendon xanthomata of the hands (A) and the Achilles tendon (B).

bicuspid valves. Aortic regurgitation is associated with subaortic stenosis associated with a to-and-fro murmur.

Hemodynamics Aortic regurgitation results in increased end diastolic volume, and occasionally in diastolic mitral regurgitation associated with an increase in diastolic left ventricular pressure. See Chap. 3 for further discussion.

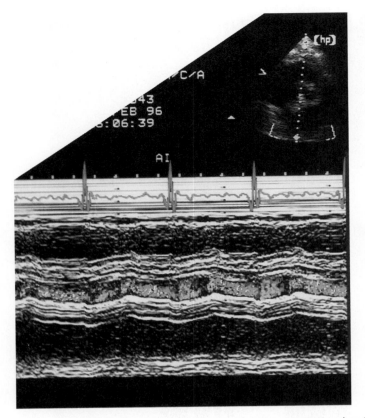

Figure 4-10 Two-dimensional and M/Q scan of aortic regurgitation showing diastolic flow. The two-dimensional image is above, across the aortic valve.

Clinical Features Patients with aortic regurgitation may be asymptomatic or present acutely with symptoms of left heart failure and syncopal attacks. Chest pain of the anginal type is frequently attributable to eccentric ventricular hypertrophy. Exertional dyspnea and fatigue are the most frequently endorsed symptoms.

Physical Signs Patients with aortic regurgitation may have a number of features reflecting high stroke volumes in systole and "runoff" in diastole: a bounding, waterhammer, or bisferiens pulse; large pulse pressure; De Musset's sign (head bobbing); Corrigan's sign (rapid rise and fall in the pulse); pulsating carotids; Traube's sign (pistol-shot pulses); Quincke's sign (subungual capillary pulsations); a hyperkinetic left ventricular impulse; and Duroziez' sign (a systolic/diastolic murmur heard over the compressed femoral artery). Of interest is the fact that the classic findings of a collapsing large pulse are not seen in acute aortic regurgitation. This is due to a low cardiac output and heart (left ventricular) failure.

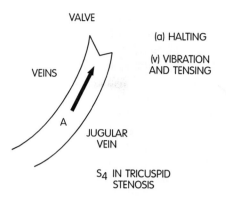

VALVE

(a) HALTING

(v) VIBRATION AND TENSING

VEINS

A

JUGULAR VEIN

S_4 IN TRICUSPID STENOSIS

Figure 4-11 Schematic diagram of tricuspid stenosis. Valve impaction is proposed mechanism of S_4.

Tricuspid Stenosis

Tricuspid stenosis (Fig. 4-11) is the thickening of the tricuspid valve, usually caused by rheumatic fever and often associated with mitral stenosis. Thus, if tricuspid stenosis is rheumatic in origin, it is often not isolated but associated with mitral stenosis. It is seen also in carcinoid syndrome, a condition resulting from tumors in the small bowel, lung, or stomach, which secrete vasoactive materials that eventually cause cardiac lesions. Right atrial tumors can simulate the physical findings of tricuspid stenosis. The neck veins and liver show prominent presystolic pulsations.

Tricuspid Regurgitation

This condition typically arises in patients as a result of right heart failure associated with pulmonary hypertension; it does not always result from disease of the tricuspid valve itself. Tricuspid regurgitation (TR) can be classified as either organic or functional (Table 4-3). It may be seen in carcinoid syndrome with or without pulmonary hypertension. Tricuspid regurgitation may occur in systemic lupus erythematosus, in substance abusers as a result of endocarditis of the tricuspid valve, or in association with Ebstein's anomaly.

Table 4-3 Classification of Tricuspid Regurgitation

Organic	Functional
Rheumatic	Secondary to right-sided failure
Carcinoid	Secondary to severe mitral disease
Bacterial endocarditis ← drug abuse	
Right ventricular infarction	
Ebstein's anomaly	

Physical Signs   Icterocyanosis of the face, systolic pulsations of the liver, and pulsatile neck veins with systolic cv-y pulsation may be present in significant tricuspid regurgitation. The systolic venous pulsation may be best seen when the clinician stands behind the patient, observing the ear lobes move slowly outward. Chest x-ray shows enlargement of the right atrium and ventricle, and prominence of the superior vena cava and azygos vein. Echocardiogram shows right atrial enlargement. Two-dimensional echocardiography enables the diagnosis to be made readily.

Tricuspid regurgitation is valuable in calculating pulmonary artery pressure using Doppler technique, which is useful in determining the degree, if any, of pulmonary hypertension. Organic tricuspid regurgitation may also occur as an isolated phenomenon with absent or minimal murmurs, or may have holosystolic, early systolic, or ejection murmurs.

Pulmonary Stenosis

Pulmonary stenosis is the narrowing of the pulmonary valve below the valve at the infundibulum or above the valve or in the branches of the pulmonary artery (Fig. 4-12). It is an unusual cause of heart disease in adults, although it is a congenital lesion.

Pathology   Pulmonary stenosis may be an isolated lesion, associated with an unrestricted ventricular septal defect (VSD), or with an overriding aorta in tetralogy of Fallot. It may be infundibular, although valvular pulmonary stenosis is 30 times as common. Combined valvular and infundibular forms are occasional occurrences.

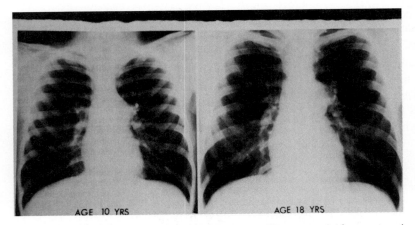

AGE 10 YRS   AGE 18 YRS

Figure 4-12   Virtually identical chest x-rays at ages 10 years and 18 years in a boy with mild pulmonic stenosis (gradient of 10 to 25 mmHg at both ages). The lung fields show normal pulmonary vascular markings. There is conspicuous dilatation of the pulmonary trunk and its left branch.

Symptoms   Patients with mild or moderate pulmonary stenosis may be asymptomatic. Severe cases may present with dyspnea, angina, and syncope. Infundibular stenosis is commonly associated with ventricular septal defects. These patients may be cyanotic intermittently. Pulmonary valvular or infundibular stenosis is present in tetralogy and pentalogy of Fallot. In Fallot's pentalogy, VSD and ASD may be present. In Fallot's tetralogy these defects are present without an atrial septal defect. In the tetralogy syndrome, i.e., tetralogy of Fallot comprising many combinations, the aorta overrides both ventricles; ventricular hypertrophy is seen and may be right-sided.

Physical Findings   Typical findings in pulmonary stenosis include a normal pulse with prominent a waves; a precordial heave; a loud, harsh midsystolic murmur; a click that disappears on inspiration; and a soft, delayed, or absent P_1. ECG usually indicates right ventricular hypertrophy. Chest x-ray often shows poststenotic dilatation of the main and left pulmonary arteries.

Pulmonary Regurgitation

Pulmonary regurgitation is present in patients with pulmonary hypertension and left heart failure associated with the Graham Steell murmur. It may occur as a complication in patients who have total correction of tetralogy of Fallot. Pulmonary regurgitation may also be encountered in idiopathic pulmonary artery dilatation. Two-dimensional echocardiography demonstrates a dilated right ventricle. Pulmonary regurgitation in a patient with left heart failure may be studied with Doppler ultrasound to determine the pulmonary artery pressure.

MYOCARDITIS AND THE CARDIOMYOPATHIES

Myocarditis is an inflammatory process involving the heart. It may be caused by infectious agents, including HIV, bacteria, fungi, rickettsiae, and spirochetes; toxic chemicals and drugs; radiation; physical agents such as heat or cold, and allergic reactions as in Dressler's syndrome. Dressler's syndrome presents as pleurisy, pericarditis, and heart failure with an elevated sedimentation rate, and is due to an autoimmune myopericarditis.

Auscultatory Findings   Auscultatory findings in myocarditis include a soft S_1, ventricular gallops, and apical systolic murmurs. In coxsackie-B and echovirus infections, combinations of myocarditis with a pericardial friction rub may coexist. Pericarditis and tamponade may occur.

The Cardiomyopathies

Cardiomyopathies, a heterogeneous group of entities, are classified into three categories: dilated, hypertrophic, and restrictive.

Dilated Dilated cardiomyopathies, often idiopathic, may occur in certain specific circumstances (e.g., pregnancy, glycogen storage disease, sarcoidosis) (Fig. 4-13). They may be ischemic due to association with valvular heart disease; are rarely congenital; and may follow myocarditis, chronic alcoholism, or cocaine addiction. Dilated cardiomyopathies also occur in collagen vascular diseases and in hemochromatosis. Auscultatory findings include a soft S_1, with S_3 and S_4 normally present, midsystolic murmur, with paradoxic splitting of S_2 (P_2A_2).

Hypertrophic Hypertrophic cardiomyopathy (HOCM) or idiopathic hypertrophic subaortic stenosis (IHSS) refer to abnormal hypertrophy of the left ventricle and septum with or without obstruction to outflow. In patients with obstruction the septum is asymmetrically hypertrophied.

Symptoms Patients may have hypertrophy of the heart and though they may present with exertional dyspnea, orthopnea, or paroxysmal nocturnal dyspnea, these patients rarely have myocardial failure. Pulsus alternans is *not* a common feature. Atrial fibrillation with embolic events occur. Sudden

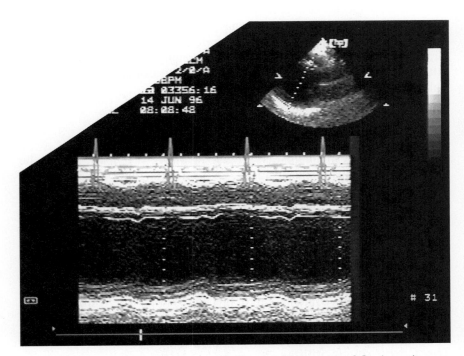

Figure 4-13 Echocardiogram of patient with dilated cardiomyopathy; 2-D echocardiogram and M-mode echocardiogram with ECG. Note the increase in the ventricle size with decreased excursion of the posterior ventricular wall and reduction of the septum markedly diminished.

death is not uncommon, especially in younger athletic patients after extraordinary exertion.

The diagnosis of hypertrophic cardiomyopathy is made by clinical examination. There is typically a bisferiens carotid pulse. The venous pressure may be elevated due to septal inflow obstructions (Bernheim's phenomenon). The apical pulse may be forceful with a presystolic impulse due to a triple-ripple S_4. A systolic thrill may be palpable.

Physical Findings Chest x-rays of patients with HOCM indicate varying degrees of cardiomegaly. Patients have thickened septa, thickened left ventricular posterior walls, and systolic anterior motion of the mitral valve impacting the septum. This motion is increased with administration of amyl nitrite, causing a loud pseudoejection click and increased loud systolic murmur. Holter monitoring is an important test to detect the presence of arrhythmias. Electrocardiographic findings may include q waves. These may be seen in myocarditis and hypertrophic cardiomyopathy and do not indicate infarction (Cardiac Pearl 47). A more detailed discussion may be found in Chap. 6 (Cardiac Pearl 95).

Pathology In patients with HOCM, the septum is asymmetrically hypertrophied and is usually one to three times the thickness of the left ventricular wall. The obstruction is worsened by factors that decrease left ventricular filling. Patients may have a family history of this disease, associated with a dominant gene with variable penetration.

Hemodynamics Ventricular contraction is initially rapid but the outflow tract is obstructed by the muscular septum and the apposition of the mitral valve, which is caused by the effect of the jet (Venturi effect). The pulse is characteristically bifid for this reason. Left ventricle relaxation is abnormal and the apical impulse may be trifid if a prominent atrial systolic wave is present.

Restrictive Restrictive cardiomyopathies are relatively uncommon and are characterized by impaired diastolic filling with preserved contractile function. Abnormal ventricular filling is commonly associated with atrioventricular valvular regurgitation. The most frequent causes of restrictive cardiomyopathies include myocardial fibrosis, *Löffler's endocarditis* (endomyocardial fibrosis with eosinophilia; a common syndrome in Africa), amyloid or iron infiltration of the heart, or connective tissue diseases (e.g., scleroderma), as well as amyloidosis and radiation damage.

Auscultatory Findings Patients frequently present with a heart that is normal in size, and with elevated venous pressure. Patients frequently have both mitral and tricuspid regurgitation murmurs and an S_3.

Physical Findings   The atria are enlarged bilaterally. Patients with inability to fill the atrium may present with symptoms and signs of pericardial constriction; indeed, the difficulty in diagnosing restrictive cardiomyopathy is its similarity to constrictive pericarditis. On cardiac catheterization, however, the absence of pericardial thickness or calcification differentiates this condition from constrictive pericardial disease.

Ascites, edema, and enlarged, tender liver may be present in patients with restrictive cardiomyopathy. Peripheral pulses are typically small. Pulmonary congestion may also be present. Echocardiographic features show diffuse low qrs voltage, nonspecific st-t changes, and conduction disturbances (atrial and ventricular arrhythmias). ECG usually indicates normal ventricular volumes, enlarged atria, shortened isovolemic relaxation time, and tricuspid and mitral regurgitation. Restrictive cardiomyopathy caused by amyloidosis is indicated by a low-voltage ECG and increased uptake of technetium-99m (^{99m}Tc) pyrophosphate. Thallium-201 scintigraphy reveals defects in the myocardial wall. Magnetic resonance imaging (MRI) is useful in showing enlarged atria and regurgitation. Cardiac catheterization shows equilibration of pressures with rapid X and Y descents in the right atrial tracing.

CARDIAC ARRHYTHMIAS

Disturbances of cardiac rhythm may be either symptomatic or asymptomatic; the latter may be detected during routine monitoring. Asymptomatic arrhythmias are not necessarily benign; they may be premonitory indicators of serious abnormalities.

Atrial Fibrillation

Atrial fibrillation (AF) is the commonest chronic arrhythmia (Cardiac Pearl 56). Atrial fibrillation occurs in pediatric cardiac syndromes such as transposition of the great arteries (TGA) or tetralogy of Fallot. In adults, atrial fibrillation may be the initial presenting sign in mitral valve disease, in thyrotoxicosis, and in atrial septal defects. Patients with atrial fibrillation may also present with enlarged left atria (e.g., in mitral stenosis and in atrial septal defect). Patients may develop atrial fibrillation following alcohol intoxication ("holiday heart") or use of recreational drugs. Atrial fibrillation may complicate Wolff-Parkinson-White syndrome, associated with Ebstein's anomaly; or may present with no evident cardiac disorder, as in lone atrial fibrillation. Atrial fibrillation may be associated with mitral valve prolapse, hypertension, or coronary artery disease. Bronchogenic carcinoma may present with atrial fibrillation associated with left atrial infiltration by tumor.

Auscultatory Findings   Atrial fibrillation is marked by a variable S_1 that is louder after a pause and which may be associated with apical systolic murmurs. Mitral regurgitation may occur during or after rapid bouts of atrial fibrillation. Atrial fibrillation sometimes complicates auscultation of the heart, for example, in patients with mitral stenosis. It is best to examine such patients in the left lateral supine position with the bell of the stethoscope at the apex with held expiration. The presystolic murmur of mitral stenosis may persist in atrial fibrillation; hence *ERUP*, not *RUP*, may be heard in the absence of atrial contraction in presystole.

Atrial Flutter and Supraventricular Tachycardia

These two rhythm disturbances are characterized by increased ($>$ 100 beats per minute) heart rates caused by rapid impulse formation. Atrial flutter is less common than atrial fibrillation and is often an unstable rhythm. In atrial flutter, sudden rate change due to transient atrioventricular block caused by carotid compression slows the heart rate and may occur with changing murmurs. Auscultatory findings in these conditions are not of great importance. Neck veins are useful in showing flutter waves. Rate change is useful for diagnosis.

Electrocardiographic strips are characteristic of supraventricular tachycardia (SVT); p waves from normal and reentrant pathways are seen before and after the qrs complex in this rhythm. Carotid sinus pressure may abolish the tachycardia in reentrant supraventricular tachycardia. In sinus tachycardia, the heart rate slows, uncovering murmurs that were previously occult.

Ventricular Tachycardia

Ventricular tachycardia is defined as three or more consecutive ventricular premature beats. It is a frequent complication of acute myocardial infarction and dilated cardiomyopathy.

Ventricular tachycardia is marked by a variable S_1 and extra sounds due to the wide qrs and atrial beats. This pattern is in contrast to supraventricular tachycardia, in which S_1 remains the same. In addition, carotid sinus pressure has no effect on ventricular tachycardia.

Atrioventricular Conduction Defects (Cardiac Pearl 84)

AV conduction defects occur within the atrioventricular node and are classified as first-, second-, or third-degree. Second-degree AV block is subclassified into Mobitz type I (Wenckebach) and Mobitz type II. The latter is almost always due to organic disease.

Right bundle branch block (RBBB) is associated with splitting of S_1 and S_2. Left bundle branch block (LBBB) is associated with a normal or soft S_1 and paradoxic splitting of S_1. Patients with AV block present with variable first sounds. Mobitz type I patients present with a softened S_1 in first-degree or second-degree atrioventricular block. Diastolic sounds are heard in patients with second-degree Mobitz type II AV block and in third-degree AV block. In Rytand syndrome, a middiastolic murmur may be heard associated with calcification of the mitral valve ring and third-degree AV block variables and diastolic murmurs. In third-degree AV block, murmurs are produced by atrial contraction, and arise from the atrial inflow tract. In sinus bradycardia, S_1 tends to be louder, and midsystolic murmurs are commonly heard. In patients with tachycardia, a tic-tac rhythm may be present. The presence of this rhythm makes it difficult to distinguish between first and second heart sounds. In third-degree heart block, a variable S_1 and double diastolic murmurs or sounds may be heard. Lyme disease is a common cause of heart block in a young person (Cardiac Pearl 29), as revealed by a variable S_1 and cannon sounds.

PERICARDIAL DISEASES

The pericardium is often involved in cardiac disease processes; it can also be affected by infections in adjacent tissues, or itself be a primary site of disease. Its importance in cardiac disturbances derives from its fibrous tissue composition. The pericardium cannot stretch rapidly to allow for severe cardiac dilatation and so tends to increase intracardiac pressure when fluid accumulates.

Friction Rubs

Two important but rare causes of pericardial friction rub are pulmonary embolus and myocardial infarction. Pericardial rubs are commonly heard in viral pericarditis. They are present in rheumatic fever and are associated with severe pain in the chest. Fibrinous pericarditis may be a feature of tuberculosis. Acute pericarditis may occur in Dressler's syndrome following a myocardial infarction, pacemaker implantation, or cardiac surgery. In this condition, patients develop a high sedimentation rate (ESR), a pericardial friction rub, and a pleural friction rub. Patients may also have signs of heart failure.

Following myocardial infarction, some patients, particularly women with hypertension, may develop pericardial rubs as a prelude to cardiac rupture and pulseless electrical activity. Such patients become suddenly dyspneic, nauseated, faint, and develop a friction rub. This condition is most likely to occur from the third to the fifth day after a myocardial infarction. Pericardial friction rubs may also be present in patients with uremia, bacterial endocarditis, or autoimmune syndromes.

Atrial Pacing

This technique has emerged as an important means of checking myocardial ischemia. Attached to some versions of the pacing device is an esophageal stethoscope, which is used for auscultating the heart as it is paced. With rapid pacing, *the murmur of mitral regurgitation tends to disappear and the murmurs of mitral and aortic stenosis get louder. Onset of atrial pacing can be easily auscultated.*

The esophageal stethoscope also is useful in detecting ischemia with associated echocardiography, in which the auscultatory findings of an S_4 and apical systolic murmur may result from a rapid-paced rate. This may be done in the operating room.

Effusion

In pericardial effusion with severe tamponade, the patient typically has cardiomegaly, positive Kussmaul's sign (an increase in jugular venous pressure during inspiration), and Broadbent's sign (retraction in the ribs with systole). Pulsus paradoxus is a classic finding. Pericardial effusion is often a sequel of radiation pericarditis or a malignant neoplasm in the pericardium (Fig. 4-14A). Figure 4-14B shows an ECHO demonstrating pericardial effusion.

Pericardial effusion is associated with softening of heart sounds and increased dullness to percussion over the precordium. As pericardial effusions accumulate, friction rubs tend to get softer and disappear. The clinical seriousness of the effusion is determined by the speed of its accumulation.

Tamponade

Pericardial tamponade typically results from rapidly developing effusions, and is characterized by a high intrapericardial pressure that restricts venous return and ventricular filling. Common causes of tamponade include neoplastic diseases, uremia, trauma, rupture of the heart or great vessels, anticoagulant therapy and radiation (Chap. 3). Occasionally, fibrinous pericarditis may evolve to tamponade.

Patients with tamponade may present with neck vein distention and pulsus paradoxus. Their ECG may show low qrs voltage with total electrical alternans, alternating amplitudes of p waves and qrst complexes. This indicates alternation of the pqrst and is thought to reflect a shifting back and forth of the heart within the pericardial sac in this condition.

Constrictive

Clinical findings in constrictive pericarditis are similar to those of restrictive cardiomyopathy; differential diagnosis is often difficult. Patients may present with either constrictive pericarditis or with effusive constrictive pericarditis. *Adhesive pericarditis,* in which the pericardium becomes fibrotic and adheres to the chest wall, may be indicated by Broadbent's sign (retraction of the ribs) and Ewart's sign (dullness on percussion below the scapula).

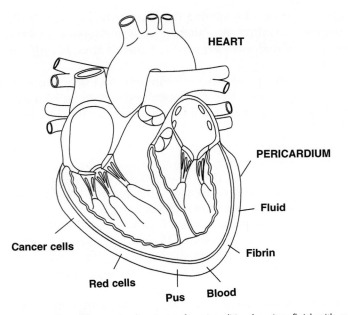

Figure 4-14 Schematic diagram of pericarditis, showing fluid with variable materials in the pericardium.

Patients may also present with pericardial rub, pulsus paradoxus and positive Kussmaul's sign. The patient may have engorged neck veins and venous descent. In patients with constrictive pericarditis, a rub is not heard. A pericardial knock in early diastole is characteristic.

INFECTIVE ENDOCARDITIS

Infective endocarditis is caused by streptococcal, bacterial, fungal, or staphylococcal inflammation of the cardiac valves. It may present as infective arteritis of a coarctation of the aorta (CoA) or a patent ductus arteriosus. Infective endocarditis may be acute or chronic, or involve native or prosthetic valves. In general, early (under 4 months) prosthetic valve endocarditis is due to *Staphylococcus epidermidis,* while fungi or other organisms may also be implicated. Late endocarditis may be due to *Streptococcus viridans.* Other organisms that involve the valves include enterococci, *Pseudomonas,* and gram-negative organisms. In general, fungal vegetations tend to be large.

Endocarditis may involve any of the left-sided valves of the heart, including the aortic, mitral, and tricuspid valves. Involvement of the pulmonic valve is, however, rare. Acute bacterial endocarditis is common in drug users, typically affects the right side of the heart, and involves the tricuspid valve. In right-sided endocarditis, although patients present with tricuspid regurgitation or stenosis, the outlook is better than in left-sided endocarditis.

Patients with infective endocarditis may develop features of pulmonary edema due to septic emboli in the lungs which lead to adult respiratory distress syndrome (ARDS). These patients are hypoxic, septic, and have right-sided murmurs.

In addition to causing systemic distress, infective endocarditis may damage valves and other cardiac tissue. Bacterial infections involving the aortic and mitral valves may cause valvular rupture and perivalvular abscesses. Extension of infection to the myocardium may be associated with Bracht-Wachter bodies, which are inclusion bodies in the intermyocardial areas. Found in the myocardium, these bodies may be associated with heart failure, heart block, as well as with myocarditis. In some cases myocardial abscesses develop, leading, in turn, to conduction disturbances or aneurysms in the sinus of Valsalva. Pericarditis may occur with subsequent suppurative pericarditis. Burrowing of the abscess into the conduction system can lead to AV block and bundle branch block. Complete heart block may occur (Cardiac Pearl 89). Patients with bacterial endocarditis or infective endocarditis may have vegetations of the valves, which in turn cause valvular stenosis. Vegetations that obstruct valvular inflow may lead to regurgitation and may cause rupture of the chordae tendineae.

Physical Findings The clinical picture is characterized by a change in murmurs and rapid development of heart failure; a patient's murmurs may seem to get louder or softer, or develop thrills that can soften and disappear over the course of a few days' hospitalization. Autoimmune manifestations such as Osler's nodes (tender, raised, bruise-like areas on the extremities), Janeway's lesions (painless erythematous rashes on palms and soles), Roth's spots (areas of retinal hemorrhage with central exudate), and petechial hemorrhages in the eyelids. The occurrence of stroke in a young febrile patient with heart murmur should prompt the diagnosis of bacterial endo-carditis (Joachim's dictum) and mandate blood cultures.

Auscultatory findings are related to the valve involved and to other cardiac structures. Embolism of a renal artery may produce a flank bruit that is louder on inspiration, and hypertension. Prosthetic valves may leak, thrombose, or become obstructed by pannus. A knowledge of baseline findings is vital in diagnosis (Chap. 4). Changing murmurs are common.

HYPERTENSION

In hypertension, elevated blood pressure may be systemic or pulmonary (Fig. 4-15). Prompt diagnosis and treatment of hypertension are vital in that the condition is synergistic with other risk factors such as diabetes or smoking.

Systemic Hypertension

Auscultatory Findings Auscultation plays an important role in diagnosing systemic hypertension. The clinician should seek to identify a secondary cause of hypertension in patients in the following categories:

1. Patients who have sudden elevations of blood pressure;
2. Younger patients with elevated blood pressure;
3. Older patients with a rising diastolic blood pressure;
4. Patients with diastolic hypertension with soft aortic regurgitation, which suggests dissection or an aneurysm, as described by Harvey. Note that an S_4 is invariably present.

Effects Hypertension may cause ventricular hypertrophy, diastolic heart failure, or aortic regurgitation; it is an important factor in causing atheroscle-rosis and dissection. Auscultatory findings are indicated.

Pulmonary Hypertension

Pulmonary hypertension may be due to left-sided failure (postcapillary), or to primary pulmonary hypertension (Fig. 4-16; Table 4-4). It may be

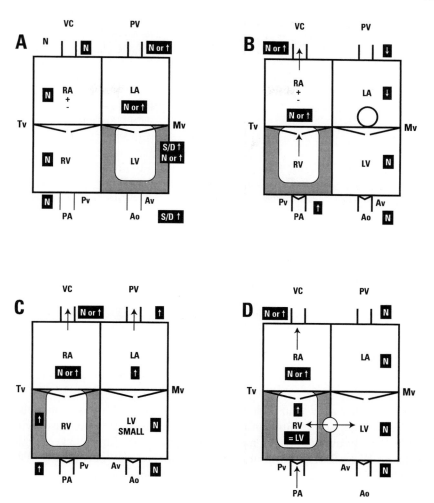

Figure 4-15 *Schematic diagrams of four forms of hypertension. A. Systemic hypertension. B. Pulmonary hypertension, precapillary. C. Pulmonary hypertension, post capillary. D. Eisenmenger VSD. VC, vena cava; RA, right atrium; RV, right ventricle; PA, pulmonary artery; PV, pulmonary veins; LV, left ventricle; LA, left atrium; A, aorta; Tv, tricuspid valve; Mv, mitral valve; Pv, pulmonary valve; Av, aortic valve.*

drug-induced, as in contraceptive or Aminorex use or with the use of other drugs. Pulmonary hypertension may be variously associated with shunts, thromboembolic states and coagulopathies, angina, and cyanosis, and may occur with signs of right-sided failure (Fig. 4-17). (Recently the fenfluramine group of drugs, used for the treatment of obesity, have been associated with pulmonary hypertension in one out of 500 cases.)

Pulmonary hypertension also may present with right heart failure. Patients, in most instances, have clinical evidence of right ventricular hyper-

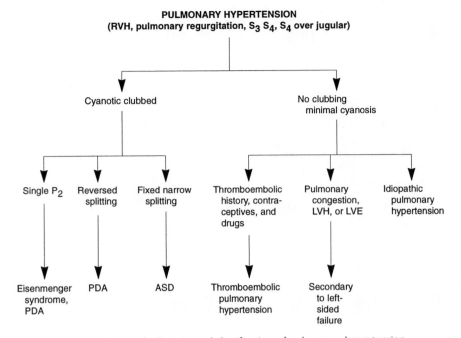

Figure 4-16 Auscultatory findings in and classification of pulmonary hypertension.

trophy, engorged neck veins, tricuspid regurgitation, and holosystolic murmur or ejection systolic murmur at the left sternal edge that increases with Carvallo's maneuver. Patients may show signs of an early click, a right ventricular S_3 or S_4. Loud pulmonary valve closure may occur early. The S_4 may be heard over the jugular veins. There are many causes and subtypes

Table 4-4 Mechanisms and Clinical Conditions Associated with Pulmonary Hypertension

Mechanisms	Clinical Conditions
Reduction in cross-sectional area of pulmonary arterial bed	Vasoconstriction ← hypoxia or acidosis
	Loss of vessels ← Pulmonary fibrosis, connective tissue disease
	Obstruction of vessels ← emboli or thrombosis
	Narrowing of vessels ← changes secondary to pulmonary hypertension
Increased pulmonary venous pressure	Left ventricular failure
	Left atrial myxoma
	Mitral stenosis
Increased pulmonary blood flow	Congenital left-to-right shunts
Increased blood viscosity	Polycythemia
Other	Cirrhosis of the liver

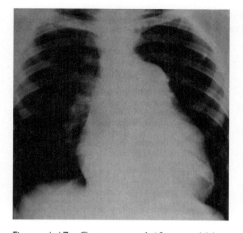

Figure 4-17 Chest x-ray of 18-year-old boy with pulmonary hypertension. The aorta is inconspicuous. The enlarged right ventricle forms an acute angle with the left hemidiaphragm, and a dilated right atrium is identified by its convex sweep along the lower right cardiac border.

of pulmonary hypertension (Fig. 4-18). Table 4-5 summarizes the auscultation of P_2 in pulmonary hypertension.

Eisenmenger Syndrome   Eisenmenger syndrome is pulmonary hypertension with a right-to-left shunt.

Eisenmenger Complex   Eisenmenger complex is congenital pulmonary hypertension and ventricular septal defect.

CARDIAC FAILURE (See Chap. 7.)

Heart failure is defined as derangement of cardiac function, leading to congestion or failure of the heart as a pump. Cardiac function may be inadequate because of dysfunction in any of four factors: (1) myocardial contractility; (2) ventricular preload; (3) afterload; (4) heart rate. Failure of the heart may be provoked by a variety of factors, including anemia, thyrotoxicosis, pregnancy, and pulmonary embolism.

Heart failure is classified into: (1) left heart failure; (2) right heart failure; (3) congestive heart failure (CHF); (4) high-output failure; and (5) low-output failure. Low output systolic or myocardial pump failure is distinguished from congestive failure or diastolic failure by their physical and auscultatory findings. Specifically, the former are characterized by small-volume pulse and soft S_1; the latter have a normal volume and pulse, but a loud S_1. S_3 and S_4 may be present in both groups of failure.

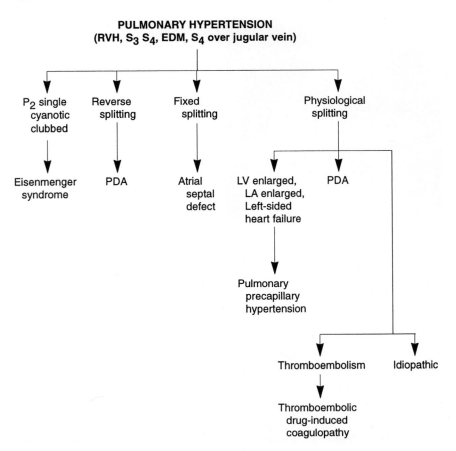

Figure 4-18 Causes and subtypes of pulmonary hypertension.

Left Heart

Left heart failure is characterized by low cardiac output and elevated pulmonary venous pressure. Patients typically complain of dyspnea. Left heart failure is associated with left ventricular dysfunction (Fig. 4-19).

Table 4-5 Auscultation of P_2 in Pulmonary Hypertension

Quality of P_2	Condition
Single P_2	Eisenmenger's complex
Physiological P_2	Eisenmenger's ductus
Physiological S_2, Narrow fixed	Ventricular septal defect
Reversed splitting	Patent ductus arteriosus
Wide splitting	Right bundle branch block ± RV failure
Reversed splitting	Left bundle branch block, LV failure
Wide splitting of A_2P_2	Pulmonary embolism and failure of RV

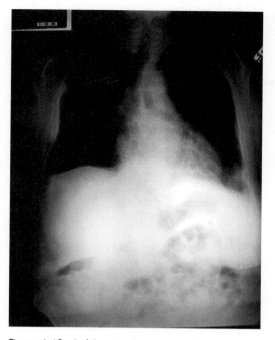

Figure 4-19   Left heart enlargement. Chest x-ray showing left ventricular and left atrial enlargement.

Right Heart

Right heart failure may be caused by pulmonary hypertension or right ventricular infarction. Patients frequently show signs of fluid retention (e.g., ascites or edema); they may complain of pain in the right upper quadrant due to a congested liver. They may also have cyanosis, angina, fatigue, a positive Kussmaul's sign, hepatomegaly, or splenomegaly.

Auscultatory findings in right heart failure include S_3 S_4 below the xiphoid process and S_4 over the jugular veins.

Congestive

Patients with CHF may have dyspnea, orthopnea, edema, anorexia, bloating, jaundice, cyanosis, elevated venous pressures, cardiomegaly or right-sided pleural effusion (Fig. 4-20). In extreme cases they may present with anasarca, cyanosis, rales throughout the chest, rhonchi, tachypnea and respiratory arrest.

Auscultatory findings in CHF include: a loud P_2, holosystolic murmurs of mitral or tricuspid regurgitation, or both. Other findings include changing murmurs, S_3 S_4, quadruple rhythm, summation gallop, basal rales, egophony, and diminished sounds over the right base.

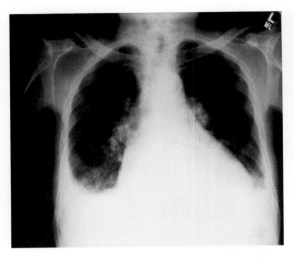

Figure 4-20 Chest x-ray showing cardiomegaly with an elongated left border indicating left ventricular hypertrophy. LA enlargement is shown by elevation of the left atrium. There is a right sided pleural effusion and small left sided effusion classic for heart failure.

High-Output

In high-output failure, cardiac pump function is inadequate due to metabolic demands or excessive requirements for increased blood flow. High-output failure is relatively uncommon but may be seen in Paget's disease, thyrotoxicosis, AV shunting, and beriberi.

Low-Output

Patients with low-output failure may present with fatigue and lethargy; in extreme cases they may have Cheyne-Stokes respiration (periodic breathing; repeated cycle of gradual increase in depth of breathing followed by gradual decrease to apnea), cyanosis, and wasting.

Auscultatory findings in low output failure may include: pulsus alternans, small pulse volume, a pulse with palpable dicrotic notch, alternating systolic blood pressures, a soft S_1, alternating loudness of S_2, and tachy- or bradycardia.

CLINICAL VIGNETTES

*The following vignettes present actual cases of patients who were affected by diseases and conditions discussed in this chapter. At the end of each case, choose the **one** answer that best describes the diagnosis indicated by the vignette.*

1. A 40-year-old male patient presented with typical angina. Exercise testing revealed pronounced ST segments and downward shift on hyperventilation. Cold pressor test was administered, placing the patient's hand in ice water while monitoring the blood pressure; blood pressure elevation signified a positive test. Following cardiac catheterization, administration of ergonovine provoked chest pain and ST segment depression.
   The diagnosis is:

   A. Coronary spasm
   B. Angina pectoris
   C. A and B.

2. A 78-year-old female patient presented with a history of radiation therapy in the chest area following mastectomy. Her venous pressure was elevated 20 mmHg. She had a positive Kussmaul's sign, with no pulsus paradoxus. Apical murmurs of mitral and tricuspic regurgitation with an S_3 were heard. The patient's heart was moderately enlarged. Moderate aortic regurgitation, a normal-looking myocardium, and short isovolemic relaxation time were present. Computed tomography showed no evidence of pericardial calcification. The patient, however, refused cardiac catheterization and myocardial biopsy.
   The diagnosis is:

   A. Restrictive cardiomyopathy
   B. Dilated cardiomyopathy
   C. Hypertrophic cardiomyopathy

3. A 67-year-old male patient presented with atrial fibrillation associated with mild mitral stenosis. He was euthyroid. Amiodarone therapy was given in full dose and cardioversion was performed successfully. Six months later, the patient, who had lost weight and suffered from tremors and fatigue, again developed atrial fibrillation.
   The diagnosis is:

   A. Spontaneous recurrence of atrial fibrillation
   B. Amiodarone-induced hyperthyroidism
   C. Coronary artery disease, causing atrial fibrillation

4. A 64-year-old female patient was seen with atrial fibrillation. She presented with a history of recurrent attacks of ascites and edema of the lower extremities. She had had paracentesis of the abdomen at least 10 times. Her edema had responded to furosemide (Lasix), a loop diuretic.

   On examination, the patient had engorged neck veins and positive Kussmaul's sign. The Y descent interruption corresponded with a pericardial knock heard in the subxiphoid area. The patient had pulsus paradoxus, which was difficult to detect on account of her atrial fibrillation.

The diagnosis is:

A. Constrictive pericarditis
B. Pericarditis
C. Tamponade

ANSWERS

1. *C. A and B.* In a 40-year-old male with exertional angina occuring at rest with the cold pressor test, *C* is the most likely diagnosis.
2. *A. Restrictive cardiomyopathy.* Moderate cardiac enlargement in the presence of aortic regurgitation and the presence of MR and TR make *A* the most likely diagnosis.
3. *B. Amiodarone-induced hyperthyroidism.* Thyroid function tests confirmed hyperthyroidism and amiodarone was discontinued.
4. *B. Pericarditis.* Chronic ascites and edema rule out constrictive pericarditis. Computed tomography indicated calcification of the pericardium, which was then surgically removed.

BIBLIOGRAPHY

Valvular Heart Disease

Aryanpur I, et al: Regression of pulmonary tension after mitral valve surgery in children. *Chest* 1977; 71:354.

Barlow JB, et al: Late systolic murmur and nonejection (mid-late) systolic clicks. *Br Heart J* 1968; 30:203.

Barnett HJM, et al: Further evidence relating mitral valve prolapse to cerebral ischemic events. *N Engl J Med* 1980; 302:139.

Bashour T, Lindsay J Jr: Midsystolic clicks originating from tricuspid valve structures: A sequela of heroin-induced endocarditis. *Chest* 1975; 67:620.

Braunwald E: Clinical manifestations of heart failure. In Braunwald E(ed): *Heart Disease.* Philadelphia, Saunders, 1988:471–484.

Braunwald E: Unstable angina. *Circulation* 1989; 80:410–414.

Breyer RH, et al: Tricuspid regurgitation: A comparison of non-operative management, tricuspid annuloplasty, and tricuspid valve replacement. *J Thorac Cardiovasc Surg* 1976; 72:867.

Bristo MR, et al: Early anthracycline cardiotoxicity. *Am J Med* 1978;65:823–832.

Bush CA, et al: Occult constrictive pericardial disease. *Circulation* 1977; 56:924.

Chuttani K, et al: Diagnosis of cardiac tamponade after cardiac surgery: Relative value of clinical, echocardiographic, and hemodynamic signs. *Am Heart J* 1994; 127:913–918.

Criley JM, et al: Prolapse of the mitral valve: Clinical and cine-angiocardiographic findings. *Br Heart J* 1966; 28:488.

D'Cruz IA, et al: Cardiac involvement including tuberculous pericardial effusion, complicating acquired immune deficiency syndrome: 25 years' experience. *J Card Med* 1984; 9:321.

Daniels SJ, et al: Rheumatic tricuspid valve disease: Two-dimensional echocardiographic, hemodynamic, and angiographic correlations. *Am J Cardiol* 1983; 51:492.

Deedwania PC, Carbajal EV: Silent ischemia during daily life is an independent predictor of mortality in stable angina. *Circulation* 1990; 81:748.

Edwards WD, et al: Active valvulitis associated with chronic rheumatic valvular disease and active myocarditis. *Circulation* 1978; 57:181.

Gaasch WH: Diagnosis and treatment of heart failure based on left ventricular systolic or diastolic dysfunction. *JAMA* 1994; 271:1276–1280.

Gooch AS, et al: Prolapse of both mitral and tricuspid leaflets in systolic murmur-click syndrome. *N Engl J Med* 1972; 287:1218–1222.

Goodwin JF, et al: Rheumatic tricuspid stenosis. *Br Med J* 1957; 2:1383.

Gottdiener JS, et al: Late cardiac effects of therapeutic mediastinal irradiation. *N Engl J Med* 1982; 306:550–551.

Hecht SR, Berger M: Right-sided endocarditis in intravenous drug users: Prognostic features in 102 episodes. *Ann Intern Med* 1992; 117:560–566.

Khandheria BK: Suspected bacterial endocarditis to TEE or not TEE. *J Am Coll Cardiol* 1993; 21:222–224.

Levine RA, et al: The relationship of mitral annular shape to the diagnosis of mitral valve prolapse. *Circulation* 1987; 75:756.

Littman D, Spodick DH: Total electrical alternans in pericardial disease. *Circulation* 1958; 17:912–917.

Mansur AJ, et al: The complications of infectious endocarditis: A reappraisal in the 1980's. *Arch Intern Med* 1992; 152:2428–2432.

Mardelli TJ, et al: Tricuspid valve prolapse diagnosed by cross-sectional echocardiography. *Chest* 1979; 79:201.

Mavissakalin M, et al: Mitral prolapse and agoraphobia. *Am J Psychiatry* 1983; 140:1612.

Mitchell AM, et al: The clinical features of aortic stenosis. *Am Heart J* 1954; 48:684.

Monane M, et al: Noncompliance with congestive heart failure therapy in the elderly. *Arch Intern Med* 1994; 154:433–437.

Oakley CM: Mitral valve prolapse: Harbinger of death or variant of normal? *Br Med J* 1984; 288:1853.

Pandian NG, et al: Diagnosis of restrictive pericarditis by 2-D echocardiography: Studies in a new experimental model and patients. *J Am Coll Cardiol* 1984; 4:1164.

Pansegrau DG, et al: Supravalvular aortic stenosis in adults. *Am J Cardiol* 1973; 31:635.

Perloff JK, Harvey WP: Clinical recognition of tricuspid stenosis. *Circulation* 1960; 22:346.

Rapaport E: Congestive heart failure: Diagnosis and principles of treatment. In Cohn JN(ed): *Drug Treatment of Heart Failure.* New Jersey, Advanced Therapeutics Communications International, 1988:127–146.

Reddy PS, et al: Cardiac tamponade: Observations in man. *Circulation* 1978; 58:265.

Reid CL, et al: Infective endocarditis: Improved diagnosis and treatment. In O'Rourk OH(ed): *Current Problems in Cardiology.* Chicago, Yearbook Medical Publishers, 1985.

Roberts WC, Perloff JK: Mitral valvular disease: A clinicopathologic survey of the conditions causing the mitral valve to function abnormally. *Ann Intern Med* 1972; 77:939.

Roberts WC, et al: Severe valvular aortic stenosis in patients over 65 years of age: A clinicopathologic study. *Am J Cardiol* 1971; 27:497.

Shah PM, Gramiak R: Echocardiographic recognition of mitral valve prolapse (abstr). *Circulation* (suppl 3) 1970; 42:45.

Shrivastava S, et al: Prolapse of the mitral valve. *Mod Concepts Cardiovasc Dis* 1977; 46:57.

Spodick DH: *Chronic and Constrictive Pericarditis.* New York, Grune & Stratton, 1964.

Spodick DH: The pericardial rub: A prospective, multiple-observer investigation of pericardial friction in 100 patients. *Am J Cardiol* 1975; 35:357.

Srebro J, Karliner JS: Congestive heart failure. *Curr Probl Cardiol* 1986; 23:1.

Stevenson LW, Perloff JK: The limited reliability of physical signs for estimating hemodynamics in chronic heart failure. *JAMA* 1989; 10:884.

Stimmel B, Dack S: Infective endocarditis in narcotic addicts. In Rahimpoola SH (ed): *Infective Endocarditis.* New York, Grune & Stratton, 1978.

Sung CS, et al: Discreet subaortic stenosis in adults. *Am J Cardiol* 1978; 42:283.

Theroux P, et al: Reactivation of unstable angina after the discontinuation of heparin. *N Engl J Med* 1992; 327:141–146.

Tornos MP, et al: Long-term complications of native valve infectious endocarditis in non-addicts. *Ann Intern Med* 1992; 117:567–572.

Trell E, et al: Carcinoid heart disease findings and follow-up in 11 cases. *Am J Med* 1973; 54:433.

Tyberg TI, et al: Genesis of pericardial knock in constrictive pericarditis. *Am J Cardiol* 1980; 46:570.

Wood P: Aortic stenosis. *Am J Cardiol* 1958; 1:553.

Wood P: Chronic rheumatic heart disease. In Wood P(ed): *Diseases of the Heart and Circulation,* 3rd ed. Philadelphia, Lippincott, 1968:690–691.

Cardiomyopathy

Abelman WH, Lorell BH: The challenge of cardiomyopathy. *J Am Coll Cardiol* 1989; 13:1219–1239.

Alexander JK: The heart and obesity. In Hurst JW (ed-in-chief): *The Heart,* 7th ed. New York: McGraw-Hill, 1990:1538–1543.

Anderson PAW: Diagnostic problem: Constrictive pericarditis or restrictive cardiomyopathy? *Cathet Cardiovasc Diagn* 1983; 9:1.

Benotti JR, Grossman W: Restrictive cardiomyopathy. *Ann Rev Med* 1984; 35:113.

Braunwald E, et al: Idiopathic hypertrophic subaortic stenosis. *Am J Med* 1960; 29:924.

Chatterjee K, et al: Hypertrophic cardiomyopathy—therapy with slow channel inhibiting agents. *Prog Cardiovasc Dis* 1982; 25:193.

D'Alonzo GE, et al: Survival in patients with primary pulmonary hypertension: Results from a national prospective registry. *Ann Intern Med* 1991; 115:343–349.

Elliott WJ: Ear lobe crease and coronary artery disease. *Am J Med* 1983; 75:1024.

Frank S, Braunwald E: Idiopathic hypertrophic subaortic stenosis: Clinical analysis of 126 patients with emphasis on the natural history. *Circulation* 1968; 37:759.

Frohlich ED: Evaluation and management of the patient with essential hypertension. In Parmley WW, et al (eds): *Cardiology,* vol. 2. Philadelphia, Lippincott, 1991:8.16–8.28.

Frohlich ED: Hypertension. In *Conn's Current Therapy.* Philadelphia, Saunders, 1993:280–296.

Frohlich ED: Pathophysiology of systemic arterial hypertension. In Hurst JW (ed-in-chief): *The Heart,* 8th ed. New York: McGraw-Hill, 1994:1391–1401.

Frohlich ED, et al: The heart in hypertension. *N Engl J Med* 1992; 327:998–1008.

Glenner GG: Amyloid deposits and amyloidosis: The B-fibrillosis. *N Engl J Med* 1980; 302:1283.

Groom D, et al: The normal systolic murmur. *Ann Intern Med* 1960; 52:134.

Grover RF: Chronic hypoxic pulmonary hypertension. In Fishman AP(ed): *The Pulmonary Circulation: Normal and Abnormal—Mechanisms, Management, and the National Registry.* Philadelphia, University of Pennsylvania Press, 1990.

Groves BM, Reeves JT: Pulmonary hypertension. In Horwitz LD, Groves BM(eds): *Signs and Symptoms in Cardiology.* Philadelphia, Lippincott, 1985:381–429.

Groves BM, et al: Acute hemodynamic effects of iloprost in primary (unexplained) pulmonary hypertension. *Semin Respir Critical Care Med* 1994; 15:230–237.

Groves BM, et al: Early diagnosis of primary pulmonary hypertension. In Wagenvoort CA, Denolin H(eds): *Pulmonary Circulation: Advances and Controversies.* Amsterdam, Elsevier, 1989:237–250.

Hall WD, et al: Diagnostic evaluation of the patient with hypertension. In Hurst JW (ed-in-chief): *The Heart,* 7th ed. New York: McGraw-Hill, 1990:1165.

Hess OM, et al: Pre- and postoperative findings in patients with endomyocardial fibrosis. *Br Heart J* 1978; 40:406.

Jamieson SW, et al: Combined heart and lung transplantation. *Lancet* 1983; 1:1130–1131.

Jervell A, Lange-Nielsen F: Congenital deaf-mutism, functional heart disease with prolongation of the QT interval, and sudden death. *Am Heart J* 1957; 54(1):59.

Joint National Committee on the Detection, Evaluation, and Treatment of High Blood Pressure. The 1992 report of the Joint National Committee on the Detection, Evaluation, and Treatment of High Blood Pressure. *Arch Intern Med* 1993; 153:154–183.

Keenan TJ, Schwartz MJ: Tricuspid whoop. *Am J Cardiol* 1973; 31:642.

Kokkinou SN, et al: Chromosomal analysis in dilated cardiomyopathy. *Circulation* 1993; 88:abstr 3078.

Kyle RA, Bayrd ED: Amyloidosis: Review of 236 cases. *Medicine* 1975; 54:271.

Larter W, et al: The asymmetrically hypertrophied septum: Further differentiation of its causes. *Circulation* 1976; 53:19.

McManus BM, et al: Hemodynamic cardiac constriction without anatomic myocardial restriction or pericardial constriction. *Am Heart J* 1981; 102:134.

Parker F: Hyperlipoproteinemia and xanthomatosis. In Callen JP (ed-in-chief): *Medicine for the Practicing Physician,* Boston, Butterworth, 1992:54.

Pinamonti B, et al: Restrictive left ventricular filling pattern in cardiomyopathy assessed by Doppler echocardiography: Clinical echocardiographic and hemodynamic correlations and prognostic implications. *J Am Coll Cardiol* 1993; 22:808–815.

Pollick C: Muscular subaortic stenosis: Hemodynamic and clinical improvement after disopyramide. *N Engl J Med* 1982; 307:997.

Rackley CE, et al: The precordial honk. *Am J Cardiol* 1966; 17:509.

Redfield MM, et al: Natural history of idiopathic dilated cardiomyopathy: Effect of referral bias and secular trend. *J Am Coll Cardiol* 1993; 22:1921–1926.

Roberts WC: Anomalous left ventricular band: An unemphasized cause of precordial musical murmur. *Am J Cardiol* 1969; 23:735.

Roberts WC, Waller BF: Mitral valve 'annular' calcium forming a complete circle or 'O' configuration: Clinical and necropsy observations. *Am Heart J* 1981; 101:619.

Rosenthal A, et al: Intrapulmonary venoocclusive disease. *Am J Cardiol* 1973; 31:78–83.

Rubin LJ, Peter RH: Oral hydralazine therapy for primary pulmonary hypertension. *N Engl J Med* 1980; 302:69–73.

Rubin LJ, et al: Treatment of primary pulmonary hypertension with continuous intravenous prostacyclin (epoprostenol): Results of a randomized trial. *Ann Intern Med* 1990; 112:485–491.

Schwartz ML, et al: Relation of Still's murmur, small aortic diameter and high aortic velocity. *Am J Cardiol* 1986; 57:1344.

Segal JP, et al: Diagnosis and treatment of primary myocardial disease. *Circulation* 1965; 32:837–844.

Siegel RJ, et al: Idiopathic restrictive cardiomyopathy. *Circulation* 1984; 70:165.

Silverberg S, et al: Pericarditis in patients undergoing long-term hemodialysis and peritoneal dialysis. *Am J Med* 1977; 63:874.

Stapleton JF, et al: Clinical pathways of cardiomyopathy. *American Heart Association Monograph No. 43.* 1974:168–178.

Stapleton JF, et al: The electrocardiogram of cardiomyopathy. *Prog Cardiovasc Dis* 1970; 13:217–239.

Steinberg EP, et al: Interventional management of peripheral vascular disease: What did we learn in Maryland and where do we go from here? *Radiology* 1993; 186L:639–642.

Stewart JR, Fajardo LF: Radiation-induced heart disease: An update. *Prog Cardiovasc Dis* 1984; 27:173.

Teare RD: Asymmetrical hypertrophy of the heart in young adults. *Br Heart J* 1958; 20:1.

Voelkel NF, Reeves JT: Primary pulmonary hypertension. In Moser KM(ed): *Pulmonary Vascular Disease.* New York, Marcel Dekker, 1979:573–649.

5

ELICITING HEART SOUNDS: TIMING, AMPLITUDE, AND PITCH

SYSTOLIC SOUNDS
First Heart Sound (S_1)
Ejection Sounds (ES)
Pulmonary Ejection Sounds
Nonejection Clicks (NECs)
Scratches
Absence of Clicks
Pseudoejection Click
Windsock Sound
Sail Sound
Pacemaker Sound and Presystolic Click of Pulmonary Stenosis

DIASTOLIC SOUNDS
Second Heart Sound (S_2)
Splitting of S_2
Single S_2
S_2 and Shunts
Malpositions of S_2 and S_1
Fourth Heart Sound (S_4)
Third Heart Sound (S_3)
Pseudo S_3

LESS KNOWN FINDINGS IN CARDIAC AUSCULTATION
Gallops
Presystolic (S_4)
Summation Gallop (Canter Rhythm)
Quadruple Rhythm
Pericardial Knock (PK)
Opening Snap (OS)
Tumor Plops
Diastolic Snaps or Clicks

PROSTHETIC VALVES
Aortic Valves
Mitral Valves

Tricuspid Valves
Repair of Mitral and Tricuspid Valves

QUESTIONS

CLINICAL VIGNETTES

ANSWERS

This chapter provides a clinical discussion of the heart sounds that were introduced in the first three chapters of this book and continues the discussion begun in Chap. 4 of the clinical issues associated with these sounds by summarizing examination techniques.

Heart sounds by definition are momentary acoustic events that are characterized by pitch, amplitude, timing, and character. They are systolic, diastolic, continuous to-fro or independent of cardiac rhythm. (Tables 5-1 and 5-2).

SYSTOLIC SOUNDS (Table 5-3)

First Heart Sound (S₁)

In listening to the normal heart at the apex using the bell of the stethoscope, one hears a dull S_1, *Lup*, followed by a sharp S_2, *dup*. The interval between *lup* and *dup* (systole) is shorter than between *dup* and the succeeding *lup* (diastole). *Lup* sounds muffled as compared to the sharper *dup* (Fig. 5-1, Table 5-1). Lup (S_1) precedes the carotid upslope dup (S_2), and is sharp and loud in the second intercostal space in normal heart rates.

In *tachycardia,* however, the timing changes. In rapid tachycardia, which occurs in shock, diastole is shorter than systole, resulting in a *tic-tac rhythm,* phonetically portrayed as Tûk'-tuk |Tûk tûk, which is in contrast to *lup-dup – lup-dup,* as indicated.

Table 5-1   Heart Sounds: Their Pitches and Character

Sound			
Name	Abbreviations	Pitches (c/s)	Character
First	S_1	100 to 120	Low
Second	S_2	120 to 150	Sharp high
Third	S_3	70 to 90	Low
Fourth	S_4	50 to 70	Low
Ejection	ES	>150	High
	OS	>150	High
Pericardial knock	PK	>150	High
Tumor plop	Plop	70 to 90	Low booming
Nonejection click	NEC	150	High
Prosthetic valve	PV	200	Sharp

Table 5-2 Timing and Amplitude of
Normal Heart Sounds

Sounds	Timing (ms)	Amplitude
S_4-S_1	4 to 120	$S_4 < S_1$
M_1T_1	20 to 40	$M_1 > T_1$
A_2P_2	20 to 60	$A_2 > P_2$
S_1-ES	40 to 100	$S_1 <$ ES
S_2-OS	60 to 120	$S_2 <$ OS
S_1-NEC	Variable	$S_1 <$ NEC
S_2-Plop	80 to 130	$S_2 <$ Plop
S_2-PK	<100	$S_2 <$ PK

Loud S_1 A loud S_1 (initial capital *Lup* = loud; lower-case *lup* = soft) is the result of an increase in M_1, T_1, or in the force of ventricular systole (Fig. 5-2, Table 5-4). Increased M_1 and T_1 occur when the mitral and tricuspid leaflets are maximally separated. This will occur with:

1. An increased gradient between atrium and ventricle
2. An electrocardiographic PR interval less than 200 ms
3. Increased flow across the mitral and tricuspid valves
4. Increased contractility of the ventricle
5. Abnormal valve leaflets (e.g., Ebstein's abnormality, mitral valve prolapse)

Thus, a loud S_1 is a feature of *Wolff-Parkinson-White syndrome* and the *Lown-Ganong-Levine syndrome,* both of which are associated with a short PR interval, usually less than 200 ms. S_1 is accentuated in *mitral* and *tricuspid stenosis,* associated with an increased gradient across the mitral or tricuspid valve, and in patients with increased *transvalvular flow,* which occurs in *ventricular septal defect, atrial septal defect, mitral valve closure,* and *tricuspid valve closure.* A loud T_1 is heard in *Ebstein's anomaly* due to increased excursion of tricuspid valve closure (sail sound). A loud S_1 is

Table 5-3 Systolic Sounds

Sound	Notes
S_1	Comprises M_1, T_1. May be single or split.
S_2	Comprises A_2, P_2. May be single or split.
Ejection sound	Vascular or valvular.
Pseudo-ejection	Occurs in idiopathic hypertrophic subaortic stenosis (IHSS) during mitral valve apposition to septum.
Pseudo S_1 pacemaker	Presystolic. Associated with intercostal contraction.
Scratch	Mean's Lerman's syndrome in thyrotoxicosis.
Nonejection click	Mitral valve prolapse, tricuspid valve prolapse.
Windsock	Associated with flail septum or closing ventral septal defect.
Sail	Associated with Ebstein's anomaly, single or split.
Pericardial	Associated with rub in systole; one, two, or three component.

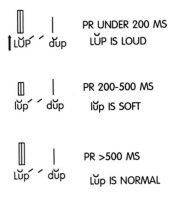

PR UNDER 200 MS
LŬP IS LOUD

PR 200-500 MS
lŭp IS SOFT

PR >500 MS
Lŭp IS NORMAL

Figure 5-1 Phonophonic representation of the PR interval and S₁ loudness.

present in patients with forceful ventricular systole during exercise, following the administration of epinephrine, and in mitral valve prolapse (Fig. 5-3). S₁ is loud in *sinus bradycardia,* as it is associated with increased stroke volume. A loud S₁ occurs in high-output states; S₁ grows louder when the patient sustains a clenched fist.

An examiner can use the loudness of S₁ to distinguish from systolic failure if cardiac output is normal in patients with diastolic failure. If cardiac output is normal in patients with diastolic failure, S₁ is normal; in hypertrophic cardiomyopathies S₁ is increased, and in dilated cardiomyopathies and following myocardial infarction S₁ is soft.

Soft S₁ (Fig. 5-4)   A soft S₁ is due to:

1.   Absent isovolumic ventricular systole.

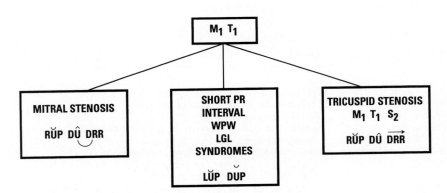

Figure 5-2   Interpretation of loud S₁. LGL, Lown-Ganong-Levine; LLSB, left lower sternal border; RLSB, right lower sternal border; WOW, Wolff-Parkinson-White.

Table 5-4   Conditions Causing Variations in S_1

Variation	Condition
	Loud S_1
Increased atrioventricular gradient	Mitral stenosis
	Myxoma
	Tricuspid stenosis
Short PR interval	Wolff-Parkinson-White syndrome
	Lown Ganong Levine syndrome
Increased blood flow	Atrial septal defect (T_1 closure)
	Ventricular septal defect (M_1 closure)
	High-output states
Increased contractility	Following or during exercise, post pause beat
	Mitral valve prolapse
Abnormal valve closure	Ebstein's abnormality
	Soft S_1
Absent isovolumic phase of ventricle	Mitral regurgitation
Long PR interval (200 to 500 ms)	
Left bundle branch block	
Decreased flow and contractility	Myocardial infarction
	Acute myocarditis
	Dilated cardiomyopathy
	Hypothyroidism
	Restrictive cardiomyopathy
Immobile valve	Mitral valve calcification

2. Prolonged PR interval (200 to 500 ms), representing delayed atrioventricular conduction.
3. A decreased flow and force of ventricular contraction, as in dilated cardiomyopathy.
4. Conditions in which the mitral valve is fibrous, calcified and immobile.

Furthermore, S_1 may be softened because of *acoustic* damping; as a result of S_1 being obscured by a long, loud murmur in aortic stenosis or mitral regurgitation; or by associated *left bundle branch block*. In addition, in mitral regurgitation, a soft S_1 may be due to the absence of isovolumic systole. A soft S_1 can be heard in diseases with prolonged PR intervals (between 200 and 500 ms), such as *first-degree atrioventricular block* and in left bundle branch block. In the case of aortic stenosis, an S_4 and absent S_1 usually indicate a transvalvular gradient of over 70 mmHg. S_1 is soft in the presence of heart failure of either the systolic or the inotropic type. Although S_1 may be normal in a *lucitropic failure* with normal cardiac contractility, it is usually barely audible in a *congestive failure* as in *dilated cardiomyopathy*. S_1 is soft in the presence of left bundle branch block or with a right ventricular pacemaker and in type B Wolff-Parkinson-White syndrome due to delayed left ventricular activation equivalent to LBBB.

Soft first sounds may occur with maximal beta-blocker therapy and in hypothyroidism. Marked reduction in intensity or absence of S_1 is seen in acute aortic regurgitation, in which LV diastolic filling causes preclosure

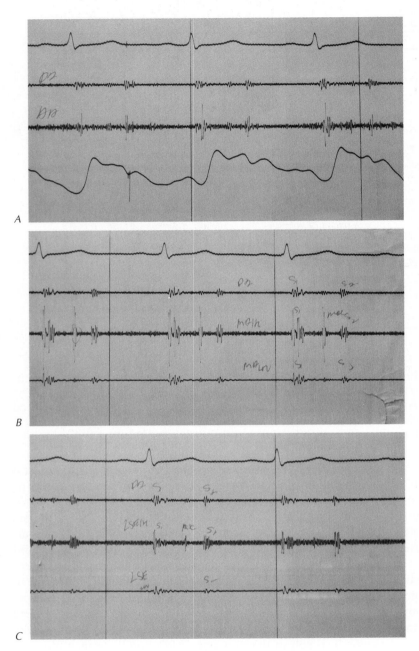

Figure 5-3   Late systolic and diastolic clicks in patient with mitral valve prolapse. A loud S_1 is seen in phonocardiograms.

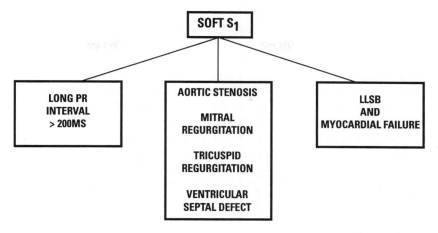

Figure 5-4   Soft S₁.

of the mitral valve (Fig. 5-5). In restrictive cardiomyopathies, S_1 is soft in part due to loss of isovolumic systole in mitral and tricuspid regurgitation, as well as to a decrease in left ventricular contractility. S_1 is thus diminished in dilated cardiomyopathies, as well as in restrictive cardiomyopathies but may be increased in hypertrophic cardiomyopathies.

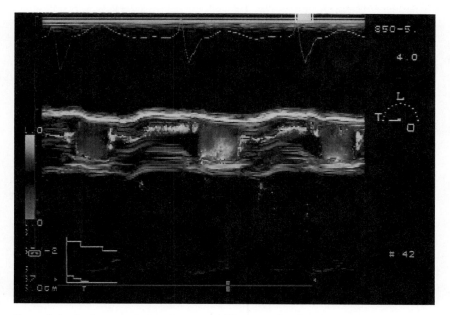

Figure 5-5   Aortic regurgitation shown on MQ screen showing severe aortic regurgitation in diastole.

Clinical Vignette

1. *First Degree AV Block.* A patient was examined by the late Paul Wood, on rounds in the United States, a male of 64 with no history of heart disease. The patient gave a history of paroxysmal atrial fibrillation and had been placed on digitalis. The patient had no complaints and was seen at a routine follow-up. On examination of the patient, he was in sinus rhythm with no elicitable abnormal findings except for the presence of a soft first sound. Dr. Wood correctly diagnosed the PR interval to be between 200 and 300 ms and made this observation before the electrocardiogram was looked at. The PR interval was in fact 300 ms and was caused by digitalis.

Comment: Paul Wood was criticized for his clinical showmanship. He was clearly teaching that the PR interval should be remembered during auscultation.

2. *Aortic Stenosis.* A 50-year-old patient with aortic stenosis was seen with a rough ejection systolic murmur, mid-systolic crescendo late peaking, best heard at the left sternal edge, somewhat musical in character. The systolic murmur heard was less prominent in the aortic area. The first sound was soft, a click was not heard, and there was an absent second sound. Left bundle branch block was present. The patient had aortic stenosis with a gradient of 100 mmHg across the valve.

Comment: An example of acoustic damping of S_2 and soft S_1 due to LBBB and the loud, long murmur preceded by S_4 indicating transvalvular gradients of 70 mmHg.

3. *Mitral Valve Prolapse and Beta Blockers.* A patient was seen on two occasions, one week apart. She was an anxious 30-year-old female with mitral valve prolapse and had been placed on beta blockers. There was a noticeable attenuation of intensity of the loud first heart sound at her second visit, probably due to the negative inotropic effect of beta blockers. This may also occur in these patients after physical conditioning.

Comment: A useful clinical end point in these anxious patients. S_1 loudness is related to DP/DT of the left ventricle.

Absence of S_1 S_1 is absent in acute aortic regurgitation due to preclosure of the mitral valve in diastole. A pseudo S_3 may be present due to preclosure of the mitral valve in early diastole. S_1 may be acoustically obliterated due to a loud, long murmur (grade VI; see Chaps. 6 and 8) in aortic or pulmonary stenosis.

    S_1 may be absent or markedly diminished in a patient with emphysema when auscultation is carried out at the apex or at the base of the heart. The heart has a vertical configuration in this condition. Hence, S_1 may be best heard below the sternum, while examining with a stethoscope positioned at the xiphoid process on the patient in held inspiration. This pushes the heart against the stethoscope. S_1 may be absent in patients with severe heart failure and bundle branch block.

Variations of S_1 (Fig. 5-6)   Regular variations of S_1 are seen in *Mobitz II type 1* or *Wenckebach heart block* (Fig. 5-7). In these diseases, the PR

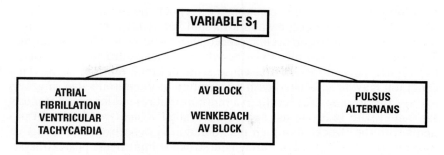

Figure 5-6   Variations of S_1.

interval is progressively prolonged and there is a corresponding progressive softening of S_1. A pause follows, and then a loud S_1 occurs, with a short PR interval. The sequence then repeats itself.

A variable S_1 is seen in *atrial fibrillation* and in *irregular tachyarrhythmias.* In fact, a variable S_1 is important in distinguishing patients with *ventricular tachycardia* from those with *reentrant supraventricular tachycardia.* A variable S_1 is an essential feature of V block grade III, with a loud intermittent *cannon sound,* "bruit de cannon."

A *premature complex* may be followed by a loud S_1 caused by *postextrasystolic enhancement of ventricular contraction* attributed to increased calcium flux into the sarcolemma.

S_1 varies in *pulsus paradoxus,* getting softer on inspiration. This can be difficult to detect, as inspiration distances the heart from the chest surface. Pulsus paradoxus is best detected by noting the effect of inspiration on blood pressure. S_1 alternates in volume in *pulsus alternans,* with an associated alternating systolic blood pressure, as detected by the stethoscope under the blood pressure cuff. In pulsus alternans, regular alternation of the pulse is elicited by light palpation at the wrist. Pulsus alternans is pathognomonic of *left ventricular pump dysfunction,* and S_2 alternans is more prominent than S_1. Unlike pulsus paradoxus, pulsus alternans shows no relationship to respiration.

In third-degree atrioventricular (AV) block, atrial contraction may immediately precede ventricular contraction and produce a booming S_1,

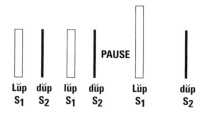

Lŭp   dŭp   lŭp   dŭp   Lŭp   dŭp
S_1 S_2 S_1 S_2 S_1 S_2

Figure 5-7   Phonophonic representation of Wenckebach rhythm; variable S_1, variable PR interval. L, loud; I, soft.

descriptively named *bruit de cannon.* (This is not to be confused with *venous cannon waves,* which occur when atria and ventricles contract simultaneously.) Atrial contraction occurs, preceding S_1, leading to what sounds like S_3 S_4, or a diastolic murmur to be heard; this atrial contraction may follow the ventricular contraction and cause a middiastolic murmur or S_3. This condition may be associated with calcification of the mitral valve ring, and in this case, atrial systole results in a murmur that resembles mitral stenosis associated with bradycardia, a condition called *Rytand syndrome.* In patients with the Brockenborough phenomenon in hypertrophic obstructive cardiomyopathy (HOCM), although the stroke volume of the postextrasystolic beat is decreased, this is not associated with a soft postextrasystolic S_1, but with a loud systolic murmur following a normal S_1. This murmur is caused by postpause augmentation of the gradient in this condition.

Split S_1   Normally M_1 precedes T_1, which is physiological. This is heard exclusively at the left lower sternal border, as T_1 is softer than M_1 (Table 5-5). A delayed T_1 may be seen in right bundle branch block, and in *Ebstein's anomaly,* in which the second component of S_1 (i.e., the *sail sound*) may be split into two sounds, producing what is termed a *trill.* The sail sound is named for its loud, flapping quality. Splitting of the S_1 is also commonly seen in Wolff-Parkinson-White syndrome type A and may be present with tricuspid stenosis because of the associated accentuation of T_1. Such splitting may also signal right atrial tumors and carcinoid syndrome. Splitting of S_1 may be useful in differentiating an opening snap from a tumor plop, in which a split S_1 is commonly heard. Reverse splitting of S_1, with T_1 preceding M_1, is rarely recognized at the bedside but can be detected on a phonocardiogram localized to the left sternal edge in left atrial myxomas, mitral stenosis, or in the presence of left bundle branch block. Reversed splitting is seen on a phonocardiogram in mitral stenosis and in left bundle branch block.

    Splitting of S_1 (M_1 T_1) is seen commonly in atrial septal defects, tricuspid stenosis, right bundle branch block, and Ebstein's anomaly, and needs to be distinguished from an S_4. There are several ways in which this can be done (Fig. 5-8).

Table 5-5   Conditions Characterized by a Split S_1

Physiological
Mitral and tricuspid S_1 (M_1T_1), heard at the left
lower sternal edge
Pathological
Right bundle branch block
Wolff-Parkinson-White syndrome
Left ventricular pacemaker
Tricuspid stenosis
Ebstein's anomaly
Atrial septal defect
Left atrial myxoma

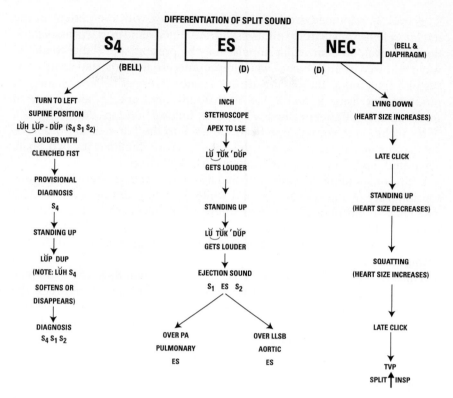

Figure 5-8 Differentiation of split heart sounds.

1. Components of a split S_1 are 20 to 40 ms apart, and best heard at the left sternal border. A split S_1 usually sounds like *Thrup*. An S_4, in contrast, is separated from S_1 and sounds like *luh-lup' dup* (S_4 S_1 S_2). For timing, see Table 5-6.

Table 5-6   Timing and Causes of Ejection Sounds

Pulmonary	Aortic
Valvular (occurs when valve opens)	
Presystolic (severe pulmonary stenosis)	Aortic stenosis
Fused to S_1 (severe pulmonary stenosis)	
After S_1 (mild to moderate)	
Vascular (occurs on full valve opening)	
Pulmonary hypertension	Systemic hypertension
Dilatation of pulmonary aorta	Dilated aorta or aneurysm
Increased pulmonary flow	Increased flow (e.g., pregnancy, high-output states)
Left-to-right shunt	

2. S_4 and S_1 combined are best heard at the apex with the patient in the left lateral position in full expiration with sustained hand grip. An associated double apical left ventricular impulse may be present, and is due to an 'A' wave followed by an 'E' wave, which represents atrial systole and ventricular systole. Examining the patient in this fashion, S_4 may be low-pitched of moderate-intensity; S_4 and S_1 are 50 to 80 ms apart and M_1 and T_1 are 20 to 40 ms apart. Phonetically, $S_4 - S_1$ is as follows: luh-lup' dup (S_4 S_1 S_2).

3. By inching the stethoscope from the apex to the left sternal border, S_4 gets softer and disappears, and the split S_1 grows louder with two finely separated, high-frequency components, M_1 T_1 THrup.

4. Sitting or standing the patient up and listening at the left sternal increases the intensity of the split first sound while S_4 disappears or is attenuated. The click sound phonetically is as follows: Lu Tuk ↑ while the split first sound is THrup.

5. A palpable presystolic impulse may be present, coinciding with S_4, enabling S_4-S_1 to be recognized.

6. The split M_1 T_1 (20 to 40 ms) is usually shorter than S_4-S_1 (50 to 80 ms).

      Using these simple rules, it is fairly easy to distinguish between the S_4-S_1 combination from M_1 T_1, and from S_1-ES. When in doubt, instruct the patient to stand up as a means of softening or eliminating S_4, and then proceed to evaluate the cause.

Ejection Sounds (ES) (Table 5-6)

Ejection sounds are auscultated using the diaphragm at the left sternal border and comprise two types: (1) *vascular* or *root*, as in *hypertension and dilation of the outflow tract;* or (2) valvular, caused by stenosis of *aortic* or *pulmonary valves.* Pulmonary ejection sounds normally precede aortic sounds. Previously known as *ejection clicks,* these are now named *ejection sounds.* They occur approximately *40 to 100 ms* after S_1 and their hemodynamic correlates have been described in Chap. 2 (Cardiac Pearl 6). Valvular ejection sounds are still sometimes referred to as clicks.

      Ejection sounds can be difficult to distinguish from split first sounds. Ejection sounds occur after S_1 and are higher pitched and louder than T_1, Lu Tuk ↑ as compared to ↑THRup↓. Ejection sounds are best heard at the left sternal edge and throughout the fourth intercostal space. These are conducted along the left sternal border and may be heard in the neck. Aortic ejection sounds or clicks may arise from bicuspid aortic valves or may be present in aortic stenosis; ejection sounds may also occur in dilated ectatic aortas or from atherosclerotic valves. It is important to note that aortic ejection sounds are best heard with the patient *sitting up* on full expiration. These sounds are not localized to the fourth intercostal space, as with the split S_1. Aortic ejection sounds usually have a wider separation from S_1 (40 to 100 ms), than a split S_1 (20 to 40 ms) (Cardiac Pearl 75).

The S_1-to-ejection sound interval is relatively constant with changes in patient position, unlike the nonejection click.

Pulmonary Ejection Sounds

Pulmonary ejection sounds due to pulmonary stenosis are localized over the pulmonary artery and disappear on inspiration. In pulmonary stenosis, these ejection sounds may be presystolic, fused with S_1, or following S_1, depending on the tightness of the valve. Pulmonary ejection sounds due to valvular stenosis get softer or disappear and occur earlier on inspiration on account of elevated right ventricular pressure, which cause valve pre-opening. Pulmonary ejection sounds that are not associated with valvular stenosis or pulmonary hypertension do not become softer during respiration. These pulmonary ejection sounds may be close to S_1, and are heard in pulmonary hypertension and idiopathic pulmonary dilatation.

In idiopathic dilatation of the pulmonary artery, pulmonary ejection sounds are associated with ejection systolic murmurs and a widely split S_2, which simulates an atrial septal defect in which the splitting of the S_2, however, is wide and fixed throughout the phases of respiration. Ejection sounds (*lu-tuk* ↑ *-dup*) are usually high-pitched and have a clicking quality.

Valvular opening sounds and root sounds in pulmonary stenosis occur early in systole as compared with valvular aortic sounds. Root sounds in pulmonary stenosis occur early, preceding S_1 in severe stenosis, but may be delayed in the presence of dilated pulmonary arteries or right bundle branch block. Vascular root sounds in hypertension are commonly delayed: (1) if the aorta is ectatic, (2) if left bundle branch block is present, or (3) with left ventricular hypertrophy with compliance abnormalities of the ventricle. These root sounds are heard relatively early in acute hypertension in the absence of left bundle branch block. Valvular sounds occur at valve opening, and vascular sounds at full opening.

Nonejection Clicks (NECs) (Fig. 5-9)

When using the diaphragm of the stethoscope at the apex, pulmonary artery (PA), and at the left lower sternal border (LLSB), nonejection clicks may be detected. Nonejection clicks and the associated late systolic murmurs that together constitute the *click-murmur syndrome* (Fig. 5-10) are associated with mitral valve prolapse and often present with chest pain, asthenia (fatigue), palpitations, spinal deformities, hypercatecholemia, anxiety, and agoraphobia. Patients may exhibit the features of Marfan's syndrome. The click and associated late systolic murmur have variable prominence in relation to each other. These are evaluated by positioning the patient so that the ventricle alters in size. Thus, having the patient stand moves the click earlier with respect to S_1; it occurs later when the patient lies down or squats (Figs. 5-5, 5-6). Systolic clicks are heard earlier when the patient

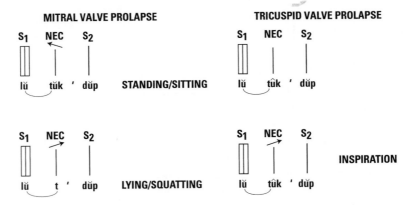

Figure 5-9 Phonophonic representation of nonejection clicks. Note "pause accent position," which shows the movement of the NEC. The heart is smaller and the NEC earlier when the patient is in the standing/sitting position. The heart is larger and the NEC later when the patient is lying supine or squatting.

does Valsalva straining and are accentuated by the patient sustaining a clenched fist. Clicks are heard in the second left intercostal space, simulating a widely split S_2 with the patient in the left-supine position only. Rarely diastolic snaps are heard (only in the left supine position) and simulate an atrial septal defect.

Electrocardiographic changes in the ST and T segments are common in patients with mitral valve prolapse. These are diastolic snaps of mitral valve prolapse and with S_2 simulate atrial septal defects. Honks or musical nonejection clicks sometimes audible without a stethoscope may take the place of clicks in mitral valve prolapse. Honks may be single or multiple; clicks may be single or multiple, systolic or diastolic. Single clicks tend to occur early and decrease when amyl nitrite is inhaled. In tricuspid valve prolapse, the nonejection click behaves similarly to mitral valve prolapse since its position varies with right-heart size. Tricuspid valve prolapse may be distinguished from mitral valve prolapse (MVP), however, by having the patient take a deep breath while sitting, which widens the interval between S_1 and the mitral or tricuspid valve click. Thus, the position of the

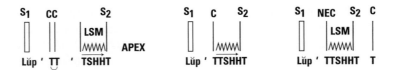

Figure 5-10 Phonophonic representation of click/murmur syndrome. Pt, patient; PA, pulmonary area; LBBB, left bundle branch block; ASD, atrial septal defect; RBBB, right bundle branch block; MR, mitral regurgitation; VSD, ventricular septal defect; HOCM, hypertrophic obstructive cardiomyopathy.

nonejection click in relation to mitral and tricuspid valve closure depends on the ventricle size, occurring early when the ventricle is small and late when it is enlarged. Nonejection sounds may be heard in the absence of prolapse in aneurysms of the atrial septum, pleural pericardial disease, and intracardiac tumors. The associated murmur in mitral valve prolapse is late, blowing, musical, or scratchy.

Scratches

These scratches, which simulate pericardial rub, are heard in systole in *thyrotoxicosis* in the so-called *Mean's Lerman's syndrome.* The cause of scratches is not yet known.

Absence of Clicks

Pulmonary   Pulmonary clicks are not heard on inspiration when auscultation is carried out over the pulmonic area in pulmonary stenosis. They reappear, however, on expiration.

Aortic   Aortic clicks are absent in aortic stenosis if the valves are immobile. These clicks may be normal or loud in mobile valves. Aortic clicks of valvular origin are absent in patients with innocent systolic murmurs and indeed offer an important means of establishing the innocence of a murmur, as described in *Still's murmur* (Chap. 2), in murmurs of straight-back syndrome, and in innocent murmurs of the right ventricular outflow tract.

Nonejection   Nonejection clicks are sometimes absent in patients with mitral valve prolapse and although clear-cut prolapse is seen in the presence of significant, late mitral regurgitation, the nonejection click may not be heard. In certain patients, standing up may cause the nonejection click to fuse with S_1; similarly, lying down makes it fuse with S_2, making the click inaudible. In some patients with mitral valve prolapse, neither click nor murmur is heard. Nonejection clicks may disappear with amyl nitrate.

Pseudoejection Click

Pseudoejection click is heard in midsystole in patients with HOCM. These patients have a long systolic murmur that precedes the click that occurs as the mitral valve impacts the septum (*systolic anterior motion*). In some patients, the click gets louder after inhaling amyl nitrite, implying that the click is produced by the slapping motion of the mitral valve against the septum, a motion that is increased by this drug.

Windsock Sound

A windsock sound is a widely split S_1 associated with the sudden slapping motion of a ventricular septal aneurysm into the right ventricle or occurs in a ventricular septal defect (VSD) that is closing. As the description suggests, the second component is dull. Slapping sounds may be due to flailing septal motion striking the right ventricle.

Sail Sound

The sail sound is caused by redundant tricuspid valve leaflets closing, tensing, vibrating, and halting in their outward excursion. This is caused by a split T_1 with a normal M_1 and a loud, split, flapping tricuspid valve closure sound. It is seen in Ebstein's anomaly, associated with a split S_1 and S_2, diastolic murmur, and a diastolic sound. A sail sound may be split causing a trill (S_1 sounds).

Pacemaker Sound and Presystolic Click of Pulmonary Stenosis

Pacemaker sound is a presystolic sound that is produced by intercostal contraction of muscles simulating a split S_1. In severe pulmonary stenosis, a click may precede S_1.

END SYSTOLIC SOUNDS (Fig. 5-11)

Second Heart Sound (S₂)

Although occurring in early diastole (Chap. 3), S_2 is a conventional systolic sound. Use the stethoscope diaphragm to auscultate the pulmonary area (PA) and aortic area (AA). S_2 is heard at the base of the heart with the diaphragm of the stethoscope (*dup-drup*), and corresponds with expiration and inspiration. It is sharp in contrast to the low-pitched S_1. Labeled "the key to auscultation of the heart" by Leatham, S_2 is caused by a complex series of events involving closure of the aortic and pulmonary valves. S_2 is normally composed of A_2 and P_2 with a 20- to 40-ms interval on inspiration (physiological splitting) (*Drup*). A_2 is louder than P_2.

In acute hypertension, rarely A_2 occurs early, paralleling the changes seen with the ejection sound (Table 5-7). In hypertension associated with left ventricular failure, left bundle branch block, aortic aneurysm, or aortic ectasia, P_2 may precede A_2, giving rise to a paradoxic second sound, cardiophonetically drUP (P_2A_2).

In pulmonary hypertension, P_2 occurs early, although in ectatic dilated pulmonary arteries or in the presence of right bundle branch block or right

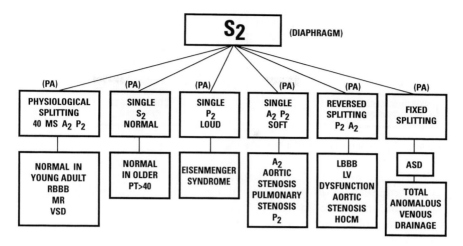

Figure 5-11 Variations in loudness and timing of S_2 in pulmonary area and aortic area.

ventricular failure, as in acute pulmonary embolism, persistent wide splitting of A_2P_2 (40 to 60 ms) occurs and P_2 is late.

Loud S_2 (Fig. 5-12)   While the aortic S_2 is heard in all four areas of the heart, pulmonic valve closure is usually heard over the pulmonary area only (Fig. 5-11). Exceptions include normotensive atrial septal defects and right ventricular enlargement, in which a loud A_2 rather than an aortic S_2 is heard at the apex and over the left chest. In a small percentage of normal patients, P_2 may be heard at the apex. Thus, P_2 is absent over all the areas of the heart except the pulmonary area, while transmission of P_2 outside of its normal location usually signifies pulmonary hypertension. Aortic valve closure is accentuated in conditions in which the valve is abnormal, such as in the presence of atherosclerosis; hence, this finding is abnormal in a young person, in whom it may be a marker of coronary artery disease. Aortic valve closure is accentuated in conditions in which the outflow tract

Table 5-7   Diastolic Sounds

Sound	Phonophonic
S_3	Dup
S_4	Luh
Pericardial knock	Dock
Mitral valve prolapse clicks or snaps	Tuk
Opening snaps	Tuk
Tumor plops	[DO8]
Sounds in Ebstein's anomaly	
Pacemaker click—presystolic	
Pulmonary stenosis click—presystolic	

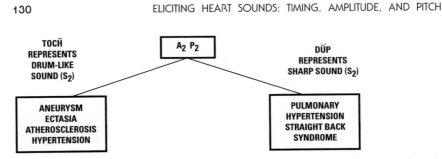

Figure 5-12   Sounds and causes of a loud S₂.

is dilated, such as in aneurysms of the aorta encountered in Marfan's syndrome and luetic aortitis. As patients age, the aorta becomes ectatic and closure of the aortic valve is associated with a loud S_2.

A_2 may have a tambour, or drumlike quality. This is probably due to resonance of the column of blood within the large aortic chamber. A loud A_2 is seen in hypertension, in coarctation of the aorta with aortic dissection or aneurysm and may occur in high-flow states such as anemia and thyrotoxicosis. P_2 may be loud over a dilated pulmonary artery or if the heart is compacted as in *straight-back* syndrome. If a tambour-quality A_2 is heard on the right third intercostal space with an early diastolic murmur in association with diastolic hypertension, this is *Harvey's sign,* which suggests an aneurysm or dissection (Cardiac Pearl 11) tök with vibration (Fig. 5-13).

Loud P_2 (Fig. 5-14)   A loud P_2 is heard in pulmonary hypertension associated with pre- or postcapillary causes, when the pulmonic valve may be atherosclerotic or diseased, and in conditions of high flow, as in the presence of shunts. Chest deformities, the straight-back syndrome and idiopathic dilatation of the pulmonary artery may accentuate P_2, which moves normally, however, with respect to A_2 on respiration. In *Eisenmenger's syndrome,* A_2 and P_2 fuse and are loud and single.

Soft A_2, P_2 (Fig. 5-15)   A soft, delayed A_2, P_2 is characteristic of aortic stenosis and pulmonary stenosis with immovable valves. The altered mobil-

MSM   A₂

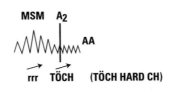

rrr   TÖCH   (TÖCH HARD CH)

HARVEY'S SIGN ON 2ND STERNAL BORDER

Figure 5-13   Phonophonic representation of an aortic aneurysm: A midsystolic murmur (MSM); a loud tambour (drumlike) A₂ followed by a diastolic murmur heard in the second right intercostal space.

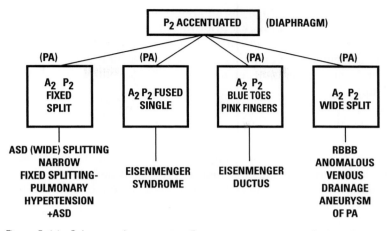

Figure 5-14 Pulmonary hypertension. Figure represents causes of a loud P_2 and its relationship to A_2 various conditions in which fixed splitting, fusion of A_2 and P_2, physiologic splitting, and persistent wide splitting are heard when the pulmonary area is auscultated with the diaphragm of the stethoscope. ASD, atrial septal defect; PA, pulmonary area; RBBB, right bundle branch block; A_2, aortic second sound; P_2, pulmonary second sound.

ity of the valves by fibrosis or calcification may cause not only delay but softening of valve closure. A soft A_2 in the presence of aortic stenosis is associated with a late A_2; hence, A_2 and P_2 may coincide, leading to a single S_2, or in more severe cases, reverse splitting of the S_2 may be present with a soft aortic component. S_2, the aortic component, thus would tend to occur

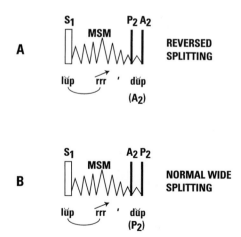

Figure 5-15 Phonophonic representation of acoustic obliteration of S_2 in aortic (A) and pulmonary stenosis (B). S_1 may be soft or absent. The systolic murmur is long in severe stenosis and peaks late.

after P_2 and S_2 may be masked by the long, late ejection murmur acoustically "running over" P_2 and ending just prior to A_2.

Thus, even as A_2 is soft in aortic stenosis with an immobile valve, a soft P_2 is found similarly in pulmonary stenosis. Delay in P_2 results in wide-splitting of S_2 and inspiration augments the A_2 P_2 split, although P_2 is soft (DR'up).

Splitting of S_2 (Fig. 5-16)

Reversed (P_2 A_2)   Reversed splitting of S_2 may occur in any situation in which the left ventricular ejection time is prolonged and A_2 is delayed. One possible example is left bundle branch block with pulmonary hyperten-sion, since A_2 is delayed and P_2 is early. Right ventricular pacing or left bundle branch block is accompanied by a prolonged ejection time and delay in conduction to the left ventricle. Reversed splitting of S_2 also is seen with right ventricular ectopic beats and type B Wolff-Parkinson-White syndrome.

Reversed splitting of S_2 is identified by listening in the second left intercostal space in inspiration and expiration. On inspiration, pulmonic closure is delayed and P_2 approaches A_2, giving rise to a single S_2, while during expiration A_2 and P_2 separate, principally due to delay in A_2 and possibly due to an early P_2. An example of this was reported in a patient with left bundle branch block and severe pulmonary hypertension.

Paradoxic splitting of S_2 may occur as a transient phenomenon in patients in whom left ventricular ejection time is prolonged due to left

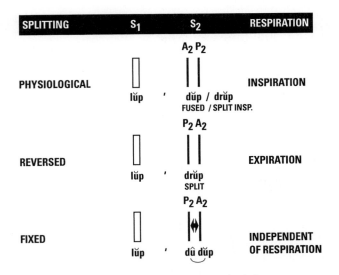

Figure 5-16   Phonophonic representation of split S_2.

ventricular dysfunction caused by ischemia. Thus, in patients who have angina, ischemia is strongly suggested by the physical findings of a transient S_4, soft S_1, paradoxic splitting of S_2, and late papillary muscle systolic murmur. These signs may be reversed by nitroglycerin or carotid sinus pressure. Paradoxic splitting is also seen in systemic hypertension, which prolongs left ventricular ejection time in heart failure.

Reversed splitting by definition relates to alterations of S_2 on respiration and must *not* be confused with paradoxic splitting. Paradoxic splitting implies $P_2 A_2$ in sequence, which may persist on expiration and inspiration.

Physiological ($A_2 P_2$)   This sound occurs in young persons in the sitting position. Decreased compliance of the pulmonary artery with respect to the aorta causes delay in P_2 with respect to A_2. Important causes for wide but physiological splitting of S_2 are right bundle branch block, mitral regurgitation, and ventricular septal defect. In these conditions, left ventricular ejection time is shortened with respect to that of the right ventricle, and A_2 tends to occur earlier. This is important in distinguishing between mitral regurgitation and HOCM. The use of amyl nitrite tends to decrease the mitral regurgitation and accentuate paradoxic splitting. Physiological wide splitting of S_2 may occur in right bundle branch block, left ventricular pacing, left ventricular ectopic beats, as well as with Wolff-Parkinson-White syndrome.

Physiological wide splitting of S_2 may be heard in conditions of volume loading or failure of the right ventricle. This splitting is due to a delay in right ventricular ejection and may occur acutely, as in pulmonary embolism. Physiological splitting of S_2 in the presence of pulmonary hypertension may be present, but the split is narrow on inspiration.

Unexplained physiological splitting of S_2 may be heard (Cardiac Pearl 9). Also, occasional splitting of S_2 is heard in the left lateral position that is not heard in the sitting position. This splitting is not physiological and may indicate mitral valve prolapse, which causes pseudosplitting of S_2 (Cardiac Pearl 45).

Physiological Pseudosplitting   Physiological S_2 pseudosplitting is absent when the patient is in the sitting position, in which a true split S_1 is often heard.

Fixed   Fixed splitting of S_2, so named because the $A_2 P_2$ sequence is heard on inspiration, expiration, or during a pause in breathing, is detected in the pulmonary area when the patient is in the sitting position. Fixed splitting of S_2 is seen in atrial septal defect, Ebstein's anomaly, Lutembacher's syndrome, and in the rare condition of total anomalous venous drainage. The $A_2 P_2$ components are widely separated and do not vary with breathing (80 to 100 ms).

Fixed splitting of S_2 relates to the enhancement of blood flow in the pulmonary circuit and the right ventricle, which delays valve closure. Fixed splitting also relates to the fact that the filled pulmonary artery does not have the capacity to increase its compliance and consequently its hangout time on inspiration. Fixed splitting, furthermore, reflects the reciprocal relationship between the left-to-right atrial shunt and right ventricular filling in inspiration and expiration, respectively; i.e., the shunt from left to right increases on inspiration, while on expiration there is a relative diminution in right ventricular filling. In noncompliant pulmonary arteries with pulmonary hypertension and atrial septal defects, P_2 occurs early leading to "close" fixed splitting. The loudness of the second component approximates A_2 in pulmonary hypertension.

Persistent Physiological Splitting, Nonfixed S_2   Wide splitting of S_2 is seen in pulmonary stenosis, which is associated with a prolonged, right ventricular ejection time. Splitting of S_2 is wide in atrial septal defect and does not often appear to be related to shunt size. The splitting relates to the dilatation of the pulmonary artery. Thus, while closure of an atrial septal defect in a child narrows the split, such closure does not narrow the split in older patients.

Wide S_2 splitting is also seen occasionally in ventricular septal defects and mitral regurgitation, and in the presence of right ventricular failure, as well as in right bundle branch block with right ventricular failure. Prolongation of hangout time due to compliance changes may cause wide splitting of S_2 in idiopathic dilatation of the pulmonary artery, and is encountered in the presence of left bundle branch block with right ventricular failure, as well as in right bundle branch block with right ventricular failure. Wide splitting in mitral regurgitation and ventricular septal defect is caused by short left ventricular ejection time and A_2.

Single S_2

In truncus arteriosus, the outflow tract comes off the single ventricle and a single S_2 is heard; in tetralogy of Fallot and in the Taussig Bing syndrome, the aorta overrides both ventricles and the S_2, which is caused by an A_2, is single and is heard at the apex.

Single S_2 is also seen in patients who have pulmonary hypertension in Eisenmenger's syndrome. In this condition, pulmonary hypertension leads to a loud S_2 that occurs early, and which is associated with a palpable P_2 over the pulmonary area. Notably, if right ventricular failure supervenes, S_2 may exhibit splitting due to increase in right ventricular ejection time.

The role of pulmonary hypertension in S_2 is of interest. While pulmonary hypertension will tend to shorten the duration between A_2 and P_2 and result in a single S_2, right ventricular failure prolongs and protracts right ventricular ejection, causing P_2 to be delayed and S_2 to split. This is often seen in patients with atrial septal defect who develop pulmonary hypertension and in whom the split narrows but remains fixed. If right ventricular failure follows, the split may increase. This could also happen if complete right bundle branch block and right ventricular enlargement or failure occur together as in pulmonary embolism. In patients with pulmonary hypertension in association with other shunts, a similar phenomenon is seen. In general, a true single S_2 is seen in patients with a ventricular septal defect and pulmonary hypertension, as in Eisenmenger's complex; normal splitting occurs in an Eisenmenger ductus; and fixed narrowed splitting is heard in Eisenmenger's syndrome and atrial septal defect. In all these conditions P_2 is accentuated.

S_2 and Shunts

Fixed splitting occurs in atrial septal defects, physiological splitting in ventricular septal defects, and reversed splitting in *patent ductus arteriosus (PDA)*. In reversed shunts (right-to-left) with pulmonary hypertension, narrow fixed splitting of S_2 is seen in atrial septal defect, single S_2 in ventricular septal defect, and usually physiological splitting in PDA with pulmonary hypertension. The loudness of A_2 P_2 gives an indication of the degree of pulmonary hypertension.

Malpositions of S_2 and S_1 (See Chap. 10.)

Malpositions of S_2 and S_1 can occur in dextrocardia and in the presence of right sided aortic arch, as in tetralogy of Fallot and Eisenmenger's syndrome. An important cause of malposition of second sounds is in both *correct transposition* and *true transposition of the great vessels,* in which aortic valve closure is heard best over the pulmonary area.

Second sounds may also be misplaced in patients with *truncus arteriosus,* depending on the type; in truncus arteriosus, second sounds are single. In a small percentage of normal patients, P_2 is heard at the apex, also in normal-pressure atrial septal defect and in abnormal chests in which a loud P_2 may result from proximity of the outflow tracts to the thorax as in straight back syndrome. Second sounds may not be heard or may be muffled in patients with chronic obstructive pulmonary disease (COPD) and emphysema, while S_2 may be displaced due to thoracic or spinal deformity. P_2 A_2 displacement is seen in Eisenmenger's syndrome as well.

DIASTOLIC SOUNDS (Table 5-8)
Fourth Heart Sound (S_4) (Fig. 5-17)

S_4 is a low-pitched sound preceding S_1, heard at the left apex or xiphoid, respective of whether it originates in the left ventricle or right ventricle.

Table 5-8   Variations of Split S_2 (S_2 A_2-P_2 or P_2-A_2)

Component	Disease/Condition	Characterization of Split
Loud A_2	Hypertension	Reversed
	Thickened, mobile valve	Reversed
	Aneurysm of aorta	Reversed
	Ectasia of aorta	Reversed; single S_2
Normal A_2	Left bundle branch block	Physiological
	Hypertrophic obstructive cardiomyopathy (HOCM)	Fixed
	Atrial septal defect with immobile valve	
Soft A_2	Hypothyroidism	
Loud P_2	Pulmonary hypertension	Fixed
	Pulmonary hypertension with atrial septal defect	Narrow, fixed
	Pulmonary hypertension with PDA	Narrow
	Pulmonary hypertension with heart failure	Wide
Normal P_2	Right bundle branch block	Physiological
	Ventricular septal defect	Physiological
	Mitral regurgitation	Physiological
	Physiological	Physiological
	Atrial septal defect	Wide fixed
	Pulmonary stenosis and tetralogy of Fallot with infundibular stenosis (not valvular)	
Soft P_2	Immobile valve	Single (no split)

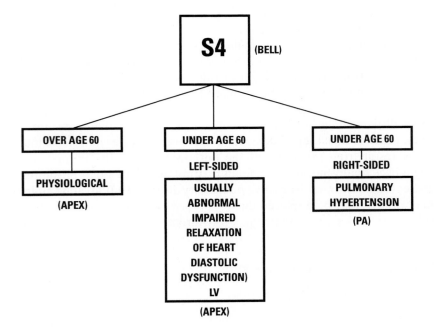

Figure 5-17   Auscultation of S_4.

S_4 is heard by using the bell with light auscultation, and with the patient in the left supine position, with fully held expiration. Phonetically, S_4 is represented as *Luh-lup/dup* and Luh coincides with the apical presystolic 'A' wave.

A low-pitched S_4 may be heard "physiologically" in older patients and may be caused by alteration in ventricular compliance. It originates from the left ventricle and is usually associated with changes in Doppler tracings arising from the left atrium. The apical impulse shows a prominent 'A' wave preceding systole that is larger than the 'E' wave seen in diastole. This Doppler finding is produced by decreased ventricular muscle compliance. In the elderly, this finding is absent in the conditioned patient (Chandraratan et al.). The prominent presystolic Doppler 'A' wave is larger than the smaller 'E' wave in diastole (abnormal A/E ratio).

When an S_4 is heard unequivocally in pregnancy, it may indicate heart failure. In this circumstance, since an S_3 is physiological in pregnancy, fourth sounds, i.e., quadruple rhythm, may be heard, or a summation gallop (*Lu-Lup', du-dup*) in which the S_4 and S_3 fuse in heart failure quadruple rhythm representing $S_1 S_2 S_3 S_4$. This so-called "train wheel" sound must be distinguished from Lu-Du-Dup, the so-called summation gallop or canter rhythm.

Ischemia provoked in a patient with coronary artery disease by sustaining a clenched fist or by isotonic exercise may become manifest as a transient S_4. Ischemia can be relieved by administering nitroglycerin and applying carotid sinus compression, or the ischemia may simply disappear when the patient rests. An S_4 should be listened for before the patient exercises on a treadmill, at the peak of exercise, and after exercise is concluded.

S_4 may be provoked when a patient is infused with saline or blood. In the presence of dilated cardiomyopathy, ventricular aneurysm, or left ventricular hypertrophy, an S_4 is often present and does not represent heart failure. In congestive failure, a soft S_1 is associated with an S_4 and an S_3. In patients with hypertrophic cardiomyopathy, diastolic failure, or hypertension with normal or high cardiac outputs, an S_4 and S_3 is often associated with an accentuated or normal S_1. An S_4 is commonly heard in hypertension.

An S_4 in aortic stenosis is commonly associated with a gradient of over 70 mmHg. The S_1 may not be readily heard under these circumstances and precedes a soft S_2. In listening to a patient being monitored with a triple-lumen catheter, the clinician can make correlations between the appearance of an S_4 and S_3, and pulmonary capillary wedge pressure. In general, fourth sounds may be heard with normal or slightly elevated filling pressure (< 15 mmHg), while in gross heart failure, third sounds are associated with filling pressures greater than 30 mmHg.

In a patient with cor pulmonale due to pulmonary embolism or respiratory failure, an S_4 is heard below the xiphoid process and indicates right ventricular failure. In tricuspid stenosis S_4 may be heard exclusively over the jugular veins and not over the heart. This may occur even in the presence of atrial fibrillation. S_4 may also be heard in a patient with pulmonary hypertension over both the heart and the neck veins.

Fourth sounds are sensitive to position and are best heard with the patient positioned left lateral supine and sustaining a clenched fist. S_4 can be distinguished from ejection sounds and clicks by standing the patient up, which tends to make S_4 grow softer or disappear as a result of decrease in preload. Right ventricular fourth sounds increase with inspiration and may be heard below the xiphoid process and over the jugular veins; these sounds are best heard with the patient in the supine position, propped up.

An S_4 in patients with hypertrophic cardiomyopathy in association with obstruction gives rise to a triple impulse at the apex. This *triple ripple* is caused by a number of factors. First there is a forcible expansion of the ventricle by atrial systole; this expansion corresponds with S_4. A rapid and slow ejection of the left ventricle causes the double impulse. This also results in a sharp upslope, or spike and dome, in the pulse wave, giving rise to the so-called pulsus bisferiens.

"Triple ripple" can be palpated with the stethoscope placed at the apex of the heart and is caused by an 'A' wave and double systolic wave seen in HOCM.

S_4 is an important manifestation of angina pectoris and should be sought after to make this diagnosis. On rare occasions, an S_4 is heard physiologically in athletes and does not signal dysfunction, although it is important in these cases to be sure that hypertrophic cardiomyopathy is not present.

Absent S_4   An S_4 disappears in a patient who develops atrial fibrillation except in the neck in tricuspid stenosis.

Third Heart Sound (S_3) (Fig. 5-18)

S_3 is caused by deceleration following rapid longitudinal elongation of the left ventricle. In young adults, tissue Doppler studies show rapid diastolic filling coincident with a high-pitched S_3; this may enable the clinician to distinguish physiological from pathological S_3 (Fig. 5-19). S_3 is auscultated with the bell of the stethoscope; the patient reclines into the left supine position, breathes out, and holds expiration.

Third sounds in general correspond to filling pressures that are 25 mmHg or higher, and may be heard in association with heart failure. As previously stated, this relationship has been clearly observed at the bedside in coronary care units in patients with triple-lumen "Swan-Ganz" catheters, which enable correlations to be made between filling pressures and heart failure. Auscultation of the heart when a patient is in sinus rhythm enables physiological correlations to be made between the presence of filling sounds (S_3 and S_4) and filling pressures. This comparison is useful when one is monitoring hemodynamics at the bedside of a patient in inten-

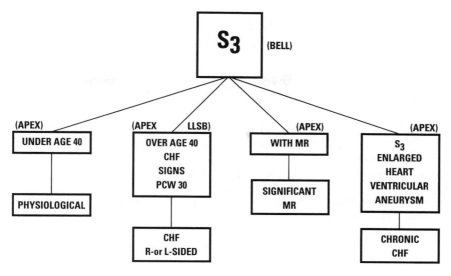

Figure 5-18   Causes of an audible S_3.

sive care. Physiological correlations may be a guide to the recurrence or regression of heart failure in patients, especially after the triple-lumen catheter is removed. Despite this, it is important to remember that an S_3

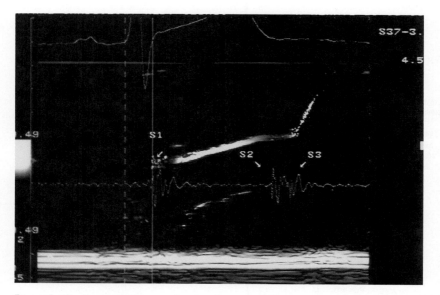

Figure 5-19   Phonocardiogram showing S_2, and an S_3 preceding peak opening of the mitral valve.

does not always designate the presence of an elevated filling pressure, but rather, reduced ventricular compliance.

A hemodynamic description of S_3 and its relationship to the rapid filling indicates that the longitudinal displacement of the ventricle halts at the peak of filling. This corresponds with S_3, as discussed in Chap. 3. Unlike S_4, third sounds may not be heard with every heartbeat.

Cardiomyopathy or Ventricular Aneurysms In chronic fibrosis or decreased compliance of the ventricle, despite decreased filling rates, as in congestive cardiomyopathy, patients may present with third or fourth sounds that persist even after heart failure has been corrected. These sounds are commonly heard in chronic ventricular aneurysms (Fig. 5-20).

High-Output States An S_3 may be heard in high-output states, such as anemic thyrotoxicosis, in the presence of arterioventricular fistulae, hypertrophic cardiomyopathies, and pregnancy. S_3 may be heard in conditions in which end systemic volumes are increased, such as valvular heart disease, systemic hypertension, ischemic heart disease, and cardiomyopathies in the absence of filling pressures exceeding 30 mmHg. Tricuspid stenosis also is associated with a loud S_3 and cor pulmonale at the left lower sternal border which increases on inspiration.

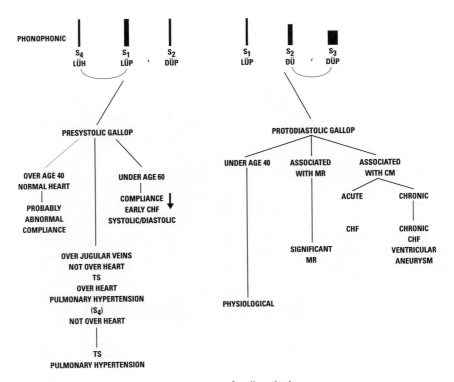

Figure 5-20 Phonophonic representations of gallop rhythms.

Aortic Regurgitation   In aortic regurgitation, pathological third sounds appear to be related to increased end systolic volume. An S_3 is an important sign that left ventricular dysfunction may have occurred and that end systolic volume has increased. S_3 is common in acute aortic regurgitation, followed by a soft S_1 middiastolic (Austin Flint) murmur and, as previously noted, an S_4 may be heard. S_1 is characteristically absent but may masquerade as an S_3. In acute aortic regurgitation, the preclosed mitral valve sound falls at S_3 and is heard (pseudo-S_3).

Mitral Regurgitation S_3 is an important sign of mitral regurgitation, but does not indicate heart failure. This, as in aortic regurgitation, has implications for treatment in considering valve replacement. S_3 indicates significant mitral regurgitation.

Physiological S_3 (See Chap. 2)   Physiological S_3 may be heard in normal patients up to age 40 in men and 45 in women. It is paradoxic that an S_3 is usually a sign of heart failure. S_3 may be normal in patients with high-output states. S_3 is high-pitched in children (*Lup-du-Dup*) $S_1|S_2\ S_3$.

Congestive Heart Failure (CHF) and Atrial Fibrillation (AF) S_3 and atrial fibrillation may occur. S_4 is absent. Thus, third heart sounds that are *not* physiological are seen in:

1. Left ventricular dilatation
2. Left ventricular failure
3. Infarct expansion
4. High-output states
5. Mitral regurgitation, hypertrophic cardiomyopathy, and ventricular aneurysm
6. Chronic ventricular aneurysms
7. Tricuspid stenosis

   Tachycardia may be followed by transient S_3. Less commonly an S_3 may follow cardioversion of atrial fibrillation.

Pseudo-S_3

Pseudo-S_3 sounds are best heard in the subxiphoid area and are associated with an increase in end diastolic volume. Thus, pseudo-third sounds are heard in patients with shunts with atrial tumors, in Ebstein's anomaly, and in mitral valve prolapse. A pericardial knock can simulate an S_3. The preclosure sound of acute aortic regurgitation may simulate S_3.

LESS KNOWN FINDINGS IN CARDIAC AUSCULTATION

1. An S_4 that may be heard over the jugular veins and not over the heart in tricuspid stenosis, with or without atrial fibrillation.

2. An S_4 that is rarely present in athletes and in four percent of normal pregnant women.

3. In terminal severe cor pulmonale five sounds may be heard below the xiphoid process (S_1 A_2 P_2 S_3 S_4), a form of quadruple rhythm in pulmonary hypertension.

4. Fixed splitting of S_2 in the left supine position, not in the sitting position, is often due to mitral valve prolapse.

Gallops (Cardiac Pearl 70) (Fig. 5-18)

Gallops are caused by left- or right-sided diastolic filling sounds. Left-sided sounds are best heard with light bell auscultation with the patients in the left supine position in held expiration. Right-sided filling sounds are best heard with the bell or corrugated variable diaphragm in the subxiphoid position with the patient in held inspiration, or at the right lower sternal border with the patient in the supine position. All filling sounds diminish with sitting or standing.

Presystolic (S_4)

Left ventricular and right ventricular gallops can be either triple or quadruple. Gallops can be presystolic (S_4, S_1, S_2); or protodiastolic (S_1, S_2, S_3). In phonetic or presystolic terminology, presystolic gallop sounds as: Luh-lup dup (S_4, S_1, S_2); protodiastolic gallop: *Lup/du-dup* (S_1, S_2, S_3). The so-called systolic gallop has been discussed previously and is due to the nonejection click present in mitral valve prolapse described by Potain.

The presystolic gallop is readily distinguished from the protodiastolic gallop visually by using two diagnostic technologies. The echocardiogram, combined with phonocardiographic recordings, shows the separation between S_3 and S_4 as the distance between the end of rapid filling and the atrial systole. This is elegantly demonstrated by color changes (blue) in the myocardial wall seen on tissue Doppler imaging with a black area (slow filling) in between (Don Michael). This period is called *diastasis*, during which only a minor amount of filling of the heart occurs. In states in which tachycardia is present, diastasis is attenuated and may disappear, resulting in an equally spaced summation gallop, which sounds as: *luh/du/dup | luh/du/dup | luh/du/dup*, also called a canter rhythm.

That this sound is more like a horse's canter rather than a gallop was wryly appreciated by Pontain in what he nevertheless termed the *bruit de galop*. However, the most effective technique is clinical, appropriate positioning of the patient with clenched fist and cardiophonetic timing. Mnemonics "Kentucky" and "Tennessee" are less helpful for the diagnosis of S_4 and S_3 gallops, respectively.

Summation Gallop (Canter Rhythm)

A *summation gallop* with tachycardia establishes that atrial systole is present, that the patient is in heart failure, and that the heart failure is more severe than in a patient who has an S_3 or S_4. Sustained clenched fist may provoke summation gallop phonetically as luh du dup, S_1 S_2 (S_3 S_4).

Quadruple Rhythm (Fig. 5-21)

To auscultate quadruple rhythm, use the bell of the stethoscope at the apex with the patient in the supine position. With treatment, the disappearance of the summation gallop coincides with some slowing of the heart and reduction of the mean pressure as recorded by a triple-lumen catheter. The *train wheel* sound (*lu/dup | du/dup*) of quadruple rhythm may result as the heart slows. This is because S_4 and S_3 separate in quadruple rhythm. The two filling sounds with tachycardia may be mistaken for mitral stenosis. As the patient's filling pressure drops further, S_4 alone may be heard; at less than 14 mmHg in the pulmonary capillary wedge pressure tracings, S_3 may disappear. Thus, the auscultatory evolution of improvement can be related to alterations in filling pressure.

   S_3 gallops are termed *protodiastolic* and usually indicate heart failure. Gallops are best heard with the bell of the stethoscope and with the patient in the left supine position. Right-sided gallops are heard best below the xiphoid process. When both S_3 and S_4 are present, S_3 is best heard at the left lower sternal border and P_2. S_4 is best heard at the apex. With right-

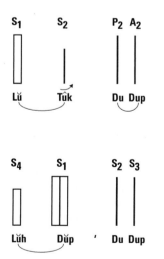

Figure 5-21 Phonophonic representation of quadruple sounds and quadruple rhythm. A. Quadruple sounds. B. Quadruple rhythm. It is important not to confuse the two.

sided gallops filling sounds are localized below the xiphoid process. The stethoscope bell is held pointing up, similar to an echo technician using a probe in a subcostal view.

Pericardial Knock (PK)

This useful physical finding strongly suggests a diagnosis of constrictive pericarditis when taken in combination with changes in the jugular venous pulse. The clinical picture is one of right-sided failure with anasarca, often with hepatomegaly and ascites. The patient usually has a normal-sized heart and engorged neck veins. A pericardial knock is best heard with the patient lying in the supine position with the head of the examining table elevated at 45 degrees; examine the venous pressure simultaneously with the pericardial knock. It is probably caused by the arrested expansion of the right side of the heart as it fills on inspiration, a phenomenon brought about by an unyielding pericardium. The high-pitched, early pericardial knock occurs in the early period of rapid-filling of the right ventricle. Combined with the increase in venous pressure on inspiration (Kussmaul's sign) and a reduction in systolic pressure (pulsus paradoxus), pericardial knock completes a triad of physical signs that signals constrictive pericarditis.

The high-pitched sound of pericardial knock has been likened by Mc-Kusick to that of a cocktail shaker. It is of interest that unlike S_3, pericardial knock occurs at the *beginning* of, and not at the *peak* of, rapid filling (Chap. 3); it cannot be recorded by an intracardiac phonocardiogram, however. The pericardial knock is therefore considered to be a mechanical phenomenon that correlates with the middle portion of the venous pressure fall rather than the trough. It corresponds to the midportion of the rapid-filling wave on the apex cardiogram (Chap. 3).

The A_2-PK delay is 100 to 200 ms. In early constrictive pericarditis, the knock occurs on inspiration only (Harvey).

Opening Snap (OS) (Fig. 5-22)

Use the diaphragm at the left sternal edge or the bell at the apex with the patient in the left supine position to auscultate for opening snap. At the apex, an opening snap may be part of a *trill* (S_2, OS, middiastolic murmur); a trill with three sounds may be heard in the pulmonary area (A_2, P_2, OS), or in the suprasternal notch. The opening snap is the high-pitched sound, vibrating and rattling in character. In the absence of complicating factors such as pulmonary or systemic hypertension, the opening snap bears a temporal relationship to A_2 (60 to 120 ms). The earlier the opening snap, the tighter the mitral stenosis.

Although opening snaps may be heard in calcified valves, these sounds are not common in patients with heavy valvular calcification and immobilization. This fact is vital in determining the feasibility of performing mitral balloon angioplasty.

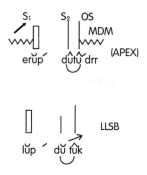

Figure 5-22 Phonophonic representation of opening snaps. OS, opening snap; LLSB, left lower sternal border; MDM, middiastolic murmur; OC, opening click; CC, closing click; MSM, midsystolic murmur; EDM, early diastolic murmur; MV, mitral valve; AV, aortic valve.

Tricuspid opening snaps follow mitral valve opening snaps. Echophonocardiographic recordings have shown that the opening snap coincides with maximum opening of the mitral or tricuspid valve. The high-pitched sound is of short duration, and best heard at the left sternal border, away from the apex, so that it can be timed accurately in relation to A_2. It is heard using the diaphragm with the patient supine with the head of the examining table elevated at 45 degrees.

In the presence of sinus rhythm, the A_2 to opening snap (A_2-OS) interval correlates with the tightness of the stenosis. Pulmonary hypertension, however, reduces left atrial flow, and thus increases this interval even in the presence of severe mitral stenosis. Thus pulmonary hypertension may result in a late opening snap. (The same increase may rarely occur in systemic hypertension with early closure of A_2, although the A_2-OS interval is usually shortened due to delay of A_2, occurring in left bundle branch block and left ventricular failure.)

In tricuspid stenosis, an opening snap may be heard and is difficult to pick out in the presence of a diastolic murmur and S_3. The opening snap increases on inspiration, follows the mitral opening snap, and is well heard in tricuspid valves that have been replaced with prosthetic valves. The sound is soft with disk valves and bileaflets, but is loud with Starr-Edwards ball valves. Opening snaps may be heard in high-output states, such as right atrial septal defects. A_2-OS intervals are lengthened by conditions that are accompanied by pulmonary hypertension. The A_2-OS duration is 15 to 120 ms. The A_2-OS interval is thus influenced by both pulmonary and systemic vascular resistance.

Tumor Plops

"Plops," sounds that reveal tumors, are usually heard early in diastole and are relatively low-pitched but loud, with a booming character in the presence of right and left atrial myxomas. Plops do not have a parallel relationship to S_1, as the opening snap does. Thus, in general a loud S_1 is associated with a loud opening snap in mitral stenosis, while the loudness of S_1 does not relate to the amplitude of the tumor plop. Middiastolic murmurs follow the plop.

Diastolic Snaps or Clicks

Diastolic snaps or clicks are often present in mitral valve prolapse. Esophageal auscultation and phonocardiograms reveal multiple snaps, which tend to disappear with the administration of amyl nitrite.

PROSTHETIC VALVES (Figs. 5-23, 5-24)

Place the ear close to, but not touching the chest to listen for the audible clicks, grade VI sounds, that sometimes signal the presence of an implanted heart device such as a prosthetic valve (Cardiac Pearl 6). Clinicians commonly encounter prosthetic valves in the mitral or aortic positions and only rarely in the tricuspid or pulmonic positions. Commonly heard sounds are of various types. General closing clicks of prosthetic valves are louder than opening clicks. Ball valves are the exception, because the opening and closing clicks are close in intensity in the mitral position but the opening click is louder than the closing click in the aortic position. This probably relates to the sharp excursion of the ball in ventricular systole with the buildup of pressure exceeding the diastolic pressure of the aorta. The closing click is coincident with S_2 and is almost as loud. A sudden absence of the sounds with an aortic ball valve prosthesis *is an acute emergency that requires immediate thrombolytic treatment or surgery.* In the mitral position, both opening snap and closing snap are about equally loud.

Aortic Valves

Listen without the stethoscope for clicks and auscultate, using the diaphragm in the left lower sternal border. When listening to ball valves in the aortic position, auscultation is best done in the sitting-up position with hands behind the patient's back. A soft, harsh systolic ejection murmur may be heard followed by a soft diastolic rumble. These are normal auscultatory findings.

If the aortic valve that is replaced is a disk, rather than a ball prosthesis, however, the auscultatory findings are notably different. With a disk, the aortic valve opening is soft and difficult to hear, while aortic valve closure is loud. A soft ejection murmur and an early diastolic murmur may be heard.

A normal aortic valve opens approximately 40 ms after S_1 and corresponds with the timing of an ejection sound. With a ball valve, by contrast, S_1 is heard in midsystole, after the normal position of an aortic ejection

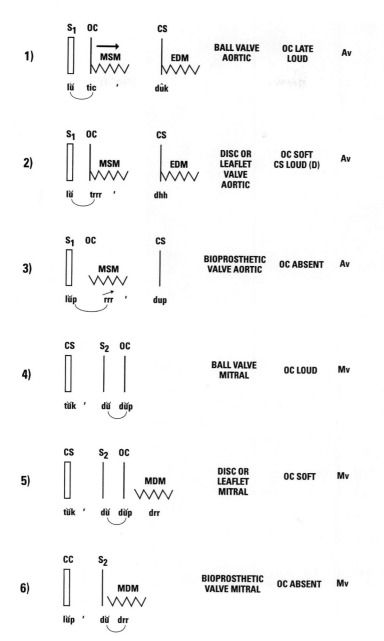

Figure 5-23 Phonophonic representation of prosthetic valves. OS, opening snap; MDM, middiastolic murmur; OC, opening click; CC, closing click; MSM, midsystolic murmur; EDM, early diastolic murmur; MV, mitral valve; AV, aortic valve.

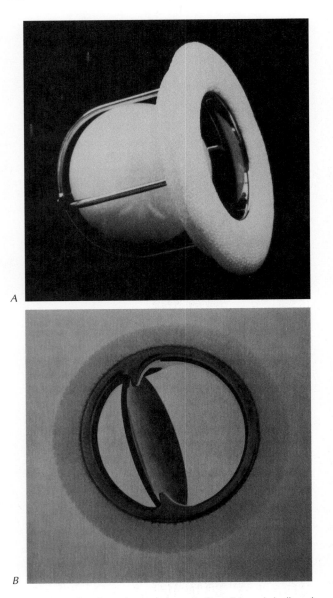

Figure 5-24 Prosthetic heart valves. *A.* Starr-Edwards ball-and-cage valve; *B.* tilting disk valve; *C.* bioprosthetic valve with stents; *D.* bileaflet valve.

click. In the case of bileaflet valves, the aortic valve closure is louder than opening of the aortic valve. The timing of valve opening corresponds with that of the disk valve and is early, occurring approximately 40 ms after valve opening. A soft ejection murmur may be heard and a diastolic murmur is not evident. With tissue valve prostheses, the aortic valve closure is

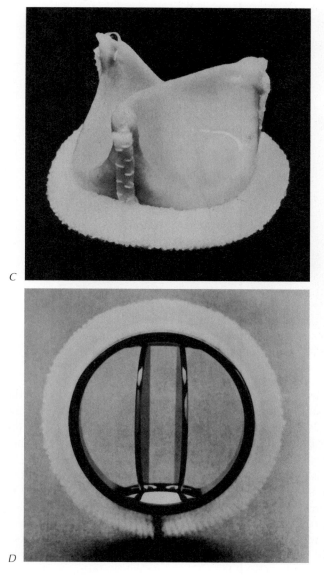

C

D

Figure 5-24   (Continued)

somewhat louder than opening of the aortic valve, which may be totally silent. A soft ejection murmur is heard with no diastolic murmur.

Mitral Valves

Auscultate for prosthetic mitral valves using both bell and diaphragm at the apex with the patient in the left supine position. Listen without the

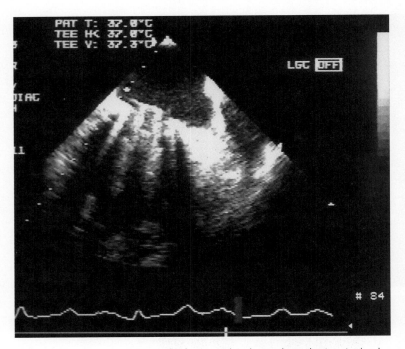

Figure 5-25 Echocardiogram of left ventricular clot and prosthetic mitral valve.

stethoscope for clicks. The opening click of a ball valve is as loud as the closing click. The A_2 interval between closing of the aortic valve and opening of the mitral valve is approximately 70 to 110 ms, corresponding to the opening snap in a patient with mild mitral stenosis. A soft systolic murmur is heard with no diastolic murmur.

In the case of disk valves, the closure of the aortic valve—synchronous with S_1—makes the soft opening of the valve difficult if not impossible to hear on auscultation. It sometimes helps to place the patient in the left lateral position and to listen at the left sternal edge, where the mitral valve opening may be heard more clearly than at the cardiac apex. A soft systolic murmur is normally heard and there is a definite short delayed diastolic rumble. The timing of the interval between aortic valve closure and mitral valve opening corresponds with the opening snap heard in a patient with moderate mitral stenosis.

In tissue valves and bileaflet valves, opening and closing snaps are heard with the closing snap being louder. The opening snap is heard best at the left sternal edge in the left lateral position. Opening snap occurs approximately 50 to 90 ms after aortic valve closure, corresponding to a patient with moderate mitral stenosis. In patients with tissue valves, the closure of the mitral valve corresponding with S_1 is louder than that of mitral valve opening. The mitral opening is audible in approximately one-half of patients and a middiastolic murmur is commonly heard with a soft apical systolic murmur.

Both aortic and mitral valves can deteriorate from a variety of circumstances. The native valves may calcify and become stenotic, valves may become regurgitant, clotting can occur, or the valves may undergo limitation of excursion. Such limitation may be due to clotting or to the growth of pannus. Vegetations may be present in the valves causing a potential source for emboli or masses.

In evaluating prosthetic valves, initial and serial evaluations by echocardiography or transesophageal echocardiography (TEE) as well as fluoroscopy are of extreme clinical importance. It is sometimes not possible to determine the significance of a single study obtained on a mitral or an aortic valve by echocardiography or TEE alone. TEE is the technique of choice in mitral and aortic valves, the caveat being that it is often useful to do a transthoracic echocardiogram as well in a patient with a mitral valve prosthesis. This particularly applies to patients in whom multiplane and biplane echocardiograms are not obtained.

Tricuspid Valves

Although patients with infected tricuspid valves sometimes have them removed or repaired, experience with replacing these valves is limited. Pulmonary valves are rarely involved, though prosthetic pulmonary valves have on occasion been used. In general, anticoagulation therapy is given to all patients having mitral valve replacements and to those with aortic valve replacements with non-bioprosthetic valves.

Repair of Mitral and Tricuspid Valves

Repair of valves, for example, with Carpentier ring, is a useful alternative in patients who have left ventricular dysfunction and whose valvular disease is such that narrowing of the valvular ring can reduce the degree of mitral regurgitation. Results in these patients are best evaluated by intraoperative TEE. Patients are placed on anticoagulant therapy for approximately 6 to 12 weeks after the procedure. Middiastolic flow murmurs are common auscultatory sequel.

Prosthetic valve endocarditis may develop within 3 months when caused by staphylococci, or later if the result of streptococci. Endocarditis associated with drug addiction may be caused by a variety of organisms and fungal infections in the immunocompromised subjects.

TRUE OR FALSE

1. A loud S_1 and tapping cardiac apex suggest mitral stenosis.
2. Reversed splitting of S_1 is heard in mitral stenosis.
3. Paradoxic splitting of S_2 is present on inspiration and expiration, while reversed splitting is present only on expiration.

4. Fixed splitting is narrow in ASD with severe pulmonary hypertension and wide in ASD without severe pulmonary hypertension.

5. An S_4 gallop is physiological in pregnancy.

6. An S_3 is a sure sign of heart failure in patients over 40.

CLINICAL VIGNETTES

The following vignettes present actual cases of patients who were affected by diseases and conditions discussed in this chapter. At the end of each case, choose the one answer that best describes the diagnosis indicated by the vignette.

1. A 29-year-old female with red hair and freckles, of Irish descent, presented with a history of palpitations. There was no other significant past history. On auscultation, S_1 was accentuated, S_2 was normal. The patient was turned to the left side and reexamined. There was a tapping apical impulse and a loud S_1 preceded by a thrill and a presystolic murmur; S_1 was followed by S_2, an opening snap, and a middiastolic murmur. The diagnosis is:

   A. Tricuspid stenosis
   B. Atrial myxoma
   C. Mitral stenosis

2. A 35-year-old Hispanic female presented with a previous history of rheumatic fever. The patient had been known to have mitral stenosis. Auscultation at the left lower sternal border revealed a middiastolic murmur preceded by a split S_1, followed by a normal S_2, and an S_3. These sounds and murmurs increased on inspiration. There was a prominent venous A wave in the neck. Auscultation over the jugular vein revealed an S_4, but an S_4 was not heard over the heart. The diagnosis is:

   A. Tricuspid stenosis
   B. Mitral stenosis
   C. Atrial septal defect

3. A male patient, age 64, was examined. He had no history of heart disease. The patient gave a history of paroxysmal atrial fibrillation and had been placed on digitalis. He had no complaints and was seen at a routine follow-up. On examination, the patient was in sinus rhythm with no abnormal findings elicited except for the presence of a loud S_1. The diagnosis is:

   A. Short PR interval, less than 200 ms
   B. Mitral valve prolapse
   C. Mitral stenosis

4. A 50-year-old patient was seen with a rough ejection systolic murmur, and a late-peaking midsystolic crescendo that was somewhat musical in character. The systolic murmur was less prominent in the aortic area. S_1 was soft, a click was not heard, and there was a paradoxically split S_2. Left bundle branch block was present. These symptoms were most like caused by:

A. Aortic valvular stenosis with Gallavardin phenomenon (severe)
B. Hypertrophic obstructive cardiomyopathy
C. Mitral regurgitation

5. An anxious, 30-year-old female patient was seen on two occasions, one week apart. An apical systolic nonejection click had been heard and she had been placed on beta-blockers. There was a noticeable attenuation of the intensity of the loud S_1 at her second visit. These symptoms were most likely caused by:

A. Lengthened PR interval
B. Mitral regurgitation
C. Effect of beta-blocker

6. A 65-year-old male was seen with a history of shortness of breath. On examination, the patient was obese with a barrel-shaped chest. The first and second heart sounds were both split with wide separation of the two components of S_2. There was no movement between A_2 and P_2 on inspiration and expiration, and A_2 was louder than P_2. The patient had an incomplete right bundle branch. The diagnosis is:

A. Atrial septal defect
B. Aortic stenosis
C. Complete right bundle branch block with cor pulmonale

7. A 20-year-old male patient was seen with a history of heart murmur. On listening at the left sternal edge, physiological splitting of S_1 was heard, while over the pulmonary area there was splitting of S_2, preceded by a grade II ejection systolic murmur (midsystolic type, no click was present). These symptoms are most likely caused by:

A. Innocent systolic murmur
B. Bicuspid valves
C. Pulmonary stenosis

8. A 30-year-old white female with a history of palpitations but with no current complaints was routinely examined. Placing the patient in the left lateral position, the examiner heard a distinct nonejection click following S_1. This was also heard in the supine position. On sitting and standing, the click appeared to disappear. On inspiration, there was a split S_1 caused by separation between S_1 and the click. The echocardiogram was consistent with the diagnosis. The diagnosis is:

A. Bicuspid valves
B. Pulmonary stenosis
C. Mitral and tricuspid valve prolapse

9. A 35-year-old male was seen with no history of hypertension. The patient had a normal habitus; examination of the heart was totally normal except for the accentuation of aortic valve closure. This was detected in the aortic area at the left sternal edge, fourth left intercostal space at the Erb's point. There were no murmurs. On exercising, and on auscultation in the left lateral position while at rest, a transient S_4 was present. These symptoms were most likely caused by:

A. Coronary artery disease
B. Tricuspid stenosis
C. Hypertension

10. A 65-year-old male patient was seen with atrial fibrillation. Auscultation revealed wide splitting of the S_2 over the pulmonary artery, accentuation of A_2 and P_2 and a loud P_2 to the apex. There was incomplete right bundle branch block with atrial fibrillation. Fixed splitting of S_2 occurred at an interval of approximately 50 ms. The diagnosis is:

A. Atrial septal defect
B. Right bundle branch block
C. Pulmonary stenosis

11. An 80-year-old female patient presented with gastrointestinal bleeding. Multiple endoscopies were unrevealing. The patient had an *anacrotic pulse* and a systolic murmur was heard over the aortic area. This peaked in late systole and S_1 and S_2 were absent. In the left lateral position, the examiner detected an S_4. The diagnosis is:

A. Pulmonary hypertension, esophageal varices and bleeding
B. Hypertrophic obstructive cardiomyopathy (HOCM)
C. Heyde's syndrome

12. A 40-year-old male presented with hypertension of 2 years' duration. He was a 20-pack-per-year smoker. On examination at the fourth left intercostal space, the patient had a grade III systolic murmur. S_1 followed by an ejection sound, and reversed splitting of S_2 with an S_4. The chest x-ray showed borderline cardiomegaly. The diagnosis is:

A. Left bundle branch block
B. Hypertension
C. Pulmonary hypertension

13. A 65-year-old female patient presented with shortness of breath. The patient was thought to have chronic obstructive pulmonary disease. On examination, the patient was in sinus rhythm with no palpable

impulses. S_1 was normal and somewhat accentuated in the fourth left intercostal space. S_2 was widely split and fixed. ECG revealed incomplete right bundle branch block. Chest x-ray showed a large pulmonary artery with pulmonary plethora. The diagnosis is:

A. Cor pulmonale, chronic obstructive pulmonary disease
B. Right bundle branch block
C. Atrial septal defect

14. A 30-year-old female patient was seen with Raynaud phenomenon and a mild degree of cyanosis and pulsating neck veins. She was in atrial fibrillation. The patient had a palpable right ventricular impulse. S_1 and S_2 were heard. *The S_2 showed narrow nonfixed splitting ($A_2 P_2$).* There was no appreciable middiastolic murmur heard on inspiration, suggesting absence of flow across the tricuspid valve. P_2 was accentuated.

   Echocardiography revealed the presence of an enlarged right ventricle; no tricuspid regurgitation was noted. Cardiac catheterization was performed, and the patient had systemic pressures in the pulmonary circuit. The diagnosis is:

A. Idiopathic pulmonary hypertension
B. Atrial septal defect with pulmonary hypertension
C. Eisenmenger complex

15. A 45-year-old female presented with syncopal episodes and had angina on exertion. A heart murmur had been previously heard. On examination, S_1 and S_2 were not audible, but an S_4 was present. There was a loud, rough, grade IV ejection systolic murmur, best heard at the left sternal edge. Pulses were anacrotic. The diagnosis is:

A. Aortic stenosis
B. Mitral regurgitation
C. Subaortic web

16. A 20-year-old male patient was seen. The patient had a long, lean habitus, including longer-than-average measurements from the pubis to the feet and from the pubis to the top of the head. The patient suffered from kyphoscoliosis, and when asked to make a fist had a thumb that protruded.

   Examination revealed a nonejection sound at the apex with a grade II midsystolic murmur. The patient was in sinus rhythm. Auscultation over the aortic area and in the right third intercostal space revealed a grade III midsystolic murmur and a loud, tambour-like, ringing aortic S_2. The diagnosis is:

A. Aortic aneurysm with mitral valve prolapse
B. Aortic stenosis

C. Aortic sclerosis

17. A 14-year-old child with moon facies was seen with a grade IV systolic murmur over the pulmonary area. There was a click preceding the systolic murmur and an S_2 was split. On inspiration the click disappeared and the split widened, although the second component of the S_2 was soft. A prominent A wave was present in the venous pulse. The diagnosis is:

A. Pulmonary stenosis
B. Idiopathic dilatation of the pulmonary artery
C. Atrial septal defect

18. A 10-year-old female patient was seen with central cyanosis. Examination revealed an ejection sound, no right ventricular heave but a palpable apical A_2. The patient was in sinus rhythm. Auscultation revealed the presence of a midsystolic murmur. The diagnosis is:

A. Pulmonary AV fistula
B. Eisenmenger syndrome
C. Tetralogy of Fallot

19. A 41-year-old Asian male who was in no obvious distress had sustained an acute anterior myocardial infarction with class IIB NYHA (New York Heart Association classification system) dyspnea on exertion. On exertion, he had a very prominent arcus cornealis, tendons xanthomata, xanthomata on his knuckles as well as in the Achilles' tendons, and examination of the heart revealed normal venous pressure, cardiomegaly with a diffuse left ventricular apical impulse, and a prominent fourth sound with a heart rate of 80 beats per minute. The patient was instructed to turn on his left side, auscultated gently with the bell of the stethoscope, asked to exhale and make a tight fist with his hands. Over the next minute, he developed an S_3 and tachycardia with a summation gallop. The patient was promptly sat up, reexamined, and found to have no filling sounds. The patient was reexamined in the left supine position and a high-pitched S_4 was heard.

    The patient did not develop shortness of breath during the time this was carried out. The diagnosis is:

A. Caused by lying on the left side
B. Occurring spontaneously
C. Induced by increased systemic vascular resistance

20. A 54-year-old female patient was seen with a history of shortness of breath. She cited a previous history of joint pains. On examination, the patient, unable to lie flat, was elevated to 45 degrees. Carotid pulses were small, the venous pressure was elevated to 10 cm above the sternal angle with a prominent A wave superimposed on a cv-y

pulsation. In the left recumbent position, the apex was not palpable. There was an impalpable right ventricle as judged by the absence of a precordial heave.

Auscultation of the apex using the bell of the stethoscope with the patient in the left lateral supine position brought out a loud S_1, a normal S_2, and a diastolic murmur that was preceded by a loud, low-pitched thud. The patient had narrow splitting of S_2 with accentuation of P_2.

Chest x-ray showed cardiomegaly with enlargement of the right atrium and a moderate degree of pulmonary venous congestion, inversion of the venous pattern, and peribronchial cuffing. ECG was unremarkable. The diagnosis is:

A. Acute mitral regurgitation
B. Mitral stenosis
C. Left atrial myxoma

21. A 23-year-old male patient was seen with a rapid onset of shortness of breath and a several-month history of heart murmur. On examination, the patient was ill looking with no congenital stigmata. An apical impulse detected on auscultation indicated a hyperdynamic impulse, left ventricular in type. The right ventricle was not palpable. Auscultation revealed the presence of an early systolic murmur and a somewhat low-pitched S_3. S_2 was widely split with a loud nonfixed P_2. The diagnosis is:

A. Mitral valve disease with endocarditis
B. Bacterial endocarditis with mitral valve disease
C. Left atrial myxoma

ANSWERS

True or False

1. *T*; 2. *F*; 3. *T*; 4. *T*; 5. *F*; 6. *F*

Clinical Vignettes

1. *C. Mitral stenosis.* The location of the murmur and the response to inspiration rules out *tricuspid stenosis (A)*. Absence of a tumor plop preceding the diastolic rumble *excludes atrial myxoma (B)*.
2. *A. Tricuspid stenosis.* The S_4 heard over the jugular veins, the increase in loudness of the sounds and murmurs with inspiration, and the normal S_2 exclude *mitral stenosis (B)* and *atrial septal defect (C)*.
3. *A. Short PR interval.* The absence of physical findings makes diagnoses *mitral valve prolapse (B)*, and *mitral stenosis (C)*, unlikely.

4. *Aortic valvular stenosis.* The character of the pulse excludes *HOCM* (*B*); the midsystolic murmur and ejection sound exclude *mitral regurgitation* (*C*).

5. *C. Effect of beta-blockers.* Beta-blockers do not *cause lengthened PR interval* (*A*); there is no holosystolic murmur with *mitral regurgitation* (*B*).

6. *A. Atrial septal defect.* Physiological splitting of S_2 is not present in atrial septal defect. The split is fixed; it does not alter with the phases of respiration. Splitting refers to the distance between aortic and pulmonic valve closure. In cor pulmonale with right bundle branch block, P_2 is accentuated, i.e., closure of the aortic and pulmonary valves, and of P_2, is louder than A_2. But physiological nonfixed splitting is present. In *aortic stenosis* (*B*) reversed splitting is present or S_2 is not heard.

7. *A. Innocent systolic murmur.* The absence of an ejection sound excludes *bicuspid aortic valve* (*B*). In pulmonary stenosis the ejection sound that is present will disappear on inspiration and hence would exclude *pulmonary stenosis* (*C*). The diagnosis clearly is that of an innocent systolic murmur.

8. *C. Mitral and tricuspid valve prolapse.* Movement of the systolic click and murmur to and from the S_1 with changes in position exclude *biscuspid valves* (*A*). A late systolic murmur and inspiratory increase of the click rule out *pulmonary stenosis* (*B*). The diagnosis is therefore mitral and tricuspid valve prolapse. Movement of the tricuspid snap away from S_1 during inspiration is characteristic.

9. *C. Hypertension.* S_4 in tricuspid stenosis is heard exclusively over the jugular veins and is not transient. An S_4 is frequently present in hypertension.

10. *A. Atrial septal defect.* The fixed splitting of S_2 excludes *right bundle branch block* (*B*) and *pulmonary stenosis* (*C*). In the latter, pulmonary valve closure is delayed.

11. *C. Heyde's syndrome.* The physical findings of an anacrotic pulse and a systolic murmur are consistent with aortic stenosis, excluding *pulmonary hypertension* (*A*). Hypertrophic obstructive cardiomyopathy is excluded by the pulse. Aortic stenosis is associated with angiodysplasia of the colon on the right side: the so-called Heyde's syndrome.

12. *A. Left bundle branch block.* Hypertension alone does not cause paradoxic splitting of S_2, excluding *B*. P_2 in Eisenmenger's syndrome and A_2 are fused, giving rise to a single S_2, excluding *pulmonary hypertension* (*C*).

13. Fixed splitting of S_2 and pulmonary plethora are inconsistent with *chronic pulmonary disease* (*A*), and *right bundle branch block* (*B*), but is characteristic of *atrial septal defect* (*C*). "Fixed splitting" means the absence of variation in the timing between aortic and pulmonary valve closure with alterations in normal respiration.

14. *A. Idiopathic pulmonary hypertension.* The absence of fixed splitting of S_2 negates *atrial septal defect (B) and Eisenmenger complex (C).*

15. *A. Aortic stenosis.* In *mitral regurgitation (B)*, S_2 is physiologically split. In *subaortic web (C)*, an aortic diastolic murmur is heard. The gradient aorta/LV in this case was over 60 mm.

16. *A. Aortic aneurysm. Aortic stenosis (B)* is excluded by the loud closure of the aortic valve. Aortic sclerosis is unusual in a 20-year-old patient. The diagnosis is, therefore, an aortic aneurysm, possibly in a patient with Marfan's syndrome.

17. *A. Pulmonary stenosis. (B) Idiopathic dilatation of the pulmonary artery is excluded by the appearance of the click on inspiration and softening of P_2, and atrial septal defect (C)* by the physiological splitting of S_2.

18. *C. Tetralogy of Fallot. Pulmonary and AV fistula (A)* is excluded by the absence of a continuous murmur and a loud P_2. The diagnosis is Fallot's tetralogy with a single S_2.

19. *C. Induced by increased systemic vascular resistance.* Filling sounds are not caused by lying on the left side, although this position may make the sounds more evident. This excludes *B* as well as *A,* for filling sounds do not occur spontaneously except in patients with ischemia.

20. *C. Left atrial myxoma.* The absence of a holosystolic murmur excludes *mitral regurgitation (A);* absence of an opening snap rules out *mitral stenosis (B).*

21. *A. Mitral regurgitation.* Endocarditis is rare in mitral stenosis, and the absence of a diastolic murmur excludes *(B).* There is no tumor plop or diastolic murmur *(C).*

BIBLIOGRAPHY

Ahuja SP, Coles JC: Further observations on the genesis of early systolic clicks. *Am J Cardiol* 1966; 17:291.

Benchimol A, Desser KB: The fourth heart sound in patients without demonstrable heart disease. *Am Heart J* 1977; 93:298.

Bonner AJ, et al: Early diastolic sound associated with mitral valve prolapse. *Arch Intern Med* 1976; 136:347.

Braunwald E, et al: Effective closure of the mitral valve without atrial systole. *Circulation* 1966; 33:404.

Caulfield WH, et al: The clinical significance of the fourth heart sound in aortic stenosis. *Am J Cardiol* 1971; 28:179.

Contro S: Ventricular gallop in mitral stenosis: Its mechanism and significance. *Am Heart J* 1957; 54:246.

Dock W: Heart sounds from Starr-Edwards valves. *Circulation* 1965; 31:801.

Dock W: Loud presystolic sounds over the jugular veins associated with high venous pressure. *Am J Med* 1956; 20:853.

Ehlers KH, et al: Wide splitting of the second heart sound without demonstrable heart disease. *Am J Cardiol* 1969; 23:690.

Estein EJ, et al: Cineradiographic studies of the early systolic click in aortic valve stenosis. *Circulation* 1965; 31:842.

Goldblatt A, et al: Hemodynamic-phonocardiographic correlations of the fourth heart sound in aortic stenosis. *Circulation* 1962; 26:92.

Gray I: Paradoxical splitting of the second heart sound. *Br Heart J* 1956; 18:21.

Grayzel J: Gallop rhythm of the heart: II. Quadruple rhythm and its relation to summation and augmented gallops. *Circulation* 1959; 20:1053.

Harris WS, et al: Modification of the atrial sound by the cold pressor test, carotid sinus massage, and the Valsalva maneuver. *Circulation* 1963; 28:1128.

Harvey WP, Stapleton J: Clinical aspects of gallop rhythm with particular reference to diastolic gallops. *Circulation* 1958; 18:1017.

Kincaid-Smith P, Barlow J: The atrial sound and the atrial component of the first heart sound. *Br Heart J* 1959; 21:470.

Kossman CE: The opening snap of the tricuspid valve: A physical sign of tricuspid stenosis. *Circulation* 1955; 11:378.

Leatham A: Splitting of the first and second heart sounds. *Lancet* 1954; 2:607.

Leatham A, Vogelpoel L: The early systolic sound in dilatation of the pulmonary artery. *Br Heart J* 1954; 16:21.

Longhini C, et al: The genesis of the opening snap in mitral stenosis: Correlations between spectral analysis and echocardiographic data. *Am J Noninvas Cardiol* 1987; 1:373.

Lopez JF, et al: The apical first sound as an aid in the diagnosis of atrial septal defect. *Circulation* 1962; 26:1296.

Luisada AA, et al: Changing views on the mechanism of the first and second heart sounds. *Am Heart J* 1974; 88:503.

Martinez-Lopez JI: Sounds of the heart in diastole. *Am J Cardiol* 1974; 34:594.

Mathey DG, et al: The determinants of onset of mitral valve prolapse in the systolic click-late systolic murmur syndrome. *Circulation* 1976; 53:872.

Minhas K, Gasul BM: Systolic clicks: A clinical, phonocardiographic, and hemodynamic evaluation. *Am Heart J* 1959; 57:49.

Mounsey P: The early diastolic sound of constrictive pericarditis. *Br Heart J* 1955; 17:143.

Mounsey P: The opening snap of mitral stenosis. *Br Heart J* 1953; 15:135.

Parry E, Mounsey P: Gallop sound in hypertension and myocardial ischemia modified by respiration and other maneuver. *Br Heart J* 1961; 23:393.

Reddy PS, et al: Normal and abnormal heart sounds in cardiac diagnosis: Part II: Diastolic sounds. *Curr Probl Cardiol* 1985; 10:36.

Shaver JA, Salerni R: Auscultation of the heart. In Hurst JW(ed): *The Heart,* 7th ed. New York: McGraw-Hill, 1990:188.

Tavel ME: The fourth heart sound: A premature requiem? *Circulation* 1974; 49:4.

Tavel ME et al: Opening snap of the tricuspid valve in atrial septal defect. *Am Heart J* 1970; 80:550.

Van de Werf F, et al: The mechanism of disappearance of the physiologic third heart sound with age. *Circulation* 1986; 73:877.

Yurchak PM, Gorlin R: Paradoxical splitting of the second heart sound in coronary heart disease. *N Engl J Med* 1963; 269:741.

Zuberbuhler JR, Bauersfeld SR: Paradoxical splitting of the second heart sound in the Wolff-Parkinson-White syndrome. *Am Heart J* 1965; 70:595.

6

SYSTOLIC AND DIASTOLIC MURMURS

SYSTOLIC MURMURS
    Mechanics of Heart Murmurs
    Classification of Murmurs
    Midsystolic Murmurs
    Holosystolic Murmurs
    Early Systolic Murmurs
    Late Systolic Murmurs
    Mitral Valve Prolapse

DIASTOLIC MURMURS
    Middiastolic Murmurs
    Early Diastolic Murmurs

OTHER MURMURS
    Changing Murmurs
    Continuous Murmurs
    To-and-Fro Murmurs
    Ectopic Bruits
    Auscultation of Bruits

QUESTIONS

CLINICAL VIGNETTES

In contrast to heart sounds, which are perceived as instantaneous transients, murmurs are protracted (150 to 250 ms) acoustic events. Murmurs are also sometimes referred to as bruits or soufflés, from the French; or susurrus, from the Latin. Murmurs are described according to their timing, loudness, or grade; quality; presence or absence of a thrill; maximum point of location; radiation; and response to dynamic techniques. A clinical auscultator needs to elicit, observe, and note each of these important features (Table 6-1).

    Additionally, the examiner must consider the physical appearance of the patient; the nature of the associated heart sounds; the cardiac impulse and venous pulse; and findings from the electrocardiogram, echocardiogram, and chest x-ray.

Table 6-1 Eponymous Heart Murmurs

Murmur	Timing	Quality	Associated condition	Maximum point
Austin Flint	Middiastolic	Low-pitched	Aortic regurgitation	Apex
Cabot	Early diastolic			Lower sternal edge
Carey-Coombs	Middiastolic		Rheumatic fever; mitral regurgitation	Apex
Cecil Cole	Early diastolic	Cooing	Aortic regurgitation	Left sternal edge, conducted to apex
Cruveilhier-Baumgarten	Continuous			
Dock's	Early diastolic		Stenoses of epicardial coronary artery disease	
Duroziez'	Diastolic			Compressed femoral artery
Gallavardin		Musical; high-pitched	Aortic stenosis	Apex; in Gallavardin dissociation, harsh systolic murmur is heard over 2 RICS
Gibson	Continuous			Pulmonary area
Graham Steell	Early diastolic	Rapid diminuendo; high-pitched	Pulmonary regurgitation	Pulmonary area; localized over pulmonary artery
Locke's			Aortic stenosis	Lower left sternal border
Mean's Learman's		Scratch		Pulmonary area; intermediate left sternal border
Still's	Midsystolic			Below nipple

SYSTOLIC MURMURS

When evaluating systolic murmurs, the clinician should first identify S_1 and S_2. S_1 is readily identified by palpation of the apex or by the carotid pulse, which are close in terms of timing. In general, S_2 is best heard at the second intercostal space (ICS) on either side of the sternum. Although it would appear to be easy to discern the dull S_1 and the sharp S_2, phonetically characterized as lup-dup (S_1-S_2), mistakes can be made in distinguishing these sounds, especially with a rapid heartbeat. In fact, S_1 is best distinguished by first identifying S_2. These are heard between S_1 and S_2.

Although, on occasion, a single sound is all that is heard, the examiner can usually discern the sounds and the timing of the murmur by routinely examining the carotid pulse, the apical impulse, and S_2.

Mechanics of Heart Murmurs

Heart murmurs are attributed to turbulence in fluids, which disturbs the normal laminar flow pattern of the blood. These turbulent currents are established by (1) obstructions to flow; (2) alteration in the size of the chamber into which blood flows; (3) valvular abnormalities that increase the velocity and volume of flow; and (4) other factors, including eddy currents, blood density and viscosity, jet impact, structural flutter, periodic oscillations and cavitation. Systolic murmurs occur between S_1 and S_2; diastolic murmurs between S_2 and S_1.

Classification of Murmurs

Note that, unfortunately, due to inexact use of terminology, incorrect terms have been used, such as *crescendo,* which indicates an increasing loudness of a murmur, *decrescendo,* which should be replaced with the word *diminuendo,* indicating a decreasing loudness of a murmur; and that the correct term for pitch change is not used herein. This word is *portamento. Portamento up* means rising pitch; *portamento down* means decreasing pitch. Acoustic damping has been previously discussed in Chap. 1. This book classifies murmurs according to nine different criteria. These include:

1. Timing
2. Phonetics
3. Point of maximum intensity
4. Loudness
5. Character
6. Radiation
7. Eponyms
8. Pitch
9. Cadence

Note that to-and-fro murmurs are not included as a category because they are a complex phonetic, i.e., the sum of 4 and 5. The above classification will apply to murmurs as described in this book. A general summary of the murmurs discussed in this chapter, arranged according to timing, can be found in Table 6-2. Their phonophonic transliterations are summarized in Table 6-3. Table 6-4 grades murmurs according to loudness.

Systolic and diastolic murmurs are deemed either innocent or pathological, signaling whether they require treatment. Noncardiac pathological

Table 6-2   Timing, Character, and Causes of Murmurs

Timing	Subtypes	Associated causes	Character
Systolic	Holosystolic		
	Mitral regurgitation		Blowing
	Ventricular septal defect		
	Tricuspid regurgitation		
	Late systolic		
	Mitral valve prolapse		Blowing
	Papillary muscle dysfunction		
	Calcification of mitral valve ring		
	Midsystolic		
	Innocent	Still's murmur	Rough or
	Ectasia of the aorta	Right ventricular outflow tract	blowing
		Pulmonary tract	
		Buzzing murmur	
		Supraclavicular	
	High-output states	Severe anemia	Rough
		Aortic regurgitation with pulmonary incompetence	
	Hypertension		
	Valvular abnormalities	Atrial septal defect	Blowing
		Other stenoses (subaortic, pulmonary, infundibular, etc.)	
		Tetralogy of Fallot	
	Early systolic		
	Acute mitral regurgitation		
	Ventricular septal defect	Acute: loud harsh early to midsystolic	Blowing
		Holosystolic	
	Holosystolic		
	Tricuspid regurgitation	With increasing pulmonary hypertension	
		Organic due to carcinoid or bacterial endocarditis	Blowing
Diastolic	Early diastolic		
	Aortic regurgitation		
	Pulmonary regurgitation	With pulmonary hypertension	Blowing
		With organic disease (carcinoid, Marfan's syndrome)	
	Supracostal ventricular septal defect and aortic regurgitation		
	Retroverted aortic cusp		
	Dock's murmur		
	Middiastolic		
	Mitral stenosis		
	Aortic and pulmonary regurgitation		Rumbling
	Ebstein's anomaly		
	Flow murmur	Ventricular septal defect	Rough
		Atrial septal defect	
		Patent ductus arteriosus	

Table 6-2   Timing, Character, and Causes of Murmurs (*Continued*)

Timing	Subtypes	Associated causes	Character
	Right- or left-sided inflow obstruction		Rough
	Mitral valve prolapse		
	Carcinoid syndrome		
	Cor triatrium		
	Ball valve clot or vegetation		
	Carcinoid tricuspid stenosis		
	Right or left atrial myxoma		
	Mitral or tricuspid valvuloplasty		
Continuous	Peak at S_2		
	Soufflé	Mammary	
		Uterine	
	Systolic accentuation		
	Fistulae	Pulmonary arteriovenous	
		Traumatic arteriovenous	
		Iatrogenic arteriovenous	
		Coronary artery venous	
	Stenosis	Carotid artery	
		Pulmonary artery branch	
		Renal artery	
	Tumors	Pulmonary hamartomas	
		Hemangiomas	
		Vascular tumors of the thyroid gland	
	Patent ductus arteriosus		
	Truncus arteriosus		
	Palliative operations in cyanotic congenital heart disease		
	Jugular venous hum		
	Aortopulmonary windows		
	Pulmonary bronchopulmonary collateral vessels		
	Cruveilheir-Baumgarten syndrome		
	Total anomalous pulmonary venous drainage		
To-and-fro	MSM		Rough and blowing in sequence
	Combinations of associated causes		
	Aortic stenosis and aortic regurgitation		
	Pulmonary stenosis and pulmonary regurgitation		
	EDM		
	Supracristal ventricular septal defects and aortic regurgitation		

Table 6-3   Categories of Heart Murmurs
and Their Associated Phonophonics

Category	Phonophonics
Midsystolic	Luh / RRR'Dup
Holosystolic	SHHH or SHHH
Early systolic	RRR / Dup
Late systolic	Lup / SHHH
Pre- and middiastolic	ERUP / DU / DRR
Early diastolic	LUP / DHHH
Continuous	RRRR

murmurs may be associated with: increased blood flow; dilated outflow tracts; abnormal valves; or interchamber communications or masses.

Midsystolic Murmurs

Midsystolic murmurs (Figs. 6-1 and 6-2) may sound early systolic if listened for at the base. This is because S_1 is soft or absent. Mid- and early systolic murmurs are diamond-shaped on phonocardiography but only the crescendo is heard. The decrescendo or diminuendo of these murmurs is not heard by auscultation, probably because of acoustic obliteration. This auditory characteristic is in contrast to the pattern of continuous murmurs, which audibly wax and wane.

Innocent Murmurs   Innocent cardiac murmurs may be heard in structurally normal hearts with normal blood flow. Innocent midsystolic murmurs are short murmurs that "keep innocent company." They are rarely heard in patients older than 20 years.

Innocent midsystolic murmurs are characterized by a pause between S_1 and the murmur and a pause between the murmur and S_2. These murmurs are not associated with a thrill; they are grade I to grade III in loudness, and are heard in the fourth left intercostal space at Erb's point in the pulmonary area (PA) and the aortic area (AA). Innocent murmurs are unassociated with clicks, ejection sounds, or other murmurs.

Table 6-4   Grading of Murmurs

I	Soft
II	Definite
III	Moderately loud
IV	Loud with thrill
V	Very loud with thrill
VI	Heard without chest contact

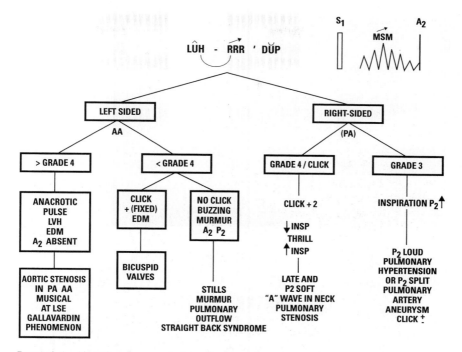

Figure 6-1 Algorithm for auscultation of midsystolic murmur.

Cardiac murmurs are not to be confused with cardiorespiratory murmurs, which are innocent noncardiac murmurs that result from the movement of inspired air. Heard during inspiration only, these murmurs stop when breathing is held.

It is extremely important for the examiner to make the positive diagnosis of an innocent systolic murmur.

Innocent systolic murmurs are of three types:

1. Still's murmur
2. Right ventricular outflow tract murmur
3. Supraclavicular murmur

Still's murmur   Still's murmur is commonly heard in children younger than 5 years old and is usually auscultable at or below the nipple. This murmur is associated with a normal S_1 and S_2. Innocent systolic murmurs are not preceded by clicks; Still's murmur has a vibrating quality and may be crackling, grunting, or twanging.

Right ventricular outflow tract murmur   Pulmonary tract murmurs are one of two kinds of innocent murmurs of the right ventricular outflow tract.

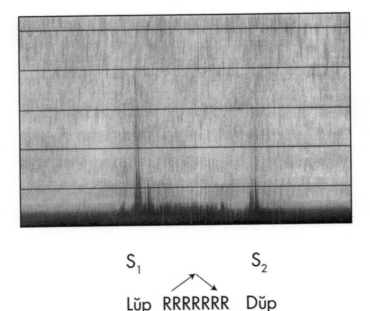

$$S_1 \qquad\qquad S_2$$

Lŭp RRRRRRR Dŭp

Figure 6-2   Acoustic spectrogram of midsystolic murmur.

Innocent pulmonary tract murmurs are detected by using the diaphragm of the stethoscope, and are midsystolic ejection in type. Unlike Still's murmur, pulmonary tract murmurs do not have a vibrating quality, and may be heard in patients of any age. The second type of innocent murmur of the right ventricular outflow tract is a buzzing murmur that may be heard in pectus excavatum and in straight back syndrome.

Supraclavicular murmurs   These are innocent murmurs heard over the clavicle, resulting from kinking of the arteries. With the aging of the population, supraclavicular systolic murmur is more commonly encountered in clinical practice. At times this murmur may be associated with pulsation above the right clavicle, due to unfolding of the aorta.

Systolic Ejection Murmurs

Aneurysms   Systolic ejection murmurs are often heard in conditions associated with dilatation of the aorta or pulmonary artery.

Aortic ectasia   Ectasia of the aorta without an aneurysm and with or without thickened nonstenotic valves is a common cause of a systolic ejection crescendo/decrescendo murmur.

Use the diaphragm for auscultation in patients with this condition. Patients with ectatic aortas have normal first and second sounds; occasionally S_2 is accentuated due to attendant valvular atherosclerosis. The aortic murmur is midsystolic ejection in type and is usually conducted into the neck, making it important to distinguish this luh rrr' dup (S_1 SM S_2) from the sounds produced by aortic stenosis or bicuspid valves. An ejection click precedes the systolic murmur and follows S_1 (Luh-tuk-dup). Similarly, a pulmonary artery with idiopathic dilatation is associated with a localized murmur, systolic in type, ejection in character, and somewhat harsh in quality. This murmur is preceded by a click and is often associated with a diastolic murmur, with wide splitting of S_2 simulating an atrial septal defect. Patients with idiopathic pulmonary artery dilatation may present with ejection sounds and midsystolic murmurs heard over the pulmonary area with wide splitting of S_2. These patients may have mitral valve prolapse or symptoms of connective tissue disorders of the Marfan type. Idiopathic pulmonary dilatation needs to be distinguished from secundum atrial septal defect, in which the wide splitting of S_2 is fixed with respiration (i.e., unaffected by breathing). The phonetic transliteration of fixed wide splitting of S_2 is luh rrr / du dup.

High-output states Systolic ejection murmurs may also be heard in high-output states. In general, outflow tract murmurs are ejection in type up to grade III and tend to be crescendo only. The phonocardiographic diamond-shaped pattern includes a decrescendo that is not audible at normal heart rates. Outflow tract murmurs should be auscultated with the diaphragm of the stethoscope; they are heard usually with an auscultatory silence between the murmur and the first and second sounds. This type of murmur includes the hemic murmur of anemia. Less commonly, an S_4 and even a thrill may be present with high-output outflow tract murmurs.

High-flow states may be caused by a number of different valvular abnormalities. Systolic murmurs that are not directly caused by either stenosis or regurgitation may be associated with conditions of increased flow. A classic example is aortic regurgitation with pulmonary regurgitation.

Apply the diaphragm to the left lower sternal border to auscultate for these murmurs. Bruits up to grade IV are crescendo in loudness and are heard on the right side. S_2 is frequently loud, snapping in character, and followed by an immediate diastolic murmur. The cardiophonics of high-output systolic murmurs are luh rrr/duh (SM S_2 DM), with the rrr representing the systolic component of the murmur, and the high-pitched duh the soft blowing, diastolic "sigh" (diminuendo in pitch and loudness) immediately following S_2.

In atrial septal defect (ASD), systolic murmurs preceded by an ejection sound are heard over the pulmonary artery, axilla, and over the sternum; because of increased pulmonary flow, this sound is also heard into the back. S_2 exhibits fixed splitting; and there is a musical or scratchy diastolic murmur heard in the lower sternal area that grows louder on inspiration as a result of the increased flow caused by functional tricuspid stenosis.

Hypertension Systemic hypertension may present with systolic ejection murmurs. This condition is auscultable with the diaphragm of the stethoscope applied to the lower left sternal border. Systemic hypertension is associated with a loud and occasional reversed splitting of S_2, and a harsh ejection systolic murmur, louder on expiration when the patient is in the sitting position. An S_4 is commonly heard. Pulmonary hypertension (hypertension within the pulmonary circulation) is associated with a short early ejection systolic murmur. This murmur is preceded by an early ejection sound localized over the second left intercostal space and followed by a single or finely split S_2 with a loud P_2. A short diminuendo early diastolic murmur may follow P_2.

Valvular abnormalities Abnormal valves are an important cause of systolic ejection murmurs. Begin auscultation by placing the ear close to the patient's chest; then use the diaphragm at the lower left sternal border. Sounds caused by valvular abnormalities are midsystolic (RRR) and crescendo as well as ejection in type. They may be associated with such nonstenotic lesions as those caused by aortic sclerosis or a calcified mitral valve ring (Fig. 6-3). The decrescendo component of these sounds, though visible on a phonocardiogram, is not audible in most cases due to acoustic obliteration. A grunting sound may be heard at the left sternal edge, or a musical

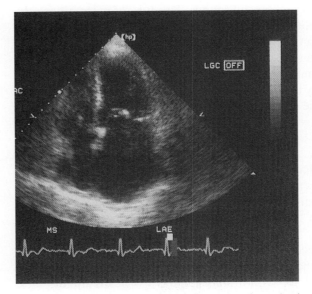

Figure 6-3   Two-dimensional echocardiogram of mitral valve calcification.

murmur reminiscent of a seagull's cry. This sound is conducted into the aortic area, where it may sound more like a puppy's whine than a seagull. Although patients with valvular abnormalities may not have either an ejection sound or reversed splitting of S_2, they may have calcification or atherosclerosis of the aortic valve or mitral valve ring. The same is not true of the pulmonary valve, in which pulmonary hypertension may be associated with abnormalities of the valve; in this case, ejection systolic murmurs are usually preceded by an early ejection sound.

It is important to distinguish between thoracic deformities and pulmonary hypertension caused by severe kyphoscoliosis, or "heart failure of the hunchback." In patients with thoracic deformities, apparent right ventricular hypertrophy is suspected on palpating the lower left sternal edge and on hearing a loud pulmonic S_2 preceded by an ejection systolic murmur over the pulmonary artery. The physiological movement of the components of the S_2, the absence of a click, and the externally visible thoracic abnormality rule out organic pathology. In pulmonary hypertension caused by severe kyphoscoliosis, on the other hand, stenotic systolic murmurs originate from the left or the right side of the heart. Keep in mind the general rule that right-sided murmurs (predominantly tricuspid murmurs) grow louder on inspiration while left-sided murmurs are better heard on expiration.

Midsystolic Stenotic Murmurs   Midsystolic murmurs are heard either with the unassisted ear or by using the diaphragm of the stethoscope. These murmurs are heard in a wide range of stenoses, including aortic, subaortic, supraaortic, idiopathic hypertrophic subaortic, pulmonary, infundibular, and branch stenoses of pulmonary arteries. Midsystolic murmurs also occur under conditions that are associated with these stenoses (e.g., tetralogy of Fallot).

Aortic Stenosis (Cardiac Pearl 92)   Physicians are likely to encounter aortic stenosis with increasing frequency as the elderly form a larger percentage of the population. Some cardiologists maintain that aortic stenosis is an inevitable development, given sufficient longevity. The combination of valvular degeneration (Mönckeberg's sclerosis) and calcification (Fig. 6-4) that causes aortic stenosis is associated with an ejection systolic murmur. In aortic stenosis, an early diastolic murmur of aortic regurgitation may also be heard (Fig. 6-5), giving rise to a to-fro murmur.

The significant auscultatory features of this condition are as follows. Loudness and the length of the murmur, not the absence of a click, correspond with the severity of the stenosis and gradient, although this correspondence is less precise than in pulmonary stenosis. The murmur of aortic stenosis is midsystolic, crescendo, in some cases musical, and associated with a thrill that radiates to the right carotid area. The murmur is represented phonetically as RRR. The musical murmur is heard close to the apex (Gallavardin phenomenon) (HMM).

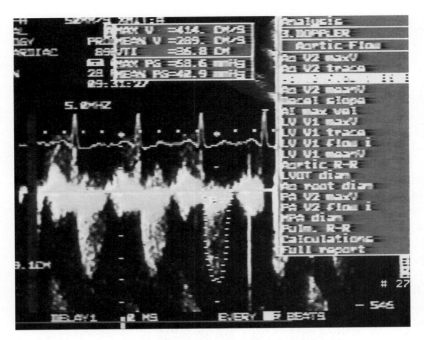

Figure 6-4 M-mode echocardiogram of aortic valve stenosis.

Mild In mild aortic stenosis the murmur is harsh, grade III-IV or louder, and there is an ejection click that may be heard also in severe aortic stenosis if the valve is mobile. Aortic valve closure is heard late, giving rise to reversed splitting of S_2 with a soft A_2 (DRup) (P_2A_2).

Moderate In moderate aortic stenosis, the murmur is longer and peaks later. If S_2 is audible at all, its reversed splitting may be obscured by its softness. This feature is particularly likely if calcification or immobilization of the aortic valve occurs. In the latter instance, the click is absent.

Severe (Cardiac Pearl 86) In severe aortic stenosis, the murmur is harsh, late-peaking, associated with a thrill, and may commence after a soft S_1. This murmur is holosystolic (persists throughout systole) with a crescendo quality that extends beyond pulmonary valve closure. The examiner should not be confused by the fact that an S_2 may not be heard at all. Note that a loud click can be heard in the presence of a mobile valve in severe aortic stenosis; and that the duration and delayed peaking in aortic stenosis is less reliable as a guide to severity than in pulmonary stenosis. S_1 is usually soft and is preceded by an S_4. This finding often denotes a gradient of less than 70 mmHg across the aortic valve. An aortic stenotic murmur may sound like a roar and may be grade VI (Table 2-3). Thus, its cardiophonetic (rrr) is rather like an early systolic murmur without an S_2, with a duration

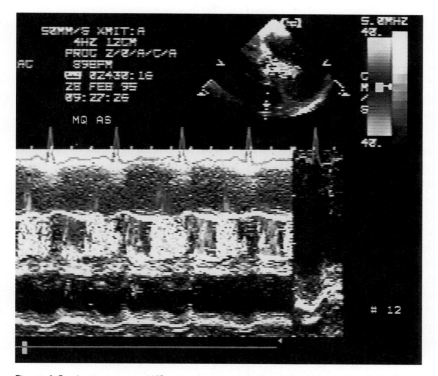

Figure 6-5 Aortic stenosis. M/Q scan showing turbulent mosaic between the valves.

that varies with severity. Occasionally, the clinician may hear a so-called Gallavardin dissociation (Cardiac Pearl 83). In this phenomenon, a high-pitched musical murmur is heard at the apex and a harsh systolic murmur is heard over the right second intercostal space (Table 6-1). In some instances of aortic stenosis, the harsh systolic murmur is unimpressive and the apical musical systolic murmur is the dominant feature (Lu-HMM'Dup), S_1 MSM S_2. In severe aortic stenosis, the systolic murmur and pulse alternate (auscultatory alternans); its phonophonic, RRR, has been likened to the growl of a dog baring its teeth. This sound is best heard to the right of the sternum, in the second right intercostal space. A significant feature of auscultatory S_2 in aortic stenosis is that it is lower in pitch, thus creating the illusion of a diamond-shaped murmur.

Pulsus parvus The primary diagnostic feature in aortic stenosis is the slow-rising small pulse that can be felt full between heartbeats and detected in the brachial and carotid arteries. The slow-rising pulse, so-called pulsus parvus or anacrotic pulse, is associated with a notch on the upslope of the slow percussion wave. In older patients, due to changed compliance in the blood vessels, the percussion wave of the pulse is large and interrupted by an anacrotic notch. Thus, it may be difficult to elicit the diagnosis of aortic stenosis in a patient in whom the pulse volume appears to be large, although the pulse wave is invariably delayed (tardus, non parvus). Occasionally, in older persons an anacrotic notch may not be readily felt on the upslope of the pulse due to Mönckeburg sclerosis. In aortic stenosis, a click precedes the murmur and there is reversed splitting of S_2 (P_2A_2). The click is absent only if the valve is immobile; hence, the click is more frequently heard in younger persons than in the elderly.

Aortic stenosis in the elderly   Aortic stenosis can be difficult to diagnose in the elderly, because S_1 is soft in this population, and the S_2 heard in the aortic area (AA) may be due to pulmonary valve closure (P_2). The examiner must therefore decide whether a diagnosis of aortic sclerosis or aortic stenosis is more appropriate. The differential diagnosis can be guided by fluoroscopic or echocardiographic determination of valvular calcification. The presence of an S_4 usually designates a gradient of 70 mmHg. S_1 is usually soft, either because of association with aortic stenosis or because of the presence of associated left bundle branch block (LBBB). The anacrotic shoulder, which should always be sought for identification, is more easily felt in the extended arm by palpating the brachial pulse while providing support to the arm. Thus, the slow-rising, full-volume anacrotic pulse characterizes aortic stenosis in the elderly.

An aortic systolic murmur in an elderly patient should point to a search for aortic stenosis. Carotid palpation of elderly patients may be difficult; carotid massage is contraindicated in these patients, in that it is a potential cause of bradycardia and asystole. Furthermore, the carotid pulse may be less accessible in a dyspneic patient.

Bicuspid valves (Cardiac Pearl 39)   Bicuspid aortic valves are a common cause of aortic stenosis in middle-aged persons. In younger patients, these are nonstenotic and noncalcific; the physical findings correspond to those that have been previously described in this book (Chap. 4).

In younger patients, it is important to detect bicuspid valves before they become stenotic (Figs. 6-6 and 6-7). A systolic ejection murmur is heard over the right side of the sternum, and there is a preceding aortic ejection sound. The detection of this click is of major importance and enables the examiner to distinguish between an innocent systolic murmur and the murmur of bicuspid aortic valves. The murmur is best heard in the right second intercostal space and may be associated with a soft immediate diastolic murmur lu tuk / duh (S_1 OS S_2 DM). It is significant that bicuspid valves are probably the most common congenital cardiac disease— occurring in 2 percent of the population—and that antibiotic prophylaxis is important in these patients. Bicuspid valves are associated with coarctation of the aorta (CoA). Soft diastolic murmurs are suspected when the sharp tup in S_2 is replaced by thh or dhh.

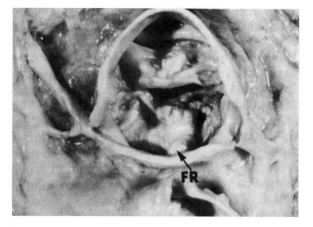

Figure 6-6 A calcified stenotic cogenitally bicuspid aortic valve. FR, false raphe. (From Am J Cardiol 1970; 26:72–83.

Congenital aortic stenosis Congenital aortic stenosis may present with bicuspid or unicuspid valves. In general, however, as compared with acquired aortic stenosis, the aortic ejection click is louder than S_1, calcification is late, and reversed splitting of S_2 is obvious because calcification has not yet immobilized the valve. Small, slow-rising pulses are characteristically

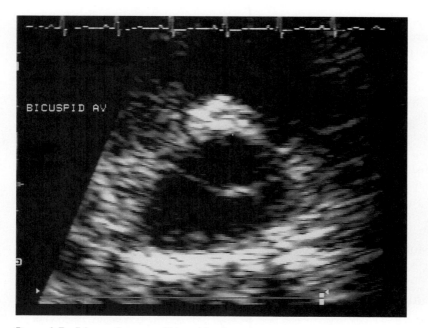

Figure 6-7 Echocardiogram of bicuspid valves.

found. The ECG shows evidence of "doming" of the valve, corresponding with the loud click. In infants, pseudoaortic stenosis due to a supravalvular xanthoma may be seen in homozygous type II hyperlipidemia. A systolic murmur, thrill, and click may be present.

Other Stenoses in the Aortic Area

Supravalvular stenosis   Supraaortic stenosis is a rare condition in which an hourglass deformity, web, or hypoplasia of the aorta (tunnel) may be present. The patient has features of so-called Williams' syndrome with hypercalcemia, mental retardation, elfin facies with pointed chin, strabismus, and thick lips. The diaphragm of the stethoscope is used to detect midsystolic murmur, heard high up under the right clavicle and often associated with a thrill. The pulse is weaker and blood pressure is lower by approximately 15 mmHg on the left arm than the right, caused by the so-called Coanda effect. In supraaortic stenosis, the ejection systolic murmur is usually heard on the right side and is crescendo and systolic. The Coanda effect is defined as streaming of blood into the left side, such that the right arm receives less blood.

Subvalvular stenosis   In patients with subaortic stenosis, the stenosis is caused by a tunnel or web. The systolic murmur is auscultable at the left sternal edge when the diaphragm of the stethoscope is used. This murmur is usually followed by a soft high-pitched diastolic murmur caused by aortic regurgitation. An ejection sound is not present.

Coarctation of the Aorta   In coarctation of the aorta (Fig. 6-8), a midsystolic murmur may be heard high over the right side of the chest, and

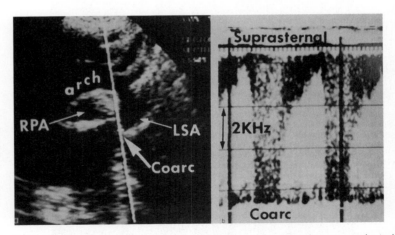

Figure 6-8 Two-dimensional and Doppler echocardiograms (suprasternal window) of coarctation of the aorta in a 10-month-old boy.

over the spine, corresponding to the second thoracic vertebra, simulating a continuous murmur. This murmur does not typically wax or wane like the murmur of a patent ductus arteriosus; it is long and may spill over S_2 into diastole. On physical examination, the features of Turner's syndrome with neck webbing may be seen. Associated midsystolic or continuous murmurs are elicited by having the patient stoop and hang the arms down in front of the body while the physician examines the shoulders, axillae, back, and supraclavicular areas for pulsation and continuous murmurs due to collaterals (Suzman's sign). This sign is also seen in tetralogy of Fallot, due to prominent intercostal arteries. Bicuspid valves with ejection sounds are an important associated abnormality in coarctation of the aorta.

Classic findings in coarctation of the aorta are a blood pressure that is lower in the left than the right arm and blood pressure in the lower limbs that is lower than normal. This so-called brachiofemoral lag may not always be present. It is important to obtain blood pressures in all four limbs. If the blood pressure in the lower limbs is slightly less than or equal to blood pressures in the right upper limb, in the setting of the clinical picture described, it is likely to indicate coarctation of the aorta. Furthermore, the peak of the femoral pulse is delayed with respect to the brachial artery, rather than the beginning of the pulse upslope. The murmur at the site of the coarctation may be continuous, late systolic and rough; or midsystolic, depending on the degree of stenosis. It is often associated with signs of bicuspid valves.

Hypertrophic Obstructive Cardiomyopathy (HOCM)   To detect hypertrophic obstructive cardiomyopathy (HOCM), use the diaphragm of the stethoscope with dynamic auscultation at the left lower sternal border. HOCM demonstrates the importance of skill in dynamic auscultation. The murmur associated with HOCM is one of two types: (1) midsystolic ejection and rough at the left sternal edge, grade III/VI; and (2) apical long systolic murmur, the murmur of mitral regurgitation associated with a pseudo-click and followed by reversed splitting of S_2. A long midsystolic ejection sound may be present, caused by systolic anterior motion of the mitral valve impacting the septum. These findings result from a systolic gradient (Fig. 6-9) across the outflow tract. The gradient is measured by Doppler and estimated by an M-mode echo, depending on the extent of valve/septal contact.

Gradients may be altered by several maneuvers and the changes in auscultatory position described in Chap. 2. These include the Valsalva maneuver, in which the patient lies supine and pushes the abdomen against the hands of the examiner while the examiner listens over the heart; or by having the patient strain, producing an immediate increase in the loudness of the murmur. Having the patient stand or inhale amyl nitrite accentuates the murmur; while having the patient squat, lie supine, or turn on the left side decreases it, as do pressor infusions (Cardiac Pearl 17).

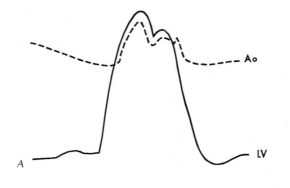

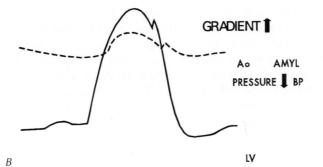

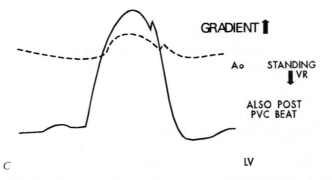

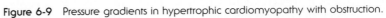

Figure 6-9   Pressure gradients in hypertrophic cardiomyopathy with obstruction.

Amyl nitrite administered during M-mode echocardiography may provoke or increase systolic anterior motion of the mitral valve, thus inducing the pseudoejection click and the long, somewhat rough systolic murmur of hypertrophic obstructive cardiomyopathy. The post pause phenomenon decreases the pulse volume and blood pressure but increases the murmur of hypertrophic obstructive cardiomyopathy.

Pulmonary Stenosis Pulmonary stenosis, like aortic stenosis, is associated with a midsystolic crescendo murmur over the pulmonary artery, a preceding ejection click, and a widely split S_2 with a soft second component caused by delayed pulmonary valve closure (Fig. 6-10). A prominent A-wave in the neck is seen. As pulmonary stenosis progresses, the click occurs earlier and fuses with S_1; in severe pulmonary stenosis it may fall before S_1. Pulmonary valve closure is absent and the harsh crescendo (RRR) murmur heard over the pulmonary artery runs the length of systole, covering A_2. The pulmonary ejection click is atypical of right-sided auscultatory events in that it disappears on inspiration. This atypicality is caused by elevation of right atrial pressure, right ventricular pressure, and partial preopening of the valves. The ejection sound or click is softened or disappears altogether. An S_4 may be present. The characteristic physical appearances are those associated with Noonan's syndrome, Williams' syndrome (Chap. 8), arterial hepatic dysplasia, and moon facies typical of pulmonary valve stenosis (Chap. 6). The murmur's grade and later peaking are related to increased gradient; the highest gradients are associated with loud murmurs and delayed peaking of the murmur in systole.

Infundibular pulmonary stenosis In infundibular stenosis, the location of the systolic murmur and thrill is in the third and fourth intercostal spaces.

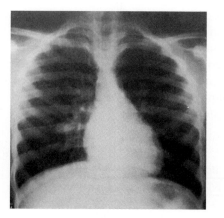

Figure 6-10 Posteroanterior chest x-ray from a 7-year-old boy with stenosis of the pulmonary arterial branches.

This location differs from pulmonary valvular stenosis in which the murmur is in the second/third interspace. A holosystolic murmur of ventricular septal defect, tricuspid regurgitation, or both are present (Table 6-5). The murmur is long and may be truly holosystolic rather than crescendo as in tetralogy of Fallot. Tricuspid regurgitation is distinguished by the duration of the murmur and its increase in time during inspiration (Carvallo's sign). Intercostal pulsations may be palpable. S_2 is single and an ejection sound is present. There is no jugular venous distention (JVD). In tetralogy of Fallot, the systolic murmur ends before S_2.

Tetralogy of Fallot   Tetralogy of Fallot is characterized by a nonrestrictive ventricular septal defect with left ventricular outflow resistance equal to or less than that of right ventricular outflow resistance. This differential produces right-to-left or biventricular shunting. Amyl nitrite may decrease the midsystolic murmur and may cause a fall in systemic blood pressure. Tetralogy of Fallot is associated with an ejection murmur often preceded by a click, and a single S_2.

Fallot's tetralogy is distinguished from infundibular pulmonary stenosis by the effect of amyl nitrite, which increases the ejection murmur in pulmonary stenosis and is not associated with an ejection sound in Fallot's tetralogy.

Pulmonary atresia S_2 is single in this condition and the murmur typically is heard high up in the second and third left intercostal spaces. It may, however, be heard in the fourth, or even the fifth, intercostal space since infundibular or subinfundibular stenosis may occur as well. A continuous murmur peaking at S_2 due to a patent ductus shunting from left to right may be heard.

In pulmonary atresia with systemic arterial collaterals, continuous murmurs may be heard due to anastomoses between bronchial arteries and pulmonary artery branches. Continuous murmurs are heard beneath the clavicle in the back or over the pulmonary area in patent ductus with pulmonary atresia. The presence of continuous murmurs over the chest wall indicates bronchopulmonary collateral and may be associated with decreased cyanosis and hypoplastic pulmonary arteries, making total correction difficult or at least more complicated.

Table 6-5   Differentiation of Pulmonary Stenosis

Pulmonary stenosis	Click	JVD	Holosystolic murmur
Valvular	+	+	−
Infundibular	−	+	+
Tetralogy of Fallot	+	−	−

Holosystolic Murmurs

Holosystolic murmurs (Figs. 6-11 and 6-12) are an important group of distinctive murmurs indicating blood flow persisting through systole. They are easily heard with the diaphragm of the stethoscope at the apex or left lower sternal border. There is no preejection period present; hence, flow occurs at the beginning of systole.

Mitral Regurgitation   Holosystolic murmurs are heard in mitral regurgitation (Table 6-6; Fig. 6-13), in which the murmur gets louder on expiration. The holosystolic murmur is blowing or musical, rarely harsh in character, often associated with a thrill. The murmur envelops S_1 and S_2, and may be associated with an S_3, which indicates that the mitral regurgitation is hemodynamically significant (Cardiac Pearl 15).

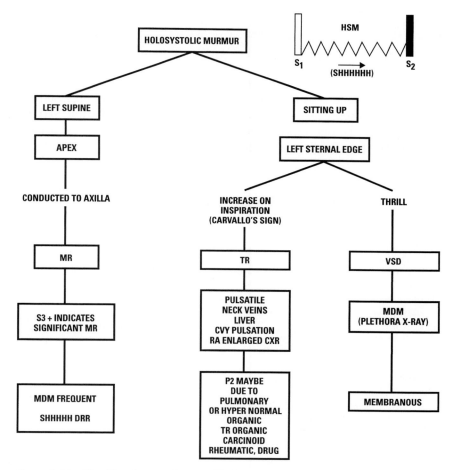

Figure 6-11   Algorithm for auscultation of holosystolic murmur.

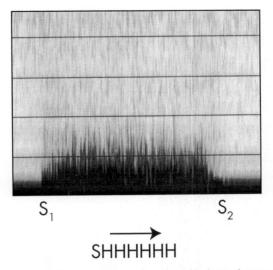

S_1 S_2

SHHHHHH

Figure 6-12 Acoustic spectrogram of holosystolic murmur.

Holosystolic murmurs are high-pitched and radiate to the axilla. Phonetically, the sound is as follows: shhh (SM S_2), with a slight crescendo at the end. In the presence of significant or severe mitral regurgitation, SHHH-DUP is heard, the dup representing S_3. Mitral regurgitation is not usually associated with an S_4, and may be heard in association with a short middias-

Table 6-6   Causes of Mitral Regurgitation

MR
  Mitral valve prolapse
  Functional
    LV dilatation
    Hypertrophic obstructive cardiomyopathy
  Rheumatic fever
  Endocarditis
    Libman-Sacks
    Infective
  Parachute mitral valve
  Left atrial myxoma (rare)
Acute MR
  Trauma
  Rupture
    Myxomatous valve
    Struts of parachute valve
    Belly of papillary muscle
      Endocardial
      Infarction
  Chordae tendineae

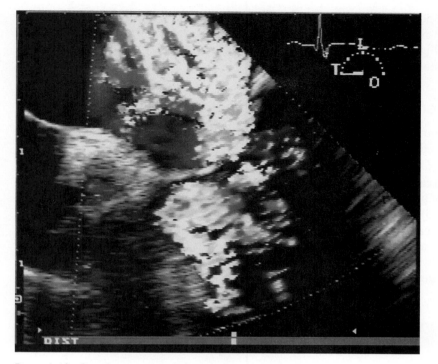

Figure 6-13 Doppler imaging of massive mitral regurgitation.

tolic murmur. Phonetically, this sounds like shhh du drrr (SM S$_2$ S$_3$ DM). A short middiastolic murmur is commonly seen in rheumatic mitral regurgitation. S$_2$ is physiologically split. In pure mitral regurgitation recorded from the apex on acoustic spectrography, S$_1$ and S$_2$ are not seen.

Ventricular Septal Defect Holosystolic murmurs in a ventricular septal defect (SHHH) may be heard at the left sternal edge in association with a thrill. The loudness of this thrill is unrelated to shunt flow. A murmur less commonly may be harsh. A systolic windsock sound splits S$_1$. There is physiological splitting of S$_2$ (DRUP). A$_2$ is louder than P$_2$. This separation distinguishes patients with VSD from those with HOCM, who have paradoxic splitting of S$_2$.

The holosystolic murmur of a ventricular septal defect may be followed by an early diastolic murmur simulating a ductus. The murmur does not peak at S$_2$. Phonic: SHHH' DHHH, not RRRR, as in a ductus with the murmur peaking at S$_2$, is seen with supracristal defects that occur most often in patients of Asian ancestry. The acoustic "covering" of S$_2$ by a crescendo murmur followed by a diminuendo is characteristic of a continuous murmur and matched by the phonocardiogram.

Tricuspid Regurgitation Holosystolic murmurs at the left lower sternal border that get louder on inspiration are caused by tricuspid regurgitation (Fig. 6-14). These murmurs may be secondary to valvular disease or heart failure.

Early Systolic Murmurs

Early systolic murmurs (Figs. 6-15 and 6-16) are listened for using the stethoscope diaphragm.

Acute Mitral Regurgitation (Cardiac Pearl 72) The early systolic murmur of acute mitral regurgitation may be caused by a number of factors (Table 6-5). This murmur can be rendered phonetically as RRR-DUP; the sound is caused by rapid elevation of left atrial pressure from S_1 to S_2 giving rise to an early systolic murmur (Chap. 3). It is followed by an audible S_3 and physiologic wide splitting of S_2. S_1 is often not heard or is soft. In acute mitral regurgitation, the direction of the jet determines the location of

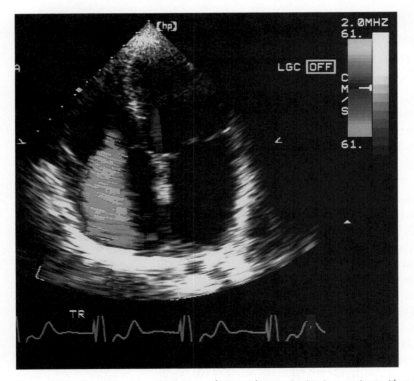

Figure 6-14 Two-dimensional imaging of tricuspid regurgitation in a patient with a dilated cardiomyopathy showing the Doppler image in the right atrium transgressing the tricuspid valve.

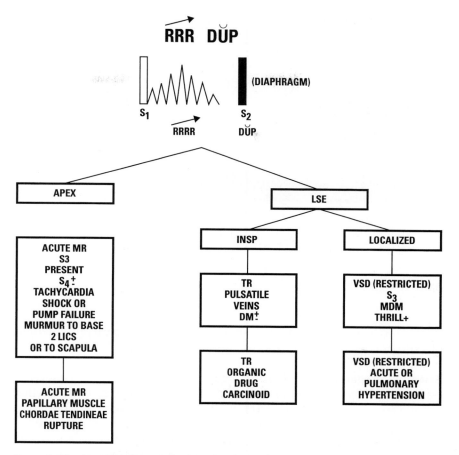

Figure 6-15   Algorithm for auscultation of early systolic murmur.

the murmur. With anterior papillary muscle belly rupture, the murmur is directed posteriorly and heard at the left scapula with postpapillary muscle belly damage. The jet directed anteriorly may manifest as a basal or "top of the head" murmur and be confused with an aortic ejection murmur. An S_3 may be heard. Early systolic murmurs are correctly diagnosed when S_1 is evident at the apex, and must not be confused with the midsystolic murmur of aortic stenosis auscultated in the aortic area. Patients are acutely dyspneic or in cardiogenic shock.

Atypical Murmurs of Ventricular Septal Defect   Other causes of early systolic murmurs include ventricular septal defects that are associated with pulmonary hypertension (Table 6-2). These apical holosystolic murmurs attenuate in duration. In tricuspid regurgitation due to carcinoid syndrome, an early or midsystolic murmur may appear on deep inspiration (Carvallo's

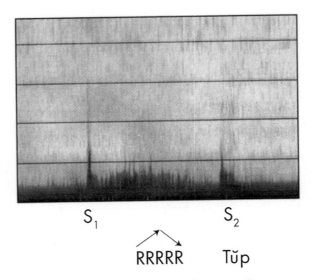

S_1 S_2

RRRRR   Tŭp

Figure 6-16 Acoustic spectrogram of early systolic murmur.

sign). Thus, midsystolic or early systolic murmurs are atypical presentations of ventricular septal defect and tricuspid regurgitation.

Tricuspid Regurgitation (Cardiac Pearl 74) Tricuspid regurgitation is characterized by a number of different types of murmurs: an early ejection systolic murmur; a holosystolic bruit; late systolic murmurs; or a bruit that ends before S_2, best heard at the left sternal edge. These different types of murmurs are all elicited by inspiration (Carvallo's sign). In severe tricuspid regurgitation, no bruit may be present. Pulsatile systolic venous waves designated cv-y and a pulsatile liver in systole may be encountered in severe tricuspid regurgitation. Rarely, pulsatile veins are seen in the scrotum. Right-sided tumors such as myxoma and lymphoma; carcinoid syndrome; Ebstein's anomaly; pulmonary hypertension; and drug-induced endocarditis, are other well-known diseases caused by tricuspid regurgitation. Tricuspid valve prolapse behaves in a similar manner to mitral valve prolapse, although the click and murmur are heard earlier in inspiration. Dynamic auscultation, however, enables the distinction to be made: The click falls earlier with sitting or standing due to decrease in heart size; it falls later on inspiration because of increased right ventricular size. The murmur in organic tricuspid regurgitation due to carcinoid is early soft systolic; in congestive heart failure, the murmur is holosystolic. Inspiration elicits the murmur.

Late Systolic Murmurs (Table 6-2)

Use the diaphragm of the stethoscope at the apex in auscultating these murmurs (Figs. 6-17 and 6-18).

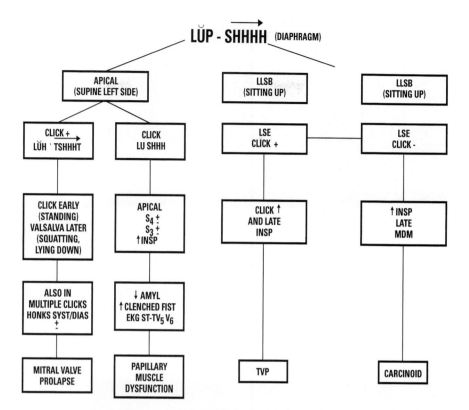

Figure 6-17   Algorithm for auscultation of late systolic murmur.

Mitral Valve Prolapse

Mitral valve prolapse (MVP) (Fig. 6-19) is the most common cause of mitral regurgitation in developed countries. A diastolic murmur in this condition is sometimes heard due to flow. The clinical features of MVP are outlined in the table.

Patients with this condition often present with anxiety as well as atypical chest pain, fatigue, and palpitations (Chap. 6). Characteristic associated findings are features of Marfan's syndrome or other forms of connective tissue disorder (e.g., Ehlers-Danlos syndrome or kyphoscoliosis of the spine). The ECG may show ST-T changes in the inferior and lateral leads (II, III, AVF, V_5, V_6).

The syndrome of mitral valve prolapse described by Barlow is now commonly recognized, and is classically associated with a systolic click and late systolic murmur, blowing in character with late peaking. Dynamic auscultation uses changes in the patient's position to alter the size of the heart (Chap. 2); this approach in turn enables detection of the motion of

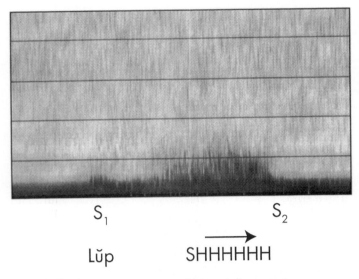

S_1 S_2

Lŭp   SHHHHHH

Figure 6-18 Acoustic spectrogram of late systolic murmur.

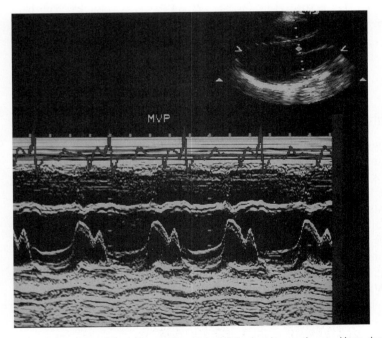

Figure 6-19 M-mode echocardiogram of mitral valve prolapse. Note the prolapse in systole.

the nonejection click and murmur. Thus, with patients in the standing position, the click and murmur tend to occur early. In the supine position and in squatting they occur late. Occasionally mitral and tricuspid valve prolapse may occur in the absence of auscultatory findings. At one extreme, MVP can be heard with a prominent click and an insignificant murmur; at the other end of the continuum, it may present with a pansystolic or holosystolic murmur and an S_3, as in mitral regurgitation. Major complications of mitral valve prolapse include ruptured chordae tendineae and acute mitral regurgitation. Embolism with a clot or vegetation lying on the valve, simulating mitral stenosis, is rare.

Echocardiographic characterization of a myxomatous appearance is important, although the diagnosis is clinical. Clicks may be single, multiple, systolic, or diastolic, and are associated with a late systolic murmur. This may be grade VI and heard as a whoop or honk. Clicks occur earlier with administration of amyl nitrite; the same drug causes multiple clicks to disappear. In other patients, clicks may be replaced by grade VI musical honks or whoops. Occasionally, the timing of clicks changes, causing split S_2 in the left lateral supine position and split S_1 in the sitting position. Clicks may masquerade as split S_2 or S_1.

Mitral Ring Calcification   Late systolic murmurs may be musical, harsh, or blowing in quality. They occur in pseudohypertrophic myopathy and in patients with inverted calcified mitral valve rings. Diabetes, hypertension, and female sex in older patients, are also associated with mitral inflow obstruction due to calcium. In these patients, AV block may occur, and atrial fibrillation is common.

Papillary Muscle Dysfunction   (Cardiac Pearl 76)
Following myocardial infarction, patients occasionally develop an apical late systolic murmur. This murmur can be represented phonetically as: Lup/shhh S_1/LSM. There is an auscultatory silence between S_1 and the late systolic murmur in papillary muscle dysfunction. On inspiration this murmur may occasionally get louder and is one of the few examples of left-sided murmurs that may become more audible on inspiration. This phenomenon is thought to be caused by the increased venous capacity of the lung and consequent reduction of left atrial pressure with increase in mitral regurgitation. The bruit may be transient during ischemia and can be made louder with the isometric exercise of sustained fist-clenching.

Aneurysms of the Ventricular Septum   These can cause late systolic murmurs that may be preceded by the windsock sound.

DIASTOLIC MURMURS

Middiastolic Murmurs (Table 6-2)

For auscultation of middiastolic murmurs (Fig. 6-20), apply the stethoscope bell to the apex and lower left sternal border. Diastolic murmurs are either

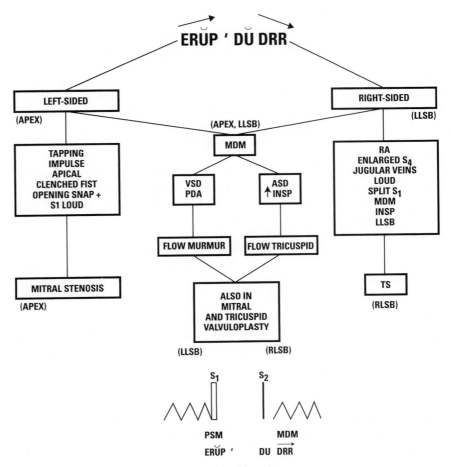

Figure 6-20 Algorithm for auscultation of middiastolic murmur.

delayed, i.e., middiastolic or presystolic with a pause after S_2; or immediate, promptly following S_2 (Fig. 6-21).

Note that diastolic murmurs are seldom innocent. The high-flow state of pregnancy is frequently associated with murmurs in midsystole and a loud S_3 simulating a diastolic murmur. A diastolic murmur in pregnancy must be considered abnormal until proven otherwise.

Flow Murmurs Increased flow antegrade or retrograde as in diastolic mitral regurgitation in the absence of stenosis of the valves may produce delayed diastolic murmurs in atrial septal defect. These delayed murmurs— louder on inspiration due to increased flow across the tricuspid valve—are musical or scratchy in character and enhanced by inspiration. They are

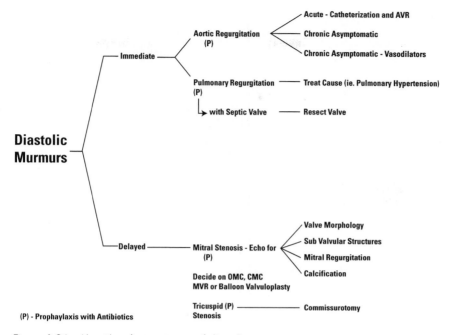

Figure 6-21   Algorithm for treatment of diastolic murmurs.

usually heard at the left sternal edge. Middiastolic murmurs may be heard in high-flow states such as ventricular septal defect as well. These are left-sided and are best heard at the apex in the left lateral position on expiration. A typical murmur of mitral stenosis is quite distinctive and extremely important to recognize. A double diastolic flow murmur may occur in atrial ventricular block.

Characteristically, diastolic flow murmurs due to shunts, whether right- or left-sided, usually indicate significant shunts. Echocardiography and contrast or color Doppler confirm the presence of shunts and allow quantification. Shunts may require coronary catheterization and surgery. Flow murmurs may also be heard following mitral and tricuspid valvuloplasty or replacement with tissue valves.

Mitral Stenosis   The clinical features of mitral stenosis are indicated in Chap. 4. Mitral stenosis is usually caused by rheumatic fever but may be seen in patients in degenerative states with calcification of the mitral valve, mitral ring, or both.

In mitral stenosis (Figs. 6-22 and 6-23), auscultatory findings may vary according to the presence of either pulmonary or systemic hypertension, or to both. Findings are also modified by atrial fibrillation, the condition

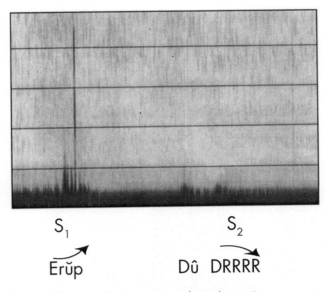

$$S_1 \qquad\qquad S_2$$

Erŭp   Dû DRRRR

Figure 6-22 Acoustic spectrogram of mitral stenosis.

of the valve, i.e., calcified or fibrotic, and by the presence of conditions such as mitral or aortic regurgitation. When mitral stenosis presents with a loud S_1 only, it is deemed silent.

In tight mitral stenosis the following are classically present: a loud S_1; a presystolic murmur; and a long diastolic murmur preceded by an opening snap (OS) with a short A_2-OS interval (50 to 70 ms). These sounds are heard in an area localized at the apex when the patient is in the left recumbent position. The apex may be displaced posteriorly by the right ventricle. The murmur of tight mitral stenosis may be audible over an area the size of an American twenty-five cent piece, as described by Osler. A thrill is associated with the murmur: ERUP' DU' DRR (S_1 S_2 MDM).

Pulmonary hypertension with right heart failure alters these physical findings, increasing the A_2-OS interval, diminishing the length of the murmur, and in extreme cases, abolishing it altogether (Table 6-7). Systemic hypertension in most cases increases the A_2-OS interval. The exception is acute hypertension in which A_2 falls late and the A_2-OS interval shortens. In long-standing hypertension with stiff left ventricles with left bundle branch block and aortic ectasia or aneurysms, A_2 falls late, hence, A_2-OS shortens. The pulmonic S_2 is accentuated and may be transmitted to the apex. In extreme cases, a loud S_1 may be all that is detected at first.

Mitral regurgitation may coexist with mitral stenosis; in fact, a blowing holosystolic murmur may be associated with a diastolic murmur. In this

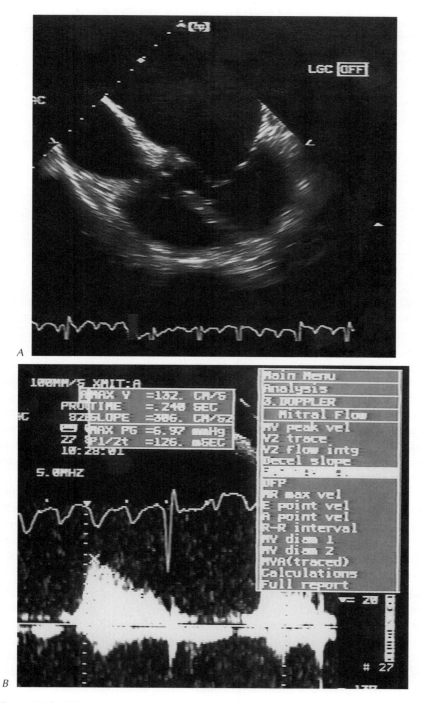

Figure 6-23 TEE (*A*) and Doppler (*B*) imaging pathognomonic of mitral stenosis. Doming of the mitral valve is seen, but no calcification, no papillary, and no chordal masses. The Doppler indicates the prolonged $t_{1/2}$ (half time) characteristic of mitral stenosis.

Table 6-7 Predominant Signs That Signal
Pulmonary Hypertension with Right
Ventricular Failure and Mitral Stenosis

Soft S_1
Increased A_2-OS interval
Right-sided failure
Loud P_2
Pulsatile liver
Ascites
Palpable spleen
Edema of the legs
Testicular atrophy
Gynecomastia
Telangiectasia
Palmar erythema
Parotid enlargement
Mitral facies

situation, if the predominant lesion is mitral regurgitation, an S_3 may be present. When the dominant murmur is middiastolic, an opening snap is usually present along with a loud S_1 and mitral stenosis is present. The pulse helps in differentiating whether mitral regurgitation or mitral stenosis is predominant; whereas a small collapsing pulse with a sharp up- and downslope is characteristic of mitral regurgitation, the pulse in mitral stenosis is, in contrast, of small volume. Occasionally a very loud diastolic murmur occurs. This murmur begins with a whine after S_2, and is caused by aortic regurgitation. It is followed by a rumbling loud middiastolic and presystolic murmur. A middiastolic murmur heard at the apex when the patient is sitting up, but not heard in the left supine position, may be a sign of an Austin Flint murmur (Table 6-1).

In mild mitral stenosis, a loud S_1 may be all that is auscultable until the patient has performed exercise and has turned on the left side, in which instance a middiastolic murmur may transiently appear. Whereas presystolic murmur is usually theoretically absent in atrial fibrillation and mitral stenosis, a transient middiastolic murmur is by no means clinically uncommon.

Pulmonary Hypertension   Auscultatory findings of mitral stenosis are attenuated in pulmonary hypertension associated with right heart failure with the: (1) decrease in the length of the murmur in middiastole; (2) prolongation of the A_2-OS interval; and (3) softening of S_1. The A_2-OS interval is invariably proportional to the left-arterial—left-ventricular (LA-LV) gradient and cardiac output, as well as to systemic vascular resistance.

In the presence of pulmonary hypertension with right ventricular failure and mitral stenosis with soft S_1 and increased A_2-OS interval, a patient may present with a range of signs including a pulsatile liver and palpable spleen; ascites; edema of the lower extremities; testicular atrophy and gynecomastia; telangiectasia, palmar erythema, and parotid enlargement. In these patients cardiac cachexia also may be present. Mitral stenosis is sometimes missed in these patients because liver failure may dominate the clinical picture.

Tricuspid Stenosis   Auscultation in patients with this condition is best done using the bell below the xiphoid process. The patient has suffusion of the face when supine, a prominent a presystolic venous wave, and split S_1 with loud T_1 best heard at the fourth and fifth left intercostal spaces. Also audible are a single S_2, and presystolic middiastolic murmurs and S_3. An S_3 is heard over the jugular veins. An opening snap may be present. The signs grow louder on inspiration. Mitral stenosis may coexist. Characteristically, inspiration (Carvallo's sign) intensifies the findings. Murmurs may be heard over the midclavicular line, due to enlarged right aorta and right ventricle. Presystolic hepatic pulsations may be present.

Differential Diagnosis of Middiastolic Murmurs

Organic pulmonary regurgitation   Organic pulmonary regurgitation is associated with a middiastolic murmur that is auscultated for using the bell over the apical pulmonary area.

Austin flint murmur   The Austin Flint murmur (Chaps. 3 and 6) is usually heard at the left sternal edge. This murmur is usually presystolic and middiastolic; the presystolic component disappears in acute aortic regurgitation. The Austin Flint murmur may be heard only at the apex with the patient in the sitting position and leaning to the left; and not heard with the patient in the left supine position.

Early Diastolic Murmurs (Table 6-2)

Early diastolic murmurs (Fig. 6-24) are listened for with the patient sitting up or in the knee-chest position (Chap. 2). The examiner uses the diaphragm to listen at the left lower sternal border, and sometimes at the right sternal border.

Immediate diastolic murmurs are an important characteristic of aortic regurgitation and pulmonary regurgitation (Fig. 6-21). Valvular aortic regurgitation normally is heard at the left sternal edge, is blowing in character, and occurs immediately after S_2 with a dual cadence, Lup/dhhh. It is accentuated by having the patient squat or clench a fist, or by administering pressors to the patient. The murmur of aortic regurgitation is characteristically early diastolic and heard at the left sternal edge, occasionally conducted to the apex (Cecil Cole murmur). The murmur may have a cooing character with a retroverted aortic cusp (Cardiac Pearl 13) or approximate the sound of

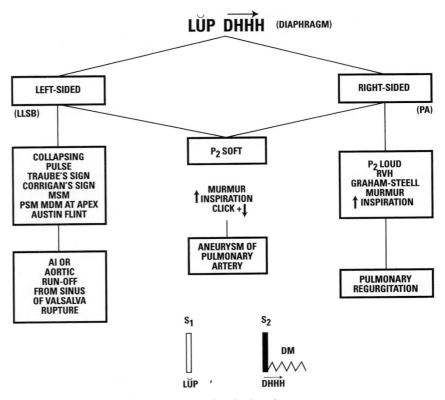

Figure 6-24 Algorithm for auscultation of early diastolic murmur.

wood being sawed. The murmur of aortic regurgitation can be associated with a middiastolic murmur, the Austin Flint murmur, and occasionally a late diastolic whoop. This murmur disappears with the administration of amyl nitrite and is not associated with a loud S_1. The presystolic component is usually heard in mild to moderate aortic regurgitation. A middiastolic murmur alone is heard in severe and acute aortic regurgitation. Occasionally a middiastolic (non-Flint) murmur is heard in aortic regurgitation down the left sternal edge. This has a triple cadence, Lup/du/dhh.

Pulmonary regurgitation is heard over the pulmonary artery and is high-pitched in pulmonary hypertension. Visible signs of aortic regurgitation include bounding pulses in the neck (Corrigan's sign); waterhammer pulses; capillary pulsation (Quincke's sign); and head bobbing (de Musset's sign). Acute aortic regurgitation may result in actual movement of the bed, observed on the ballistocardiogram.

McCusick first described the characteristic spectrograms of retroverted aortic valve cusp. In this condition, S_1 is soft, characteristically, and followed by midsystolic murmurs that may be as loud as grade IV, and rarely associated with a thrill giving rise to a to-and-fro murmur. These murmurs are distinguished from aortic stenosis by the character of the pulse; collapsing (rapid up- and downslope) in retroverted aortic valve cusp as distinct from anacrotic in aortic stenosis. S_2 is loud but may become soft in severe aortic regurgitation.

Acute Aortic Regurgitation (Cardiac Pearls 73, 77) Phonetically, acute aortic regurgitation (AR) sounds as follows: RRR' DH DU' DRR (SM S_2 DM). The RRR represents the early Austin Flint murmur. S_1 is absent.

Acute aortic regurgitation (Fig. 6-25) may occur as a result of infective endocarditis in a native or prosthetic valve; prosthetic valve dehiscence; or traumatic rupture. Acute AR constitutes a medical emergency. Phonetics are useful in diagnosing acute aortic regurgitation with subtle presentation. S_1 is absent. LUP'-DHH is replaced by RRR' DU DUP (MSM S_2 S_3), heard best at the left sternal border. The Austin Flint middiastolic murmur lup' du drr may be heard. DUP is caused by preclosure of the mitral valve (Chap. 3).

In severe aortic regurgitation, preclosure of the mitral valve occurs with characteristic echocardiographic findings. S_1 is soft to absent, and an Austin Flint murmur in late or middiastole is usually present. An S_3 is present, and is due to mitral valve preclosure in a patient who is critically ill. The murmur of aortic regurgitation is best heard with the patient sitting

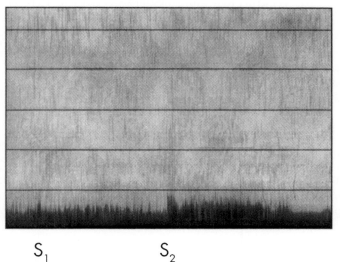

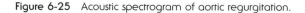

Figure 6-25 Acoustic spectrogram of aortic regurgitation.

up, with hands behind the back or over the head. As the patient is in full expiration, the examiner uses the diaphragm of the stethoscope for auscultation.

Aortic regurgitation is more prominent when the patient makes a clenched fist, and is reduced with the administration of amyl nitrite. The aortic regurgitation murmur is occasionally middiastolic at the left sternal border, and at the apex (Austin Flint) where it may be best heard. In aneurysms, it may be best heard in the right first intercostal space (Harvey's sign).

Pulmonary Regurgitation   Pulmonary regurgitation is seen with severe pulmonary hypertension or may be encountered in idiopathic dilatation of the pulmonary artery or as a result of valvular endocarditis. The murmur, called the Graham Steell murmur (Table 6-1) is localized over the pulmonary artery and may or may not be associated with a click. A Graham Steell murmur rarely grows louder on inspiration, is high-pitched, and has a rapid diminuendo quality. Doppler readings correlate well with the clinical findings and enhance diagnostic precision. This is especially so when Doppler measurement is combined with transesophageal echo (TEE). Graham Steell murmurs are preceded by a loud P_2.

Patients with organic pulmonary regurgitation due to valve disease not due to pulmonary hypertension have a murmur over the pulmonary area that is typically a triple cadence with a middiastolic blow (lup du dhh), not unlike mitral stenosis. These patients may have accentuation of the murmur on inspiration or with amyl nitrite, indicating the right-sided origin. P_2 is soft or absent. The typical murmur is early diastolic in pulmonary hypertension (Graham Steell).

Although the condition itself rarely requires treatment unless the valve is a focus for septic embolization, the pulmonary hypertension associated with the condition should be treated.

OTHER MURMURS

Changing Murmurs

Changing murmurs are a common feature encountered in alterations in high-output states, as in anemia, thyrotoxicosis, and pregnancy. In the treatment of hypertension with failure, a mitral regurgitation murmur may be detected that disappears as the blood pressure is controlled. Conversely, mitral systolic murmurs may diminish or disappear in shock or severe heart failure, due to poor flow. Innocent murmurs do not change to any degree, while the middiastolic murmur characteristic of acute rheumatic fever (Carey-Coombs) and mitral regurgitation are characteristically evanescent.

Murmurs may alter their characteristics in acute myocarditis and acute endocarditis, as well as in patients with cardiac tumor. Mechanical factors such as clots, tumors, vegetations, pannus, or valve damage can cause changing murmurs. Musical murmurs may change in character from day to day.

The importance of using notation, i.e., phonoacoustograms, to record murmurs is that this enables the clinician to recognize changes over time. Murmurs change when hemodynamics alter the factors causing the murmurs.

Continuous Murmurs

Continuous murmurs (Figs. 6-26 and 6-27) occur in systole and diastole, are phonetically sounded as RRRRR, and peak at S_2, acoustically obliterating it. The causes of continuous murmurs are listed in Table 6-2.

Patent Ductus Arteriosus   The murmur of a patent ductus arteriosus (PDA) (Fig. 6-28) is physiological at birth, systolic in timing, and disappearing on about the third day of life. In the adult this murmur results from shunting of blood from the aorta through an open passage into the pulmonary artery, close to the subclavian artery. The single most important point about the murmur is that its maximum intensity is centered around S_2.

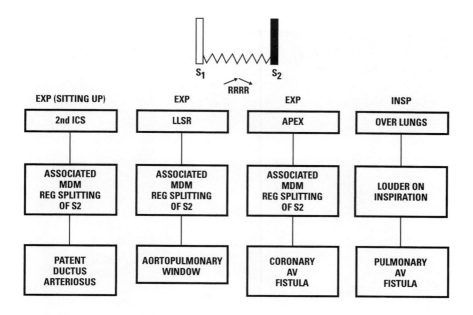

Figure 6-26   Algorithm for auscultation of continuous murmur.

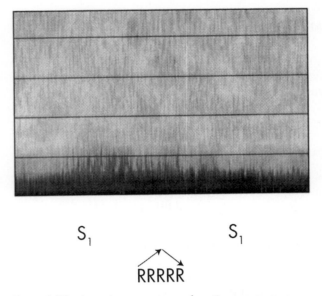

S_1 S_1

RRRRR

Figure 6-27 Acoustic spectrogram of continuous murmur.

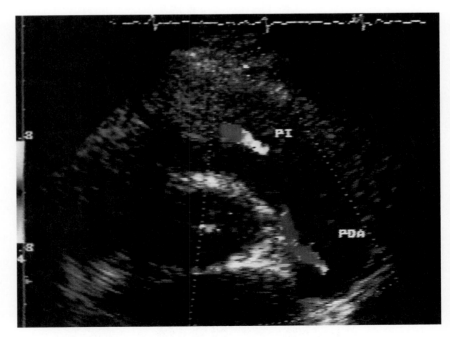

Figure 6-28 Doppler imaging of patent ductus arteriosus.

The murmur is heard in systole and diastole. Isometric exercise (e.g., fist clenching) prolongs the murmur even further into diastole.

The murmur of patent ductus arteriosus is heard in the second left intercostal space and is localized. Its associated features include vigorous arterial pulsations over the carotids and the presence of a wide pulse pressure. In neonates, elevated resistance in the pulmonary circuit leads to the presence of a midsystolic murmur in this area. Midsystolic murmurs are distinguished from ejection murmurs, which are usually heard over the carotids. A continuous murmur of a ductus arteriosus causes increased flow through the lungs and enlarges the left atrium, thus leading to a delayed diastolic flow murmur arising from increased blood flow across the mitral valves. This murmur is a result of excessive flow and is best heard in the left lateral position on full expiration with the bell of the stethoscope.

Clearly, the more obvious the collateral flow, the rosier the patient's complexion, and the more likely that the flow through the pulmonary artery is significant. In severe pulmonary artery atresia, the patent ductus alone may maintain flow through the pulmonary circuit through one or both branches of the pulmonary artery. Notably, the presence of continuous murmurs over the chest, representing bronchopulmonary anastomosis, is inversely related to the degree of cyanosis in a child with pulmonary atresia. Surgery to correct this condition is less promising than for pulmonary artery atresia.

The natural history of patent ductus arteriosus murmur, if it leads to pulmonary hypertension, is such that over a period of years, it may attenuate and eventually become a systolic murmur peaking late in systole that may disappear altogether in the presence of severe pulmonary hypertension. The systolic murmur starts soft, is loudest at the closure of the aortic valve, and then gradually grows softer. In pulmonary hypertension, reversal of flow may occur in the ductus; this leads to cyanosis of the toes and fingers of the left hand with clubbing and relative sparing of the right upper extremity. These patients have palpable S_2s with normal splitting and have pulmonary hypertension with a reversed ductus. This condition is sometimes called Eisenmenger's syndrome with reversed flow through a ductus arteriosus, to distinguish it from Eisenmenger's complex, which describes a ventricular septal defect in association with pulmonary hypertension and a reversed shunt. In contrast, patients with Taussig-Blalock syndrome, double outlet syndrome, and transposition with patent ductus arteriosus, shunt through their ductus into the feet and have reversed differential cyanosis with pink toes and blue fingers.

Jugular Venous Hum A jugular venous hum, resulting from abnormal flow in the jugular veins, is heard as continuous murmurs in the supraclavicular area and is common in pregnancy. The clinician examining the patient's neck should not confuse jugular venous hum with an arteriovenous fistula or some other form of arteriovenous communication. A diagnosis is readily made by auscultating over the right clavicle and turning the neck to one side, which may increase or abolish the hum. Placing the index finger over the vein above the murmur extinguishes it. A jugular venous hum is a normal physiological finding. Jugular venous hums, first described by Pontain in 1867, are universal in children and have been heard in healthy adults as well. Intensity can vary from faint to being auscultable without a stethoscope.

Dynamic auscultation can alter jugular venous hum; deep inspiration may augment it. In addition, the supine position and Valsalva maneuver are useful in reducing the intensity of deep venous hums or abolishing them. Although the hum is continuous and unassociated with the presence of an S_1 or S_2, it is typically louder in diastole than in systole.

Aortopulmonary Window An aortopulmonary window is a low-lying communication (described as a "window") between the aorta and the pulmonary arteries. Austin in 1830 described the first known case of aortopulmonary window. The murmur is usually continuous but is heard best in the third or fourth intercostal space. This condition occurs commonly in males, in contrast to patent ductus arteriosus, which is more common in females. In rare cases, heart failure can result. Aortopulmonary windows also can cause pulmonary hypertension with a syndrome similar to patent ductus arteriosus. With aortopulmonary window, however, the reversal of the shunt causes central cyanosis in the entire body, rather than differentially, as in patent ductus arteriosus.

Largely on account of the fact that aortopulmonary windows are nonrestrictive and associated with elevated pulmonary vascular resistance, continuous murmurs are less commonly heard. On occasion, murmurs may be absent in the presence of significant pulmonary hypertension; and a single S_2 may be heard with a Graham Steell murmur. With significant pulmonary hypertension, right ventricular hypertrophy, A waves and central cyanosis develop. In infancy, as with the shunt in ventricular septal defects, heart failure can occur. In both patent ductus arteriosus and in aortopulmonary windows, patients are acyanotic. Bounding arterial pulses and wide pulse pressures are not features of a ventricular septal defect, which can be confused with this condition. Two-dimensional echocardiogram confirms the diagnosis. Color Doppler, as well as Doppler imaging, allows accurate localization. The use of the intravascular Doppler wire may help localize the site of the shunt.

Arteriovenous Fistulae

Coronary arteriovenous fistulae These are commonly seen in patients with shunts between the coronary artery and coronary veins, and at the origin of the left coronary arteries from the pulmonary artery. This condition rarely occurs iatrogenically, but is seen on occasion with severe angina resulting from the so-called "steal syndrome." Incidence is about the same in males and females. In these fistulae, a continuous murmur exists from birth and is heard at the apex. The majority of patients are symptomatic and may present with effort dyspnea, congestive failure, angina, and myocardial infarction. The patient's growth is usually not affected, and the pulses are normal in an acyanotic patient. Sudden death may supervene at any age, although patients are known to have survived into their late 60s. On occasions where the arteriovenous fistula drains into the atrium or coronary sinus, atrial fibrillation may herald the onset of congestive failure.

The location of the murmur varies and may be heard in the right lower sternal border, just across the midline in the subxiphoid area; at the apex; or at the upper mid-left sternal border. These locations correspond with the artery involved—usually enlarged—and the vein or right-sided chamber into which it drains. As in patent ductus arteriosus, increased flow into the right side of the heart produces a middiastolic murmur across the mitral or tricuspid valves. The Valsalva maneuver (Phase 4; see Chap. 2) may cause the arteriovenous murmur to soften as pressures in the right side of the heart rise.

Pulmonary arteriovenous fistulae   Pulmonary arteriovenous fistulae cause central cyanosis and digital clubbing. They present with continuous murmurs located anywhere in the lungs. The murmur gets louder on inspiration, in contrast to the continuous murmurs described earlier in this chapter. The diagnosis can be made by injecting contrast material into the right side of the heart, as is done in echocardiography, and following the time course of the contrast. Delayed return of contrast material to the left atrium is strong evidence of bronchopulmonary anastomosis. This differs from the immediate appearance of contrast material in the left atrium in a patent foramen ovale. This process is well demonstrated with a contrast agent such as Albuminex. Pulmonary arteriovenous fistulae are frequently associated with hereditary capillary telangiedema (HCT) seen in the tongue, skin, and angiomas in organs such as the liver (Cardiac Pearl 26). Cyanosis may occur and treatment is by embolization of the fistulae.

Collateral Vessels

Intercostal collateral arteries   Suzman, the South African cardiologist, described a sign in which patients who are asked to bend down with their arms hanging at their sides, show collateral arteries around the shoulders, along the right and left sternal borders, and, less commonly, over the upper abdominal walls. Continuous murmurs may be heard over these collateral vessels, with axillary palpable pulsations in coarctation of the aorta and in extreme tetralogy of Fallot.

Bronchopulmonary collateral vessels   The bronchial arteries may anastomose with the central pulmonary artery; or it may enter the lung parenchyma and branch within it with no connections. These collateral vessels give rise to continuous murmurs. Collaterals are seen in pulmonary atresia and the anastomoses provide collateral to the lung. Bronchopulmonary collaterals can be auscultated anywhere over the lungs and give rise to continuous murmurs. Intercostal pulsations may occur (Suzman's sign).

Pulmonary Branch Stenosis   In pulmonary branch stenosis seen in the rubella syndrome, systolic murmurs extend into diastole. They are heard in the axillae or over the lung.

Mammary Soufflé   Continuous murmurs are heard late in pregnancy anywhere over either breast. This so-called mammary soufflé, literally "puff" in French, has a tendency to be loud in the second or third right or left intercostal space on either side bilaterally. The murmur begins after a gap following S_1 and runs throughout systole. The pitch may be relatively high, but the murmur is not musical. Mammary soufflé is best heard when the patient is supine and may vanish when the patient sits up. The murmur's intensity is not affected by the Valsalva maneuver, although local compression can eliminate the murmur. The loudness may vary from time to time. Although the murmur of patent ductus arteriosus may be simulated, the mammary soufflé peaks earlier. Continuous murmurs over the uterus are heard in normal pregnancy.

Anomalous Coronary Arteries   Continuous murmurs are extremely important as a sign of anomalous coronary arteries.

Dock's murmur   Dock's murmur (Table 6-1) is an early diastolic murmur that is heard with stenoses of epicardial coronary artery disease. Anomalous origin of the coronary arteries and the pulmonary artery may occur with involvement with the left main, right, left anterior descending, or left circumflex coronary arteries. The associated murmurs are localized over the precordium and are early diastolic.

Anomalous origin of the left main coronary artery   Anomalous origin of the left main coronary artery is detected in infancy. A small percentage of affected children reach adulthood because of effective intracoronary collaterals. Patients present with papillary muscle dysfunction, mitral regurgitation, congestive failure, and the typical auscultatory findings of these conditions. In the presence of anomalous origin of the left coronary artery to the pulmonary artery, a loud continuous murmur is heard along the sternal border or at the base, reflecting retrograde flow through intracoronary anastomoses, connecting left and right coronary arteries. A mitral regurgitation murmur and an S_3 may be present, as well as cardiomegaly. Angiography of the right coronary artery demonstrates extensive collateralization to branches of the left main coronary artery and opacification of the pulmonary artery. These patients have a high incidence of sudden death; surgical correction is recommended.

Anomalies of the right coronary artery   Anomalies of the right coronary artery from the pulmonary artery may occur. The condition presents with dyspnea or angina.

Anomalous origin of the left anterior Descending Artery   The left anterior descending artery may arise anomalously from the pulmonary artery, with origin of the right and circumflex coronary arteries from the appropriate sinus of Valsalva. Patients with this condition have severe myocardial ischemia, mitral regurgitation, papillary muscle dysfunction, and may have continuous murmurs. The degree of sensitivity of this sign is low, however, especially in young patients. These murmurs may be heard over pancreatic tumors or hepatomas, as well as over the overly large heart.

Anomalous origin of the circumflex coronary artery   Anomalous origin of the circumflex coronary artery appears to be a benign condition. Coronary arteries may arise aberrantly from the aorta.

Anomalous origins of coronary arteries in the sinus of valsalva   Occasionally, the left main coronary artery arises from the right sinus of Valsalva. These anomalies, although sometimes responsible for sudden death, are not associated with distinct physical signs. Similarly, the right coronary arteries may arise aberrantly from the left sinus of Valsalva. The condition may be associated with myocardial ischemia and heart block.

Other Continuous Murmurs   Other causes of continuous murmurs include total anomalous pulmonary venous drainage, a small atrial septal defect, portal venous collateral over the abdomen, renal artery stenosis, severe iliac stenosis, bruits over vascular thyroid glands, vascular tumors (e.g., hemangiomas), and aortic coarctation. Continuous murmurs are also seen in Cruveilhier-Baumgarten syndrome due to portacaval connections in Laennec's cirrhosis. The murmur of coarctation and other stenotic murmurs may be continuous in tight obstructions, late systolic in intermediate cases, and midsystolic in mild stenosis. Continuous venous bruits are heard over the fontanelle in infancy. Carotid-cavernous sinus fistulae may cause continuous murmurs, as well.

To-and-Fro Murmurs (Table 6-2)

By definition, to-and-fro murmurs are midsystolic and early diastolic murmurs with a gap in systole between them and augmentation of the diastolic component (Fig. 6-29). To-and-fro murmurs are usually caused by rupture of a mycotic aneurysm in a sinus of Valsalva into the right atrium or the right ventricle, and less commonly by rupture into the left atrium. The clinical picture is one of rapidly developing failure in a patient who has a to-and-fro murmur with diastolic attenuation. Ventricular septal defects of the supracristal type may cause atypical to-and-fro murmurs; these are holosystolic and early diastolic murmurs (SHHH / DHHH). A ductus is characterized by a continuous murmur with systolic accentuation with peaking of the murmur at S_2, obliterating S_2. Phonetically, this murmur is represented by RRRRR. In contrast, luh/du/dhh (S_1 MSM S_2 EDM) designates the presence of a to-and-fro murmur that can also be heard with a combination of conditions listed in Table 6-2. S_2 (DU) is heard distinctly and separately from LUP and DHH.

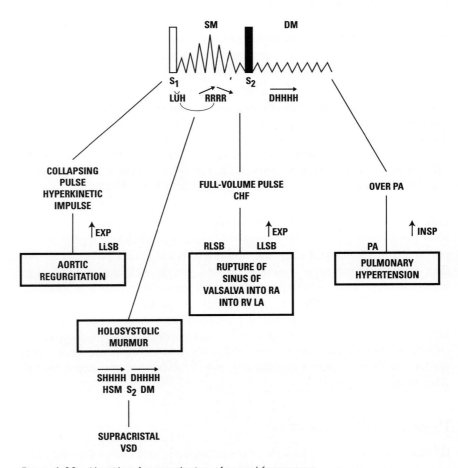

Figure 6-29 Algorithm for auscultation of to-and-fro murmur.

BRUITS

Ectopic Bruits

Ectopic bruits are heard over the carotid arteries and are important in the diagnosis of carotid stenosis. These sounds may be brought out by rotation of the neck and by auscultation. Ectopic bruits in older patients and those with transient ischemic attack (TIA) or stroke may suggest carotid stenosis; hence murmurs of this type provide strong reason to perform a Duplex Doppler study to detect obstructions in the carotid arteries that may presage stroke.

There has been an extensive amount written about bruits in the abdomen in general; they may denote stenoses in arteries, such as the celiac or mesenteric arteries, or may be present over abdominal aneurysms. The degree of sensitivity and specificity of this sign is low, however.

Bruits over the flanks are even more unpredictable. These may be heard over pancreatic tumors or over hepatomas.

Arteriovenous bruits may be heard over the spleen, over the liver, and may be part of the picture of the Osler-Rendu-Weber syndrome. It is evident that extraneous bruits are important to listen for on a regular basis.

Auscultation of Bruits

For the most effective detection of bruits, listen to the heart, both carotid arteries, over the abdomen, and to both femoral arteries. Continuous bruits are heard over arteriovenous fistulae and become discontinuous as the fistula clots. The absence of bruit should alert one to the possibility of an obstructed arteriovenous fistula. The high prevalence of innocent bruits (7 to 31 percent) in younger age groups dictates that in normotensive asymptomatic individuals, no further investigation is warranted. In patients with signs of renovascular hypertension, there is a high specificity of systolic bruit, in particular of systolic and diastolic bruits. Subsequent investigation should consider renovascular hypertension; a captopril renogram or angiogram should be performed. Auscultation of the abdomen in young patients is often negative. Signs of possible renovascular disease or renal artery embolism in older patients include systolic and diastolic bruits, diastolic hypertension, renal failure of unexplained origin, and atrial fibrillation with sudden development of hypertension.

In general, renal artery bruits are high-pitched systolic and diastolic and may be accentuated with inspiration. Renovascular disease bruits are localized in 70 percent of patients with fibromuscular disease and in 43 percent of patients with atherosclerotic disease. Bruits over the head may be accentuated by compression of the opposite carotid artery.

TRUE OR FALSE

1. Papillary muscle dysfunction may lead to a variety of systolic murmurs, holosystolic, late, or ejection.

2. Tricuspid regurgitation murmurs are not always holosystolic but are accentuated by inspiration.

3. The middiastolic bruit of atrial septal defect is decreased with inspiration.

4. The click murmur syndrome may be due to tricuspid valve prolapse.

5. In mitral regurgitation and ventricular septal defect, S_4 is rare.

6. S_1 and S_2 may both be absent in severe aortic stenosis, listened to at the apex.

7. Systolic and diastolic murmurs are heard in both aortic stenosis and aortic regurgitation but are differentiated by the pulse.

8. An Austin Flint murmur in acute aortic regurgitation is presystolic.

9. Pulmonary regurgitation murmurs are all named Graham Steell murmurs.

10. Organic pulmonary regurgitant murmurs may be middiastolic.

11. A patient with a patent ductus arteriosus with a reversed shunt presents with clubbed cyanotic toes and pink nails on the right hand, while a patient with transposition with a patent ductus or Taussig-Bing syndrome presents with cyanosed fingers which are clubbed and pink toes.

12. Continuous murmur over the abdomen may be due to portal venous collaterals caused by the Cruveilhier-Baumgarten syndrome.

13. An ectopic murmur heard over the aorta or the flanks in a young patient is unlikely to be of clinical significance.

14. Patent ductus arteriosus with reversed shunt may present with cyanosis of the toes and of the left arm and the absence of a systolic murmur with a loud P_2.

15. Truncus arteriosus is an important cause of continuous murmur. S_2 is single.

CLINICAL VIGNETTES

The following vignettes present actual cases of patients who were affected by diseases and conditions discussed in this chapter. At the end of each case, choose the single answer that best describes the diagnosis indicated by the vignette.

1. A 30-year-old female was referred with a heart murmur. Examination revealed a grade III buzzing ejection systolic murmur at Erb's point associated with physiological wide splitting of S_2 with a loud P_2 ($P_2 > A_2$). With the patient in the sitting position, a right ventricular impulse was felt and an S_3 was heard at the apex. The patient had pectus excavatum with no evidence of pulmonary hypertension or cor pulmonale and straight back syndrome.
   The diagnosis is:

A. Atrial septal defect
B. Straight back syndrome
C. Pulmonary hypertension

2. A 54-year-old male patient had a large, pulsatile bulging mass about the size of a watermelon on his chest. There was, in fact, no sternum; the bone had been eroded by an underlying aneurysm. Overlying it was a loud systolic murmur and a peculiar S_2, phonetically like toh (tock, a guttural 'ch' as in German ich), giving the murmur a tambour quality followed by an early diastolic murmur. The chest x-ray indicated calcification of the ascending aorta.
    The diagnosis is:

A. Marfan's syndrome, with aneurysm
B. Syphilitic aneurysm
C. Dissecting aneurysm

3. On examination, a 30-year-old female patient had an ejection systolic murmur of grade III intensity preceded by an ejection sound over the second right intercostal space. On second examination on the following day, after the patient had received a transfusion, no murmur or ejection sound was audible. The pulse had decreased in rate and volume from the previous day.
    The diagnosis is:

A. Bacterial endocarditis
B. Hemic murmur
C. Bicuspid valves

4. A 60-year-old male patient was seen in his hospital room. He had presented with angina, and had given a history of coronary artery bypass surgery. On auscultation, the patient had delayed pulses and a systolic murmur over the aortic area in the right second intercostal space. This patient was in heart failure; the a systolic murmur (grade II) was not impressive, but the anacrotic pulses, single S_2, calcification of the valves, and subsequent echocardiogram with Doppler confirmed the diagnosis.
    The diagnosis is:

A. Aortic stenosis
B. Aortic sclerosis
C. Hemic murmur
D. All of the above

5. A 75-year-old male patient was examined who had hypertension and a midsystolic murmur over the chest with an accentuated single P_2. The patient's toes were clubbed and cyanotic. The left hand was clubbed and less cyanotic while the right hand was normal. The patient

had pulsating neck veins, accentuation of pulmonary valve closure with close physiological splitting, diminished pulses in the left arm and lower extremities.
The diagnosis is:

A.   Eisenmenger ductus arteriosus
B.   Eisenmenger syndrome with atrial septal defect
C.   Eisenmenger complex

6.   A 50-year-old male patient presented with hypertension. Examination revealed large bounding upper extremity pulses with a low blood pressure in the legs. The patient had robust upper truncal development but thin lower limbs. Auscultation indicated the presence of a grade III systolic murmur, ejection in type, over the aortic arch, preceded by a click, and a continuous murmur at the back in the midline close to the spine. Brachiofemoral lag was present. An angiogram was performed.
The diagnosis is:

A.   Bicuspid valves
B.   Coarctation of the aorta
C.   Both of the above

7.   A female patient, aged 75, developed sudden chest pain with some ECG changes indicating ST segment elevation in V_2 and V_3. The patient was examined prior to administration of nitrites. This examination revealed sharp bisferiens [double impulse] carotid pulses and a long apical crescendo harsh systolic murmur located at the left sternal edge. The murmur was heard only when the patient was asked to sit up. S_2 had reversed splitting.
The diagnosis is:

A.   Impending myocardial infarction
B.   Hypertrophic obstructive cardiomyopathy (HOCM)
C.   Mitral regurgitation

8.   A 56-year-old male patient was seen with chest pain and acute failure after shoveling eight inches of wet snow off his driveway. Auscultation revealed an early systolic murmur at the apex with a loud S_3. The patient was immediately scheduled for surgery. The ECG did not show signs of infarction, and no thrill was felt.
The diagnosis is:

A.   Acute mitral regurgitation
B.   Acute ventricular septal defect with myocardial infarction
C.   Dissecting aneurysm

9.   A 6-year-old female patient was examined. She had strikingly sharp facial features, lean long fingers, and a deformed chest. Auscultation

revealed an apical, late systolic murmur with two or three clicks preceding the murmur.
The diagnosis is:

A. Mitral valve prolapse
B. Marfan's syndrome
C. Both of the above

10. A female patient, age 30 years old, presented with few symptoms except a history of fatigue. After conducting formal auscultation, the examiner asked the patient to stand and touch her toes 10 times, and lie down between each attempt. The examiner then turned the patient on her side, auscultated the apex with the bell of the stethoscope and could hear phonetically a rrup' du drrr (S_1 S_2 DM), rrup' du drrr, rrup, rrup. Thus, the diastolic murmur, which is represented by the drrr, provoked by exertion, disappeared after the first two beats of auscultation, replaced by Tup-S_2.
The diagnosis is:

A. Mitral stenosis
B. Physiological S_3
C. Pericardial knock

11. A 70-year-old female patient presented with complete heart block and a diastolic murmur. The chest x-ray showed calcification of the AV ring. The echocardiogram showed no masses and a normal mitral valve.
The diagnosis is:

A. Rytand syndrome
B. Mitral stenosis
C. Left atrial myxoma

12. A 60-year-old male patient developed a diastolic murmur (new) 2 weeks after cardiac surgery. He was febrile and had a history of prostatitis. The murmur evolved over the next few days; a loud systolic murmur and an S_3 were present with an absent S_1 and an apical middiastolic murmur. P_2 was slightly accentuated. An echocardiogram was ordered.
The diagnosis is:

A. Acute aortic regurgitation
B. Pulmonary regurgitation
C. Vegetation in mitral valve

13. A 31-year-old female was seen during her eighth month of pregnancy. A loud continuous murmur was heard over the left breast in the left intercostal space. The patient was found to lose the murmur with stethoscope compression.
The diagnosis is:

A. Patent ductus arteriosus
B. Mammary soufflé
C. Aortopulmonary window

ANSWERS

True or False

1. *T*; 2. *T*; 3. *F*; 4. *T*; 5. *T*; 6. *T*; 7. *T*; 8. *F*; 9. *F*; 10. *T*; 11. *T*; 12. *T*; 13. *T*; 14. *T*; 15. *T*.

Clinical Vignettes

1. *B, Straight back syndrome.* A buzzing ejection systolic murmur, not associated with fixed splitting of S_2, would tend to rule out *A*. The absence of right ventricular enlargement, although a right ventricular impulse was felt, in the presence of pronounced pectus excavatum makes the diagnosis of right ventricular enlargement difficult. Thus *B, straight back syndrome with physiological wide splitting of S_2, P_2 louder than A_2, is* the most likely diagnosis.

2. *B, Syphilitic aneurysm.* A pulsatile mass on the front of the chest would rule out a dissecting aneurysm. A differential diagnosis between syphilitic aneurysm and an aneurysm associated with Marfan's syndrome is difficult to make; however, a rapidly expanding aneurysm that has eroded into the sternum would tend to favor syphilitic aortitis and aneurysm. The linear calcification in the ascending aorta is a further point.

3. *B, Hemic murmur.* The absence of sepsis in a patient who is not obviously ill and cessation of the murmur after a transfusion would make *B* the likely diagnosis, i.e., hemic murmur caused by anemia.

4. *A, Aortic stenosis.* The diagnosis in this patient with delayed pulses and a systolic murmur over the aortic area rules out aortic sclerosis and a hemic murmur. The diagnosis of aortic stenosis is clinically made and can be confirmed by echocardiography.

5. *A, Eisenmenger ductus arteriosus.* The characteristic findings in this case, of clubbed and cyanotic toes in the presence of relatively pink fingers on the right hand with the absence of clubbing, point to *A*, a diagnosis of reversed ductus arteriosus. In Eisenmenger syndrome, S_2 exhibits fixed splitting. In Eisenmenger complex, a single S_2 is heard. Physiological splitting of S_2 is present in Eisenmenger syndrome with ductus arteriosus.

6. *C, Both of the above.* The physical findings are consistent with the presence of coarctation of the aorta. An ejection sound or click in early end systole makes the likelihood of bicuspid valves high. The correct answer is therefore *C*.

7. *B, Hypertrophic obstructive cardiomyopathy (HOCM).* Reverse split-
    ting of S_2 in association with a sharp pulse and a long apical systolic
    murmur (not harsh and crescendo in type) located at the left sternal
    edge, make *B* the likely diagnosis. *A* and *C* do not have any features
    consistent with the findings in this case. In mitral regurgitation, S_2 is
    physiologically split.

8. *A, Acute mitral regurgitation.* The presence of an early systolic murmur
    at the apex with acute heart failure excludes *C. A* and *B* are possibilit-
    ies. The presence of a loud S_3 and the absence of electrocardiographic
    evidence of myocardial infarction make *A* the likely diagnosis. The
    absence of a thrill is a further point against a ventricular septal defect.

9. *C, Both of the above.* The patient in question had features of both
    Marfan's syndrome and of mitral valve prolapse. The correct answer
    is therefore *C.*

10. *A, Mitral stenosis.* The presence of a middiastolic murmur provoked
    by exertion, isotonic or isometric, makes the diagnosis of mitral steno-
    sis very likely. The evanescent quality of the murmur is consistent
    with a diagnosis of early mitral stenosis. Pericardial knock is an early
    sound, not a murmur; and a physiological S_3 is a sound.

11. *A, Rytand syndrome.* In this patient, the presence of complete heart
    block, a middiastolic murmur, and calcification of the mitral valve
    ring make the diagnosis of *A, Rytand's syndrome,* the most likely. The
    clinical findings do not suggest mitral stenosis or left atrial myxoma.

12. *A, Acute aortic regurgitation.* The development of an early diastolic
    murmur in this patient two weeks after cardiac surgery suggests early
    infective endocarditis. Pulmonary regurgitation is unlikely. P_2 is not
    accentuated. A typical Graham Steell murmur with rapid decrescendo
    is not heard. An apical middiastolic murmur suggests an Austin Flint
    murmur. There is no indication of a vegetation in the mitral valve.
    The absence of S_1 and the presence of an S_3 are characteristic of regur-
    gitation.

13. *B, Mammary soufflé.* The continuous murmur heard over the left
    breast in a pregnant female, and obliterated by pressure, makes *B* the
    most likely diagnosis.

BIBLIOGRAPHY

Systolic

Allen H, et al: Significance and prognosis of an isolated late systolic murmur: A 9-
    to 22-year follow-up. Br Heart J 1974; 36:525.

Amidi M, et al: Venous systolic thrill and murmur in the neck: A consequence of
    severe tricuspid insufficiency. J Am Coll Cardiol 1986; 7:942.

Barlow JB, et al: Late systolic murmurs and non-ejection ('mid-late') systolic clicks.
    Br Heart J 1968; 30:203–217.

Barlow JB, et al: The significance of late systolic murmurs. Am Heart J 1963; 66:443–452.

Braunwald E, et al: Part III. The circulatory response of patients with idiopathic hypertrophic subaortic stenosis to nitroglycerin and to the Valsalva maneuver. Circulation 1964; 29:422–431.

Bruns DL, Van der Hauwaert LG: The aortic systolic murmur developing with increasing age. Br Heart J 1958; 20:370.

Cassidy J, et al: The effect of isometric exercise on the systolic murmur of patients with idiopathic hypertrophic subaortic stenosis. Chest 1975; 67:395–397.

Criley JM, et al: Prolapse of the mitral valve: Clinical and cine-angiocardiographic findings. Br Heart J 1966; 28:488–496.

DeLeon AC Jr, Harvey WP: Pharmacological agents and auscultation. Mod Concepts Cardiovasc Dis 1975; 44:23–28.

DeLeon AC, Jr: "Straight Back" Syndrome. In Leon DF, Shaver JA(eds.) American Heart Association Monograph No. 46, Physiologic Principles of Heart Sounds and Murmurs. New York: American Heart Association, 1975:197–208.

DePace NL, et al: Acute severe mitral regurgitation: Pathophysiology, clinical recognition and management. Am J Med 1985; 78:293.

Dohan MC, Criscitiello MG: Physiological and pharmacological manipulations of heart sounds and murmurs. Mod Concepts Cardiovasc Dis 1970; 39:121–127.

Fischer ML, et al: Hemodynamic responses to isometric exercise (handgrip) in patients with heart disease. Br Heart J 1973; 35:422–432.

Fontana ME, et al: Functional anatomy of mitral valve prolapse. In Leon DF, Shaver JA(eds.) American Heart Association Monograph No. 46, Physiologic Principles of Heart Sounds and Murmurs. New York: American Heart Association, 1975:197–208.

Fontana ME, et al: Postural changes in left ventricular and mitral valvular dynamics in the systolic click-late systolic murmur syndrome. Circulation 1975; 51: 165–173.

Fontana ME, et al: The varying clinical spectrum of the systolic click-late systolic murmur syndrome: A postural auscultatory phenomenon. Circulation 1970; 41:807–816.

Freeman AR, Levine SA: Clinical significance of systolic murmurs: Study of 1000 consecutive 'non-cardiac' cases. Ann Intern Med 1933; 6:1371–1385.

Gallavardin L, Racault P: Le souffle de retrecissement aortique peut changer de timbre et devenir musical dans sa propagation apexienne. Lyon Med 1925; 135:523–529.

Hancock EW: Differentiation of valvular and supravalvular stenosis. Guys Hosp Rep 1961; 110:1–30.

Karliner JS, et al: Hemodynamic explanation of why the murmur of mitral regurgitation is independent of cycle length. Br Heart J 1973; 35:397–401.

Kligfield P, Okin P: Effect of ventricular function on left ventricular ejection time in aortic stenosis. Br Heart J 1979; 42:438–441.

Kramer DS, et al: The post extrasystolic murmur response to gradient in hypertrophic cardiomyopathy. Ann Intern Med 1986; 104:772–776.

Leatham A: The spectrum of ventricular septal defect. In Leon DF, Shaver JA(eds.) American Heart Association Monograph No. 46, Physiologic Principles of Heart Sounds and Murmurs. New York: American Heart Association, 1975:135–138.

Leatham A: Systolic murmurs. Circulation 1958; 17:601.

Leatham A, Segal BL: Auscultatory and phonocardiographic findings in ventricular septal defects with left-to-right shunt. Circulation 1962; 25:318–327.

Leatham A, Vogelpoel L: The early systolic sound in dilation of the pulmonary artery. Br Heart J 1954; 16:21–33.

Leon DF, et al: Effect of respiration on pansystolic regurgitant murmurs as studied by biatrial intracardiac phonocardiography. Am J Med 1965; 39:429–441.

Leonard JJ, Shaver JA: Acute mitral insufficiency. Hosp Pract May 1985:75–96.

Levine SA, Likoff WB: Some notes on the transmission of heart murmurs. Ann Intern Med 1944; 21:298.

Linhart JW, Razi B: Late systolic murmur: A clue to the diagnosis of aneurysm of the membranous ventricular septum. Chest 1971; 60:283.

Morrow AG, et al: Severe mitral regurgitation following acute myocardial infarction and ruptured papillary muscle. Circulation 1968; 37 & 38 (suppl 2):124–132.

Movitt E, Gasul B: Pure mitral insufficiency of rheumatic origin in adults. Ann Intern Med 1953; 38:981.

Nellen M, et al: Effects of prompt squatting on the systolic murmur in idiopathic hypertrophic obstructive cardiomyopathy. Br Med J 1967; 3:140–143.

Paley HW: Left ventricular outflow tract obstruction: Heart sounds and murmurs. In Leon DF, Shaver JA(eds.) American Heart Association Monograph No. 46, Physiologic Principles of Heart Sounds and Murmurs. New York: American Heart Association, 1975:107–121.

Perloff JK: Clinical recognition of aortic stenosis: The physical signs and differential diagnosis of the various forms of obstruction to left ventricular outflow. Prog Cardiovasc Dis 1968; 10:323–352.

Perloff JK: Recognition and differential diagnosis of pulmonary stenosis. In Segal BL, et al(eds): The Theory and Practice of Auscultation. Philadelphia, Davis, 1964.

Perloff JK, Harvey WP: Auscultatory and phonocardiographic manifestations of pure mitral regurgitation. Prog Cardiovasc Dis 1962; 5:172–194.

Perloff JK, et al: Systemic hemodynamic effects of amyl nitrite in normal man. Am Heart J, 1963; 66:460–469.

Rackley CE, et al: The precordial honk. Am J Cardiol 1966; 117:509–515.

Reddy PS, et al: Cardiac systolic murmurs: Pathophysiology and differential diagnosis. Prog Cardiovasc Dis 1971; 14:1–37.

Rios JC, et al: Auscultatory features of acute tricuspid regurgitation. Am J Cardiol 1969; 23:4–11.

Roger H: Recherches cliniques sur la communication congenitale des deux coeurs par l'inocclusion du septum interventriculaire. Bull Acad Med (Paris) 1879; 8:1074–1189.

Ronan JA, et al: Systolic clicks and the late systolic murmur. Am Heart J 1965; 70:319.

Segal BL, Likoff WB: Late systolic murmur of mitral regurgitation. Am Heart J 1964; 67:757.

Sharpey-Schafer EP: Effects of squatting on the normal and failing circulation. Br Med J 1956; 1:107–104.

Shaver JA: Heart murmurs: Innocent or pathologic? I. Hospital Medicine June 1982; 18:13–31.

Shaver JA: Heart murmurs: Innocent or pathologic? II. Hospital Medicine June
    1982; 18:13–22.
Shaver JA: Systolic murmurs. Heart Dis and Stroke 1993; 2:9–17.
Shaver JA, et al: Clinical presentation and noninvasive evaluation of the patient
    with hypertrophic cardiomyopathy. In Shaver JA, Brest AN(eds): Cardiomyop-
    athies: Clinical presentation, differential diagnosis, and management. Philadel-
    phia, Davis, 1988:149–192.
Stefadouros MA, et al: Paradoxic response of the murmur of idiopathic subaortic
    stenosis to the Valsalva maneuver. Am J Cardiol 1976; 37:89–92.
Steinfeld L, et al: Late systolic murmur of rheumatic mitral insufficiency. Am J
    Cardiol 1975; 35:397.
Sutten GC, Craige E: Clinical signs of severe acute mitral regurgitation. Am J
    Cardiol 1967; 20:141–144.
Tavel ME: Innocent murmurs. In Leon DF, Shaver JA(eds.) American Heart
    Association Monograph No. 46, Physiologic Principles of Heart Sounds and
    Murmurs. New York: American Heart Association, 1975:102–106.
Tavel ME, et al: Late systolic murmurs and mitral regurgitation. Am J Cardiol
    1965; 15:719.
Vogel JH, Blount SG: Clinical evaluation in localizing levels of obstruction to
    outflow from left ventricle. Am J Cardiol 1965; 15:782–792.

Diastolic

Bousvaros G: Response of phonocardiographic and hemodynamic features of mitral
    stenosis to inhalation of amyl nitrite. Am Heart J 1962; 63:101.
Chen CC, et al: Variable diastolic rumbling murmur caused by floating left atrial
    thrombus. Br Heart J 1983; 50:190.
Craige E, Millward DK: Diastolic and continuous murmurs. Prog Cardiovasc Dis
    1971; 14:38–56.
Criley JM, Hermer HA: The crescendo presystolic murmur of mitral stenosis with
    atrial fibrillation. N Engl J Med 1971; 285:1284–1287.
Criley JM, et al: Mitral stenosis: Mechanico-acoustical events. In Leon DF, Shaver
    JA(eds.) American Heart Association Monograph No. 46, Physiologic Princi-
    ples of Heart Sounds and Murmurs. New York: American Heart Associa-
    tion, 1975:149–159.
Criley JM, et al: Mitral valve closure and the crescendo presystolic murmur. Am
    J Med 1971; 51:546.
Fortuin N, Craige E: On the mechanism of the Austin Flint murmur. Circulation
    1972; 45:558.
Green EW, et al: Right-sided Austin Flint murmur: Documentation by intracardiac
    phonocardiography, echocardiography and postmortem findings. Am J Cardiol
    1973; 32:370.
Harvey WP, et al: 'Right-sided' murmurs of aortic insufficiency. Am J Med Sci
    1963; 245:533–543.
Hurst JW, Cobbs BW: Diastolic rumbles. Bull Emory Univ Clin 1963; 2:69.
Killip T III, Lukas DS: Tricuspid stenosis: Clinical features in 12 cases. Am J Med
    1958; 24:836–852.
Leatham A: Rheumatic aortic incompetence with delayed diastolic murmurs on
    auscultation. Proc R Soc Med 1950; 43:309.50.

Paul MH, et al: Congenital complete atrioventricular block: Problems of clinical assessment. Circulation 1958; 18:183.

Perloff JK: The Clinical Recognition of Congenital Heart Disease, 3rd ed. Philadelphia, Saunders,1987:244.

Peters MN, et al: The clinical syndrome of atrial myxoma. JAMA 1974; 230:695.

Ravin A, Darley W: Apical diastolic murmurs in PDA. Ann Intern Med 1950; 33:903–914.

Runco V, Booth RW: Basal diastolic murmurs. Am Heart J 1963; 65:697.

Runco V, Levin HS: The spectrum of pulmonic regurgitation. In Leon DF, Shaver JA(eds.) American Heart Association Monograph No. 46, Physiologic Principles of Heart Sounds and Murmurs. New York: American Heart Association, 1975:175–182.

Rytand D: An auricular diastolic murmur with heart block in elderly patients. Am Heart J 1946; 32:579.

Sakamoto T, et al: The point of maximum intensity of aortic diastolic regurgitant murmur. Jpn Heart J 1968; 9:117–133.

Sanders CA, et al: Tricuspid stenosis: A difficult diagnosis in the presence of atrial fibrillation. Circulation 1966; 33:26–33.

Sangster JF, Oakley CM: Diastolic murmur of coronary artery stenosis. Br Heart J 1973; 35:840.

Schrier V, Vogelpoel L: The loud musical diastolic murmur of an abnormal rheumatic chorda. Am Heart J 1960; 22:403.

Schrier V, Vogelpoel L: The loud musical diastolic murmur of an abnormal rheumatic chorda. Am Heart J 1961; 62:315.

Segal JP, et al: The Austin Flint murmur: Its differentiation from the murmur of rheumatic mitral stenosis. Circulation 1958; 18:1025–1033.

Shaver JA: Diastolic murmurs. Heart Dis and Stroke 1993; 2:98–103.

Stoman G, Wee KP: Isolated congenital pulmonary valve incompetence. Am Heart J 1963; 66:532.

Tavel ME, Bonner AJ: Presystolic murmur in atrial fibrillation: Fact or fiction? Circulation 1976; 54:167.

Ueda H, et al: 'Silent' mitral stenosis: Pathoanatomical basis of the absence of diastolic rumble. Jpn Heart J 1985; 6:206–219.

Continuous

Campbell M, Deuchar DC: Continuous murmurs in cyanotic congenital heart disease. Br Heart J 1961; 23:171.

Fowler NO, Geause R: The cervical venous hum. Am Heart J 1964; 67:135.

Groom D, et al: Venous hum in cardiac auscultation. JAMA 1955; 155:639.

Hurst JW, et al: Precordial murmurs during pregnancy and lactation. N Engl J Med 1958; 259:515.

Jones FL: Frequency, characteristics and importance of the cervical venous hum in adults. N Engl J Med 1962; 267:658.

Keith JD, et al: Complete anomalous pulmonary venous return. Am J Med 1954; 16:23.

Muir CS: Coronary arteriovenous fistula. Br Heart J 1960; 22:374.

Myers JD: The mechanisms and significance of continuous murmurs. In Leon DF, Shaver JA(eds.) American Heart Association Monograph No. 46, Physiologic

Principles of Heart Sounds and Murmurs. New York: American Heart Association, 1975:202.

Spencer MP, et al: The origin and interpretation of murmurs in coarctation of the aorta. Am Heart J 1958; 56:722.

Tabatznik B, et al: The mammary souffle of pregnancy and lactation. Circulation 1960; 22:1069–1073.

To-and-Fro

Chow LC, et al: Accurate localization of ruptured sinus of Valsalva aneurysm by real-time two-dimensional Doppler flow imaging. Chest 1988; 94:462.

Gleason MM, et al: Ruptured sinus of Valsalva aneurysm of right sinus Valsalva: An unusual cause of right ventricular outflow obstruction. Am Heart J 1985; 109:363.

Kronzon I, et al: Non-invasive diagnosis of left coronary arteriovenous fistula communicating with the right ventricle. Am J Cardiol 1982;49:1811–1813.

Minkoff SM, et al: Rupture of an aneurysm of the sinus of Valsalva into the right atrium. Am J Cardiol 1967; 19:278–284.

Peters P, et al: Doppler color flow mapping detection of ruptured Valsalva aneurysm. J Am Soc Echo 1989; 2:195.

7

AUSCULTATION IN CRITICAL CARE

CHEST PAIN
   Cardiac/Vascular Sources
   Pulmonary Sources of Chest Pain
   Gastrointestinal Sources of Chest Pain
   Musculoskeletal Sources of Chest Pain

HEART FAILURE
   With Myocardial Infarction
   Other Causes
   Emergency Treatment of Heart Failure

CARDIAC ARREST

SHOCK
   Clinical Evaluation of Shock
   Hypovolemic Shock
   Cardiogenic Shock
   Myocardial Rupture
   Pseudoaneurysms
   Obstructive Shock
   Neurogenic Shock
   Septic Shock

SUBSTANCE-RELATED CARDIAC EMERGENCIES
   Drugs of Abuse
   Prescription Medications

TRAUMA
   Blunt Trauma
   Ventricular Contusion

POST-TRAUMATIC RUPTURES (AORTA/HEART)

VASCULAR TRAUMA
   Coronary Arteries

    Carotid and Femoral Arteries
    Valves

DISSECTING HEMATOMA OR ANEURYSM

PENETRATING INJURIES OF THE HEART

VASCULAR EMERGENCIES
    Rupture of Abdominal Aneurysm
    Systemic Embolism
    Deep Venous Thrombosis

Since the mid-1960s, emergency and critical care medicine have become specialties in their own right. The contemporary cardiologist called to the emergency department or the intensive care unit now works with physician assistants, nurses, paramedics, and others who have received advanced training in critical care assessment and treatment.

The cardiologic evaluation of the patient in emergency and critical care settings has devolved into a state of patient inspection with a battery of tests and acute intervention. The result is that clinicians rarely use the stethoscope; and then, for example, only to confirm the placement of an endotracheal tube or to evaluate lung sounds. The art of auscultation has for the most part been devalued and put aside as difficult to carry out in this environment. These attitudes have led to the virtual demise of auscultation in the critical care milieu.

The cardiologic evaluation of patients in emergency and critical care settings is, however, complicated by several factors. One is noise pollution, which was briefly discussed in Chap. 1, but is especially prevalent in emergency settings. In the emergency room itself, extraneous noise is typically produced by staff and patient traffic; while in intensive care units, such monitoring devices as respirators and pumps create an auditory environment antagonistic to effective auscultation.

The second factor that frequently complicates the cardiologic assessment is an incomplete patient history; in many cases the critical care patient is unconscious or otherwise unable to speak, and the clinician may have to rely on information obtained from family members or friends, emergency workers, or bystanders.

The third factor is urgency. The quest for efficiency and speed in examination, diagnosis, and treatment of emergencies leads to greater reliance on specialized tests and equipment. Paradoxically, the consequent deemphasis on auscultation and other basic aspects of clinical evaluation deprives patients of an optimal analysis of their clinical condition, and increases the cost of care by overreliance on a preconceived battery of tests.

It is, however, precisely in the urgent and emergent environment of critical care settings that clinical skills are put to greatest use. Cardiovascular crises, which require a particularly high level of clinical competence, are among the most common problems encountered in these settings. Thus skill in auscultation, despite the difficulties, remains as crucial in the emergency department or intensive care unit as it is in any aspect of medicine. This chapter will discuss auscultation in the context of the most common presenting problems in emergency and critical care settings.

These are emergencies that are seen with salient clinical and auscultatory findings. Table 7-1 is a summary of these findings with appropriate tests and treatment.

CHEST PAIN

Giving top priority to patients presenting with chest pain is essential. Differential diagnosis of chest pain is crucial in emergency medicine because of the frequency of the presenting complaint; the range of possible causes, some life-threatening; and the potential clinical and economic consequences of misdiagnosis. Specifically, 5 million people are seen in emergency rooms with chest pain per annum. Of these, 1 to 1.5 million have myocardial infarctions (MI), 1 million unstable or accelerated angina, and 3.5 million chest pain labeled "rule out myocardial infarction" (ROMI). A variety of conditions, major and minor, fall within this residual category.

Chest pain may arise from four major sources: (1) cardiac/vascular, (2) pulmonary, (3) gastrointestinal, and (4) musculoskeletal. The differential diagnosis relates to the character, nature, severity, location, provoking or precipitating factors, relieving and exacerbating factors, radiation, duration, and previous history of the chest pain; as well as to such accompanying signs as shock, heart failure, dyspnea, and diaphoresis.

Cardiac/Vascular Sources

Cardiac/vascular causes of chest pain need to be considered first in the differential diagnosis because of the potential seriousness of their outcomes.

Myocardial Infarction   Patients with acute myocardial infarction (MI) develop chest pain, often occurring in the small hours of the morning, and lasting longer than 1 h. They often delay their arrival in the emergency room by an average of 2 to 4 h. The pain of MI, although characteristically described as "crushing," located retrosternally, and radiating across the chest, may be atypical and mimic indigestion. The pain of acute MI is characteristically *not* relieved by nitroglycerin, in contrast to anginal pain. A minority of patients, diabetics in particular, may present with painless myocardial infarction with such ischemic equivalents as dyspnea or arrhythmias.

Table 7-1 Auscultatory Findings Associated with Chest Pain Encountered in the Emergency Room

Cause	Findings	Actions
Mitral valve prolapse	Nonejection clicks Late systolic murmur	ECHO Possible valve replacement

Hypertrophic obstructive
    cardiomyopathy (HOCM)
	Atrial fibrillation
	Ventricular arrhythmias
	Bisferiens carotid pulse
	Triple ripple
	Loud S_4, pseudoejection
	    click
		ECG
		ECHO
		Beta-blocker
		Surgical consult

Acute PE presenting with
    pericarditis or pleuritis;
    inferior wall ECG changes
    caused by PE rather than
    infarction
	Ejection click
	Loud P_2, late
	Wide physiologically split S_2
	S_4
		ECG
		Chest x-ray
		D-dimer test
		ABGs
		V/Q scan
		Pulmonary angiogram
		Heparin
		Thrombolytics
		Surgical consult

Patients with MI and
    dissecting aneurysms;
    dissection in coronary
    artery as well as aorta
	Faint early diastolic
	    murmur
	S_4
	Diastolic hypertension
		Enzyme test
		ECG
		Chest x-ray
		ECHO

Pericarditis	2 to 3 friction rubs	Rule out AMI, PE Sedimentation rate ECHO, TEE Skin test Resting ECG
Pleurisy	Friction rub	Skin test ECHO Chest x-ray V/Q scan
Pneumothorax	Amphoric breath sounds Shifted sounds	Chest x-ray Drain or tap fluid under water seal
Mediastinal pneumothorax	Crunch	Surgical referral
Air embolism	Mill wheel murmur	Turn patient on left side Aspiration
Aortic dissection	Early diastolic murmur Loud A_2 Re-entrant bruit	Surgical consult, TEE Beta-blocker
Intraaortic hematoma	Murmurs not heard	

Musculoskeletal causes of
    chest pain
	Findings dictated by
	    condition; often no
	    systemic cardiac findings
		Treatment dictated by
		    condition

The electrocardiogram of a patient with MI shows ST segment elevation in two adjacent leads or in two leads taken from a similar area of the heart. New bundle branch block may be present without interpretable ST segments, but with characteristic auscultatory signs (soft S_1, paradoxical splitting of S_2, and S_4).

Other Acute Coronary Syndromes   In the differential diagnosis of chest pain, the pain of angina differs from that of myocardial infarction in several respects. Patients frequently describe it as "squeezing," "burning," or "like indigestion." Anginal pain is characteristically not sharply localized, often brought on by exertion, and is usually relieved by nitroglycerin.

Patients diagnosed with unstable angina, Prinzmetal's angina, or accelerated angina are usually admitted to the hospital for evaluation by electrocardiography, enzyme tests, echocardiography, or scintigraphy. Clinical examination of symptomatic patients may reveal auscultatory signs of ischemia (S_4, S_3, and soft S_1). These signs are evanescent, are corrected with nitroglycerin, but may recur. This applies to apical late systolic murmurs as well.

ROMI   Because of the importance of ruling out myocardial infarction as a cause of chest pain, a large percentage of patients with thoracic complaints may be placed initially in the category of "rule out myocardial infarction." At present, chest pain centers in the United States triage these patients according to the pretest probability of heart disease. The relevant factors are listed in Table 7-2. A variety of protocols are then used in diagnostic assessment of ROMI patients. Standardization of both triage criteria and procedures awaits further development, as these protocols have significant variations.

Table 7-2   Factors Used in Determination of Pretest Probability of Cardiac Ischemia

Genetic	Gynecologic
Family history of cardiac ischemia	Use of oral contraceptives
Patient History	Menopause
Previous heart disease	Cardiovascular
Previous coronary artery disease	Strokes/TIAs
Lifestyle	Hypertension
Smoking	Claudication
Cocaine usage	Loud A_2 in young patients
Type A personality (hostile)	Blood
External Features	Polycythemia
Tophi	Hyperlipidemia
Ear crease	Hyperuricemia
Xanthelasma	Elevated LPa
Ochronosis	Other Syndromes
Truncal obesity	Diabetes

Dissecting aneurysm and intraaortic hematoma   In patients with dissecting aneurysms, the pain is sudden and severe, often described as "tearing"; it radiates into the back and is often intractable. It is typically associated with a history of hypertension or Marfan's syndrome.

Auscultatory findings in dissecting aneurysms consist of a loud A_2, an early diastolic murmur at the left sternal border, and a reentrant bruit over the spine or back (Fig. 7-1). Reentrant murmurs are heard over the midline in the back. Diastolic hypertension may be present. Aortic regurgitation murmurs may be soft, and heard on the right side (Cardiac Pearl 11/ Harvey's sign).

Tamponade may occur in patients with dissecting aneurysms due to dissection of the right coronary artery. Tamponade may be associated with inferior wall myocardial infarction and extravasation of blood into the pericardium due to right coronary arterial dissection. A rub and pulsus paradoxus may be heard.

Dissecting hematomas do not present with auscultable signs. Transesophageal echocardiography (TEE) can identify hematomas. They do not possess reentrant tracts or an intimal tear in the aortic wall. Patients may develop dissecting hematomas in the descending aorta secondary to trauma.

Pericarditis   Patients with pericarditis should be examined carefully to rule out pulmonary embolus (PE) or acute MI. Clinically diagnosed pericarditis mandates an electrocardiogram, chest x-ray, echocardiogram, sedimentation rate test, white blood cell count (WBC), complete blood count (CBC), cardiac enzymes, D-dimer test, serological tests, and blood gases. Pericarditis in myocardial infarction may be an ominous sign of *cardiorrhexis* (cardiac rupture), with nausea, faintness, and sudden dyspnea. Cardiac arrest with pulseless electrical activity (PEA) may follow. Cardiorrhexis (Fig. 7-2), hemorrhagic pericarditis from anticoagulant medication, or *Dressler's syndrome* (Chap. 4) may present with pericardial friction rubs.

Morton's syndrome   This condition describes chest pain associated with superficial thrombophlebitis.

Pulmonary Sources of Chest Pain

Pleurisy   Patients with pleurisy (inflammation of the pleural tissue) commonly present in the emergency department with fever, chest pain, and a

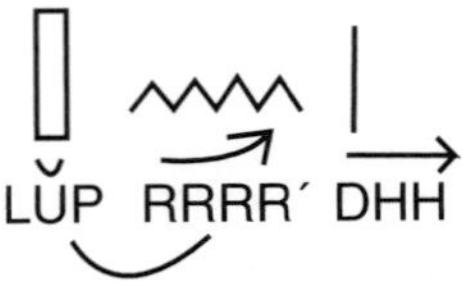

Figure 7-1 Phonophonic representation of auscultatory findings in dissecting aneurysms. Early diastolic murmur, loud A_2 (Harvey's sign).

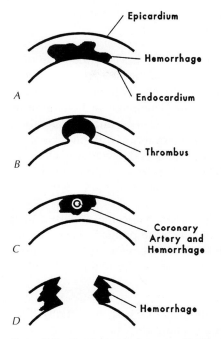

Figure 7-2 Cardiorrhexis. Rupture of left heart following myocardial infarction. A. The wall of the heart with an impending rupture and a hemorrhagic infarct. B. Increasing necrosis. C. Complete hemorrhage and necrosis. D. Complete dehiscence. The blood that egresses in this fashion may be walled off to form pseudoaneurysms; they may also cause tamponade and sudden death. These changes may be serially seen on echocardiography.

loud friction rub. The pain of pleurisy is typically worse on inspiration. The rub may be audible, pleural, or pleuropericardial.

The diagnosis is made after pulmonary embolism—which may present with the same symptoms—is ruled out. Pleurisy may be the first manifestation of tuberculosis or an autoimmune disease; or it may overlie an area of pneumonia. Pleurisy is a frequent sign of Dressler's syndrome (Chap. 4).

Pneumothorax Pneumothorax is defined as accumulation of air in the pleural space or mediastinum; it is categorized as spontaneous or traumatic. Pneumothorax typically occurs as a complication of chronic obstructive pulmonary disease (COPD), asthma, tuberculosis, cystic fibrosis, and *Pneumocystis carinii* pneumonia (in HIV patients). The patient may have severe chest pain and shortness of breath. Amphoric breathing (amphora-flask; high-pitched bronchial breathing) may be heard over the pneumothorax along with diminished breath sounds. Patients with tension pneumothorax may be in shock with displaced chest organs and mediastinum. Tension pneumothorax should be suspected in patients with severe tachycardia, hypotension, and mediastinal shift. Shock is caused in these patients by a moving mediastinum (so-called "mediastinal flap").

Acute Pneumomediastinum   Pneumomediastinum is a condition that may occur as a complication of spontaneous pneumothorax. A "crunching" sound is heard and chest crepitus may be palpable. Patients may present with shock, and a history of excessive vomiting. There may be hematemesis due to esophageal tears in the *Mallory-Weiss syndrome* (mucosal laceration of gastroesophageal junction). Patients may be cyanotic with physical findings of a pleural effusion. If pneumomediastinum is detected, the clinician should consider postemetic rupture of the esophagus (Boerhaave's syndrome).

Bornholm Syndrome (Pleurodynia)   Bornholm syndrome is caused by a viral infection that resembles pleurisy, in which the patient has chest pain in the area of diaphragmatic attachment. Epidemic pleurodynia is caused by coxsackieviruses B1 to B5. There are no physical findings relevant to the heart.

Pulmonary Embolism   Pulmonary embolism (PE) is potentially life-threatening. Pulmonary emboli may arise from thrombi in the venous circulation, from tumors that have invaded the venous circulation, or from other sources (e.g., air, amniotic fluid, or foreign material injected into the veins). More than 90 percent of pulmonary emboli, however, originate from deep venous thrombi, most often in the calves. No single sign or symptom is sufficient to confirm the diagnosis of PE, although patients commonly present with dyspnea, cough, hemoptysis, diaphoresis, and anxiety in addition to the chest pain (which is often pleuritic). Patients with PE may also present with pulmonary infarction, tricuspid regurgitation, acute right heart failure, tachypnea, or a history of pain and swelling in one leg.

Auscultation of patients with PE often indicates an S_3 in the tricuspid or subxiphoid area. Wide splitting of S_2 and a loud P_2 may be heard. An S_4 may be heard over the jugular veins and subxiphoid area. A holosystolic murmur of tricuspid regurgitation or right ventricular S_3 and S_4 may be auscultable. Rubs may be present, either pleural, pericardial, or both.

Although laboratory findings are not diagnostic of PE, measurement with a pulse oximeter may indicate a degree of desaturation, which is difficult to correct with a standard dose of oxygen. The ECG may reveal signs of inferior wall myocardial infarction; it may be confused with classic findings of Q waves in III, but not in AVF; S in I; and ST-T changes and right bundle branch block (RBBB) in precordial leads. Venous pressure may be elevated. Because PE is often associated with deep venous thrombi, it is important to remove any casts or splints on the lower extremities and examine them for deep venous tenderness and a positive Homan's sign (pain in calf with forcible dorsiflexion of foot).

Acute Air Embolism (Cardiac Pearl)   Acute air embolism (Fig. 7-3) may occur in female patients who present with sudden collapse following insufflation of the Fallopian tubes that may inadvertently introduce air into the veins. A swishing "millwheel" murmur is characteristic of acute air embolism. This noisy murmur occurs in both systole and diastole. Patients with acute air embolism are moved *immediately* into the left supine position to prevent pulmonary air embolism and shock until the air is aspirated.

Gastrointestinal Sources of Chest Pain

Gastrointestinal disorders causing chest pain are less likely to represent serious emergencies, but may complicate the diagnosis nonetheless. It has been estimated that as many as 25 percent of patients complaining of chest pain have gastroesophageal reflux disease (GERD). Clinicians should inquire about a sour or acid taste in the mouth in order to rule out GERD. Gall bladder disease and pancreatitis may simulate myocardial ischemia, with associated nonspecific electrocardiographic changes.

   Esophageal spasm is frequently confused with angina because it may cause substernal pain that may be relieved by nitrates. Patients with acute cholecystitis, pancreatitis, or esophagitis may have symptoms that mimic as well as precipitate angina. Esophagitis is typically exacerbated by recum-

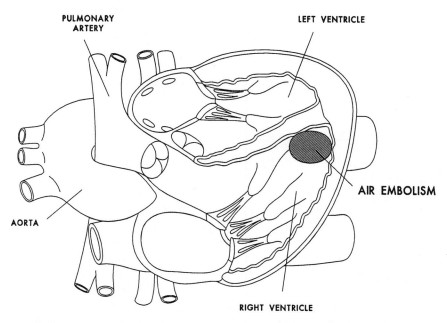

Figure 7-3 Air embolism. The heart is shown in the left lateral position, which allows the air trapped in right ventricle to lie against the chest wall and not embolize into the lungs.

bency. Patients with possible GI disorders who complain of chest pain should be evaluated by a gastroenterologist.

Musculoskeletal Sources of Chest Pain

Musculoskeletal causes of chest pain are characterized by pain that is reproduced by palpation of the patient's chest wall. In addition to rib fractures caused by trauma, musculoskeletal causes of thoracic pain include herpesvirus infections and reflex pain syndromes.

Tietze's Syndrome Tietze's syndrome, sometimes called *anterior chest wall syndrome,* is caused by inflammation of the costochondral junctions, which may be warm, swollen, and red. The patient may experience diffuse chest pain that can be reproduced by local pressure.

Herpes Zoster and Radiculitis Herpes zoster can produce chest pain from intercostal neuritis that mimics angina. The unilateral skin rash enables the diagnosis to be made.

Shoulder-Hand Syndrome Shoulder-hand syndrome is a form of reflex sympathetic dystrophy that may cause pain in the shoulder frequently described as "burning" or "aching." Shoulder-hand syndrome is common after neck or shoulder injuries and following myocardial infarction. There are no systemic symptoms in reflex sympathetic dystrophy.

HEART FAILURE

Heart failure may develop suddenly in previously asymptomatic patients; it may also present as an acute exacerbation of preexisting heart disease.

With Myocardial Infarction

Heart failure may be caused by right ventricular infarction, by a large initial infarction, by extension of a preexisting recent infarction, or may arise de novo. Patients with right heart failure present with a positive Kussmaul's sign, tricuspid regurgitation, an S_4, pulsus paradoxus, and evidence of inferior myocardial infarction. Echocardiographic changes of ST elevation in precordial leads on the right side may be present. Acute heart failure associated with a thrill at the left sternal edge, holosystolic in character, usually suggests a ventricular septal defect (VSD). A friction rub and sudden nausea are premonitory signs of sudden collapse, pulseless electrical activity (PEA), and cardiorrhexis. In bundle branch block, wide physiologic splitting of S_2 (RBBB) and S_1, or paradoxic splitting of S_2 may be heard (LBBB) with soft S_1. Heart block may occur with characteristic auscultation findings (Chap. 4). The progressive nature of filling sounds as it relates to pressure inside the heart has been discussed in detail in Chap. 5.

Other Causes

Heart failure may result from a variety of other causes and is characterized by gallop rhythm, S_3, or quadruple rhythm. These abnormalities may be found in cardiomyopathies; valvular emergencies; acute stenosis or regurgitation due to infection; tumors; and rupture. Such abnormalities may be caused by drug overdose, acute myocarditis, pulmonary embolism, arrhythmias, or acute hypertension. Auscultatory findings are important in making the diagnosis. Myocardial failure is associated with a soft S_1 and pulsus alternans Chap. 8. Cardiophonetics are described in Chap. 4.

Emergency Treatment of Heart Failure

Heart failure may be the incident cause for admission to the emergency department. Patients may present with increasing shortness of breath, frank pulmonary edema, and incipient respiratory failure. These patients should be evaluated immediately with a pulse oximeter, chest x-ray, and echocardiogram. Oxygen is administered. Furosemide (Lasix) may need to be given intravenously. The patient is placed on an intermittent Doppler blood pressure recording machine (Dinamapp); or arterial lines are placed, with or without a triple-lumen pulmonary flotation catheter.

In acute cases, patients require immediate treatment in the presence of respiratory failure. If indicated by poor blood gas results or inadequate ventilation, the clinician should intubate the patient immediately. Auscultation findings may be difficult to perform on account of secretions and tachypnea. The use of angiotensin-converting enzyme (ACE) inhibitors and beta-blockers has been demonstrated to be effective in heart failure. Digoxin (Lanoxin) is used to treat atrial fibrillation.

CARDIAC ARREST

This condition occurs in a variety of circumstances. The underlying electrocardiographic signs are part of the diagnostic picture that determines the best treatment strategy. Standard protocols are used depending on the rhythm and the cause of the arrest. Auscultation indicates either no heart sounds or profound bradycardia. Cardiac arrest may follow cardiac rupture or tamponade.

SHOCK

Shock is a critical state that occurs when the circulation of arterial blood cannot meet the metabolic needs of body tissues. It is characterized by peripheral hypoperfusion, oliguria, low blood pressure, low cardiac output, pallor, cold extremities due to vasoconstriction, and altered mental status. The skin is typically cool and moist.

Shock may be classified as hypovolemic, cardiogenic, obstructive, neurogenic, mechanical (e.g., in valve malfunction and tamponade), septic, and anaphylactic (Table 7-3).

Clinical Evaluation of Shock (Fig. 7-4)

Hypotension may be a physiologic phenomenon as long as perfusion of tissues is maintained. Thus, the signs of shock in a hypotensive patient are decreased skin and muscle temperature, diaphoresis and dysfunction of the kidneys, as well as altered mental status. These are signs of tissue hypoperfusion (Chap. 8).

Hypovolemic Shock

Hypovolemia is associated with dry tongue and mucous membranes, reduced ocular tension, loss of body weight, and tachycardia without the presence of S_3 or S_4 filling sounds in the recumbent state.

Hypovolemic shock results from decreased intravascular volume. Loss of blood and other fluids is often obvious, but may also be due to "third

Table 7-3 Types of Shock and Common Causes

Type	Cause(s)
Hypovolemic (volume loss)	Blood loss
	Trauma
	GI bleeding
	Hemolysis
	Plasma loss
	Burns
	Loss of fluid/electrolytes
	Vomiting/diarrhea
	Hyperosmolar states
	"Third spacing"
Cardiogenic (elevated filling pressures)	Right ventricular infarction
	"Pump failure"
	Valvular dysfunction
	Ventricular rupture (wall, septum, or valve)
Obstructive (elevated filling pressures behind obstruction	Pericardial disease
	Pulmonary hypertension or emboli
	Atrial myxoma
	Atrial or mitral stenosis
	Ball valve clot
Septic (low systemic vascular resistance)	Gram-negative bacteremia
Neurogenic (vasomotor paralysis)	Stroke
	Spinal cord injury
	Vasodilator drugs
Anaphylactic (histamine shock)	Exposure to allergen (medications, foods, serum, animal venom)

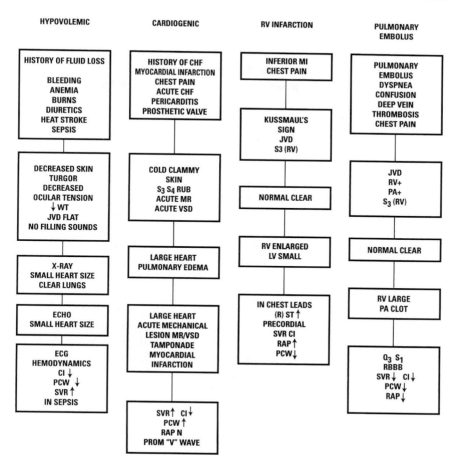

Figure 7-4 Auscultatory and other clinical findings in hypotension and shock. CHF, congestive heart failure; MI, myocardial infarction; RV, right ventricle; LV, left ventricle; JVD, jugular venous distension; WT, weight; MR, mitral regurgitation; VSD, ventricular septal defect; PA, pulmonary artery; ECG, electrocardiogram; CI, cardiac index; PCW, pulmonary capillary wedge; SVR, systemic vascular resistance; RAP, right atrial pressure; RBBB, right bundle branch block.

spacing" (collection of blood/fluid within dilated capillaries of internal body cavities). Hyponatremia causing hypovolemia may be associated with cramps, postural hypotension, and tachycardia, as in Addison's disease.

Hypotension occurs in hypovolemic shock when fluids lost are not replaced. Hypotension due to anemia (from blood loss or hemolysis) is associated with pallor and air hunger. Hemolysis with anemia may present with jaundice. In anemia, a high-output state with loud S_1 and ejection sounds and midsystolic murmurs may be present, as well as an S_3. In patients with hypovolemia due to anaphylaxis, urticaria, swelling of the tongue, or tachycardia induced by epinephrine treatment may be present. Left ventricular hypovolemia is due to right ventricular infarction associated with inferior myocardial infarction. The venous pressure is elevated and Kussmaul's sign may be present. A right ventricular S_3 and S_4 associated with a tricuspid regurgitation murmur may be heard. Pulsus paradoxus may simulate tamponade.

Cardiogenic Shock

Patients in cardiogenic shock have the classic appearance of shock: confused mental state; cold, clammy extremities and thighs; oliguria; pallor; and severe hypotension (below 80 mmHg systolic pressure). Characteristic hemodynamics may include the "gap phenomenon," i.e., disparity between intraarterial pressure and the palpated cuff pressure. Patients with triple-lumen flotation catheters in the pulmonary capillary wedge position may show a prominent V wave, which is suggestive but not pathognomonic of acute ventricular septal defect. Simultaneously, oxygen saturation of mixed venous blood (SvO_2), as well as pulmonary arterial blood, may indicate a left-to-right shunt due to ventricular septal defect.

In right ventricular infarction associated with inferior myocardial infarction, the wedge pressure is low, the right atrial pressure is high, and the right atrial/left atrial pressure ratio is 0.8 or higher. Signs of right ventricular infarction include: venous distention, Kussmaul's sign, right-ventricular, S_3, or S_4, tricuspid regurgitation, and pulsus paradoxus simulating tamponade.

In myocardial infarction, four causes of cardiogenic shock can be distinguished, each with specific clinical signs:

1. A large area of recent myocardial ischemia or infarction in a previously normal-sized heart.
2. A small new area of myocardial infarction in a patient with a previous infarction or terminal cardiomyopathy, previously associated with cardiomegaly.
3. Right ventricular infarction, with its special features.
4. Mechanical defects, including septal rupture; rupture of the left ventricular free wall leading to pseudoaneurysm; and rupture of the papillary muscle belly.

Until recently, cardiogenic shock has had an extremely high mortality rate. Recognition of its causes, however, and the development of specific corrective measures have improved the prognosis for most patients.

Myocardial Rupture

Echocardiography alone is often diagnostic in patients with myocardial rupture. The echocardiogram may show actual dehiscence by echo and signs of tamponade. In myocardial rupture, complete rupture of the ventricular free wall usually results in immediate death. A pseudoaneurysm, however, may appear clearly on echocardiogram after an albuminex injection. Pseudoaneurysms have a narrow-neck connection to the left ventricle caused by rupture of the wall into the pericardial sac, constituting a "blind alley" into which blood is pumped. Tamponade is an occasional occurrence. Auscultation may reveal the presence of a rub preceding rupture or a to-and-fro murmur heralding a pseudoaneurysm.

Patients with myocardial rupture are treated promptly by surgery, those with ventricular septal defects or papillary muscle ruptures by inserting an intraaortic balloon pump, arterial lines, and a triple-lumen catheter for hemodynamic monitoring. Medications may include dopamine (Intropin), dobutamine (Dobutrex), and amrinone (Inocor). Optimizing the patient's respiratory status and treating the cause of respiratory derangement is essential. In the event of massive infarction caused by an obstruction to a proximal artery, angioplasty with or without stenting takes precedence over thrombolytic drug therapy. In acute ventricular septal rupture or mitral regurgitation due to ruptured papillary muscle, surgery is indicated urgently, and prolonged diagnostic cardiac catheterization avoided. Right ventricular infarction is treated with fluids, administration of dobutamine, and an intraaortic balloon. This combination is useful in all cases except in acute aortic regurgitation. Tamponade is treated by paracentesis and surgery. Prosthetic valve thrombosis requires thrombolysis or surgery; septic valves are replaced. Valve clicks may not be evident.

Pseudoaneurysms

Pseudoaneurysms are false or incomplete aneurysms of the ventricle which may present postinfarction or post trauma. They develop when incomplete or gradual rupture of the myocardium is sealed off by the pericardium. Dissecting aortic aneurysms are pseudoaneurysms which may present with aortic regurgitation; with murmurs over the subclavian and carotid arteries; or with murmurs over the back. Continuous murmurs may be audible on auscultation. Pseudoaneurysm of the left ventricle may be present with a to-and-fro murmur and if large with shock.

Obstructive Shock

When obstructive shock is caused by tamponade, tension pneumothorax, or massive pulmonary embolism, it is an emergency requiring immediate treatment. In obstructive shock due to pulmonary embolism, the patient is tachypneic with cyanosis, arterial oxygen saturation, and rapid pulse. Venous pressure is elevated with a loud P_2. Right ventricular filling sounds may be evident with a site of deep venous thrombosis in the thigh. In tamponade, evaluation of venous pressure and pulsus paradoxus is present with tachycardia and tachypnea. Examination of the patient in the right supine position may be helpful in accentuating right-sided auscultatory findings.

Other causes of obstructive shock include myxomas and malfunctioning prosthetic valves. In the latter condition, clicks may not be evident on auscultation, or a new murmur may be present. In valvular dysfunction due to endocarditis, changing murmurs may appear. In myxomas and ball valve clots, examination in the lateral positions may provoke the signs.

Neurogenic Shock

In stroke, hypotension may be associated with raised intracranial pressure. *Cheyne-Stokes respiration* (Chap. 8) and *Biot's respiration* (irregular respiration) may be present. Also, bruits may be heard over the carotid arteries and atrial fibrillation may be present. The clinician should auscultate carefully for neck bruits, valvular murmurs, atrial septal defects, or intracardiac shunts. Stroke patients often have a history of hypertension or valvular heart disease.

Patients with spinal cord injuries may also present with neurogenic shock.

Septic Shock

Patients with sepsis (gram-negative bacteremia) may present with fever and chills, restlessness, changes in mental status, hypotension, and shock. The extremities are typically warm. The drop in blood pressure and associated oliguria resemble the features of cardiogenic shock. Sepsis may originate in other body systems, particularly the lungs, gastrointestinal tract, and genitourinary system; but may also be derived from infected surgical incisions and IV lines.

Auscultatory findings and cardiovascular symptoms in septic shock may include bounding pulses, a loud S_1, pericardial rubs, murmurs, heart failure, and tachycardia. There may also be decreased filling pressure and hypovolemia. Patients with sepsis are treated with aggressive fluid replacement with volumes as high as 3 L/h. Drug therapy usually includes steroids and antibiotics. Placement of arterial lines is necessary for hemodynamic monitoring. Intubation may be required in patients with respiratory failure. The auscultatory findings in high output states (Chap. 6) and in heart failure (Chap. 4) may be evident.

SUBSTANCE-RELATED CARDIAC EMERGENCIES

Drugs of Abuse

Drug overdose—particularly with cocaine—is a frequent cause of admission to the emergency department with acute cardiac and respiratory failure.

Highly cardiotoxic, cocaine may cause coronary artery spasm, myocardial infarction, end heart failure, cardiomyopathy, or endocarditis. Plasma cocaine levels are not proportional to central nervous system (CNS) effects, but are elevated. In chronic users, a dilated cardiomyopathy with heart failure may be the mode of presentation. Treatment includes rehabilitation of patients and possible referral for transplantation. Regression of heart size and heart failure may occur, if consumption ceases.

Alcohol is cardiotoxic and may cause a high-output state, hypertension, a filling sound, S_3, S_4, and loud S_1 and S_2. In exceptional cases, beriberi with high-output failure may develop in malnourished patients. Jugular venous distention (JVD), tachycardia, edema of the legs, and the absence of albuminuria are also associated with beri beri due to alcohol consumption. Recognition of the signs of alcohol abuse is important, particularly for patients living alone or in nursing homes.

Abuse of injected drugs can also lead to infective endocarditis of the right heart. Endocarditis in turn may produce septic pulmonary emboli that are carried to the lungs. Respiratory and cardiac failure with tricuspid regurgitation may result. Tricuspid regurgitation murmurs may be ejection, holosystolic, or barely audible, depending on the lesion and the relative right ventricular pressures.

Prescription Medications

Medically administered drugs that may cause cardiac disorders include some cytotoxic agents [e.g., doxorubicin (Adriamycin)] that can cause arrhythmias and intractable heart failure. Pleural or pericardial effusions and rubs may be caused by such drugs as hydralazine (Apresoline) or procainamide (Pronestyl). In some cases patients may develop cardiac dysfunction from hypersensitivity to penicillin or sulfonamides. Anorexiants such as fenfluramine (Pondimin) or Aminorex may cause pulmonary hypertension. 5-Fluorouracil may cause coronary spasm pain and an S_4 may be present.

TRAUMA
Blunt Trauma

Focal blunt trauma may be the cause of chest pain in patients presenting in the emergency room. A common source is the impact of the steering wheel on the driver's chest in automobile accidents. Pain from blunt trauma can usually be reproduced by pressure on the chest wall. In blunt trauma to the chest, it is vital for internists and other specialists in the emergency department to determine the presence of myocardial trauma.

Traffic accidents causing trauma may have immediate or delayed medicolegal consequences. Trauma is the leading cause of death in patients under 40 in the United States.

Ventricular Contusion

Right Ventricle   Right ventricular contusion is the most common traumatic injury to the chest. Associated auscultatory findings may include a new murmur of tricuspid regurgitation or a pericardial rub. Patients with ventricular contusion may have few symptoms; the diagnosis is made by electrocardiography, echocardiography, scintigraphic testing, and clinical examination. Occasionally, the injured myocardium may be "stunned" and nonfunctional; right heart failure may then develop. This sequela is associated with a right ventricular gallop, positive Kussmaul's sign, and pulsus paradoxus.

In general, ventricular contusion does not require diagnostic testing beyond an ECG, chest x-ray, and transthoracic echocardiogram in the absence of heart failure, tamponade, acute myocardial infarction, enzyme elevation, or hemodynamically significant arrhythmias.

Left Ventricle   Traumatic injury of the left ventricle may be worse in diastole and may lead to a true aneurysm or a pseudoaneurysm. Typical signs consist of to-and-fro systolic and diastolic murmurs. These abnormalities may develop for the first time following the injury and are related to the ingress and egress of blood though the aneurysm. In transmural injury following trauma to the chest, development of a true ventricular aneurysm with symptoms of heart failure may occur. The apical impulse is widely felt, and an S_3 and S_4 may be heard. Ventricular aneurysms are usually evident on echocardiography, although some cases may require transesophageal echocardiography using a multiplane probe to outline the extent of the aneurysm.

Commotio Cordis   Traumatic injury to the myocardium may lead to arrhythmias, causing premature beats or heart block. When the chest injury is severe, sudden death may occur with no postmortem evidence of cardiac contusion. This phenomenon is called *commotio cordis*, and may be associated with fatal arrhythmias. Commotio cordis probably causes sudden myocardial stunning.

POST-TRAUMATIC RUPTURES (AORTA/HEART)

The aorta or ventricle may rupture as a result of trauma, either at the root or at the level of the ligamentum arteriosum, and result in exsanguinating hemorrhage. Intramural hemorrhage into the aortic wall may occur with or without subsequent dissection into the aortic lumen. Thus, aortic diastolic murmurs may be heard; and pulses may not be present in all four limbs. Occasionally, trauma to the aorta may extend to the carotid arteries, causing hemiplegia. Myocardial trauma may present several months later. Rupture of the heart may present as a true or pseudoaneurysm months after the traumatic event (Fig. 7-5).

VASCULAR TRAUMA

Coronary Arteries

Trauma to the coronary arteries may lead to acute myocardial infarction. Injury may cause a coronary arteriovenous fistula to produce a continuous murmur. The location of this murmur depends on the artery involved: In the left anterior descending coronary artery the murmur is located at the apex; in the circumflex coronary artery it is at the back; in the right coronary artery it is heard to the right of the sternum.

Carotid and Femoral Arteries

Injuries to the great vessels of the body (the carotid or femoral arteries) may lead to arteriovenous fistula formation, false aneurysms, and dissections. Trauma to the carotids may cause stroke, while injury to the femoral arteries may cause gangrene.

Valves

Injuries to the pulmonary, aortic, tricuspid, or mitral valves may result from either blunt or sharp trauma to the chest. In penetrating injuries, the ventricular septum may be damaged. The characteristic murmurs of acute mitral regurgitation, which may be early systolic, may be heard locally at the apex, or conducted to the back or front of the chest. In patients with mitral regurgitation, an S_3 and possibly an S_4 may be heard. The aortic, mitral, and tricuspid valves may develop acute endocarditis with vegetation.

In severe traumatic aortic regurgitation, an acute systolic and diastolic murmur may be heard in association with a soft or absent S_1, an S_4, and an S_2. Traumatic pericarditis may present with a friction rub. A friction rub, however, may also signal the rupture of a cardiac chamber.

Trauma to the chest may result in an aortopulmonary fistula between the aorta and the pulmonary arteries or other adjacent structures. Auscultatory findings may include a to-and-fro murmur with accentuated diastole, if a fistula is connected to a right-sided structure, the left atrium, and the left ventricle. The precise location of the murmur depends on the position of the fistula.

Penetrating wounds of the aorta may cause pericardial tamponade or mediastinal hematomas. Recent advances in surgical technique have improved the prognosis for these patients.

DISSECTING HEMATOMA OR ANEURYSM

Dissecting hematomas or aneurysms frequently occur below the subclavian artery [Type III (Fig. 4-8)]. They are recognized by urgent transesophageal echocardiography (TEE) or computed tomography, which enable a rapid diagnosis to be made.

PENETRATING INJURIES OF THE HEART

In pericardial penetrating wounds involving the myocardium, these wounds may remain open, resulting in bleeding during diastole as well as systole. They may spontaneously close rapidly due to contraction of the heart with apposition of muscle fibers; or lead to scars, pseudo- or true aneurysms, and arrhythmias. Pericardial wounds may remain open, allowing blood to drain into the pleural space. Even if they seal, however, clotting may cause tamponade in the pericardium. Signs of tamponade may appear with rapid accumulation of 600 to 1000 cc of blood in the pericardial space. This causes signs which include cold, clammy skin and elevated venous pressure. More subtle signs include muffling of cardiac sounds, with pulsus paradoxus.

Penetrating injuries to the ventricular septum or cardiac valves may produce ventricular septal defect or valvular insufficiency. Small cardiac wounds may bleed relatively slowly and cause hemopericardium. Hemo-

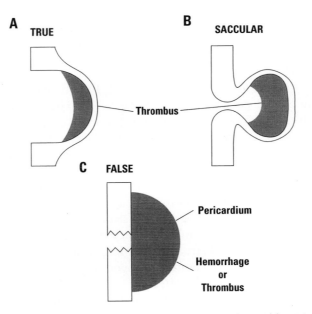

Figure 7-5 Three types of dissecting aneurysms. In type I the point of origin is in the ascending aorta; in type II, it is circumferential; in type III, it originates beyond the subclavian artery.

pericardium should be suspected in any penetrating wound of the chest, neck, or upper abdomen, especially the precordium; 60 to 80 percent of patients with this condition die shortly after injury because of cardiac tamponade or bleeding. Blood pressures are difficult to elicit in severely hypotensive patients.

Determining central venous pressure (CVP) in the absence of heart failure is the most reliable test for determining whether blood loss, tamponade, or both are causing shock. The zero level for the manometer used to measure central venous pressure should be at the midaxillary level; its saline column should fluctuate during respiration. A CVP of about 12 (cmH_2O) at the time of admission that rises indicates tamponade. Tamponade can also develop with low venous pressures. In suspected tamponade, chest x-rays are of little value, and echocardiography is essential.

VASCULAR EMERGENCIES

Rupture of Abdominal Aneurysm

Rupture of an aneurysm is a medical emergency and may require immediate surgery. The condition may be detected by the presence of a tender expansive abdominal mass and overlying systolic murmur. Physical signs are discussed in Chap. 4. Angiography and computed tomography of the abdomen are appropriate diagnostic tests. Chronic vascular insufficiency may have been present with abdominal pain and malabsorption. Signs of tendon xanthomata may be present, because these aneurysms are associated with type II hyperlipidemia.

Systemic Embolism (Cardiac Pearl 53)

Systemic emboli may cause stroke or gangrene of the bowels and extremities. The heart must be examined carefully for valvular disease, endocarditis, and atrial fibrillation. Surgical intervention is the usual treatment, with the possible exception of obstruction to blood vessels in the extremities. In these cases, invasive catheterization, ultrasound, or laser wires may be used to cause thrombolysis. Systemic anticoagulation may be needed. *Livedo reticularis* is an uncommon microembolic skin disorder producing mottled discoloration of the skin of the extremities. No specific auscultatory findings are present. Atrial fibrillation and auscultatory findings associated with the cause may be present, as in mitral stenosis.

Patients may present with carotid or overlying bruits, tenderness over superficial arteries in the head, atrial fibrillation, findings associated with valvular heart disease, changing murmurs, hypertension, dissection, early diastolic murmurs, and left-to-right shunts.

Embolism from the right side (paradoxic emboli) may occur through a patent foramen ovale, incomplete closure of an atrial septal defect, right-to-left shunts, ventricular septal defect, patent ductus arteriosus, or carotid disease. Cardiac valvular disease or masses and aortic dissection may also permit emboli to cause strokes. Atrial fibrillation is commonly associated with these conditions.

Deep Venous Thrombosis

Deep venous thrombosis may be present with classic signs as described in Chap. 8. The diagnosis is made by Doppler ultrasound, venography, and ventilation/perfusion (V/Q) scan. A ruptured Baker's cyst may simulate deep venous thrombosis; a history of arthritis in the same leg may assist in differential diagnosis. No specific auscultatory findings are present.

TRUE OR FALSE

1. Intraarterial pressure recorded by a sphygmomanometer is always equal to that obtained by an arterial line.
2. Right ventricular contusion may resemble right ventricular infarction in clinical presentation.
3. Patients with blunt trauma of the chest without evident cardiac abnormalities should be discharged from the hospital after a chest x-ray and an electrocardiogram are negative; and then evaluated as outpatients.
4. Patients with cardiac arrest who have overdosed on tricyclic antidepressants should not be given sodium bicarbonate during CPR.
5. A patient presenting to a tertiary care center with cardiogenic shock from myocardial infarction should be treated with thrombolytic therapy rather than angioplasty.
6. A patient with a prosthetic valve and shock should be evaluated by angiography first with a view to determining the cause of the problem.
7. In a patient with recurrent pulmonary emboli, important consideration should be given to the use of a Greenfield filter or umbrella or Birds Nest filter in the vena cava.
8. In a patient presenting with acute pericarditis and acute myocardial infarction, pulmonary embolism should always be ruled out as the cause of the pericarditis.
9. Evaluation of a thrombosed prosthetic valve is done by fluoroscopy, echocardiography, and listening for clicks.
10. A precordial thrill and early systolic murmur suggest an acute ventral septal defect.

CLINICAL VIGNETTES

The following vignettes present actual cases of patients who were affected by diseases and conditions discussed in this chapter. At the end of each *case, choose the **one** answer that best describes the diagnosis indicated by the vignette.*

1. A 35-year-old male presented with severe lower chest and abdominal pain. On clinical examination, he had the features of long, lean fingers and a history of dislocated lenses in his eyes. The relative who accompanied him had similar features. The patient's span was greater than his height. His ears were somewhat misshapen. His upper trunk was shorter than his lower trunk, measured from his occiput to his pubis and from his pubis to his feet. The test of choice in this acutely ill patient would be:

A. CT scan
B. Transesophageal echocardiogram
C. Cardiac catheterization

2. A 60-year-old male patient presented with severe chest pain, shortness of breath, and history of arthroscopy. A tight bandage had been placed over his leg. The patient was tachypneic with a gray complexion. Venous pressure was elevated to 15 cm from the phlebocentric axis. On auscultation, a right ventricular S_4 was heard; P_2 was loud and S_2 widely split. The right ventricle was palpable. The D-dimer test result was elevated. The patient's ABGs were abnormal, indicating acute respiratory alkalosis.
The diagnosis is:

A. Acute myocardial infarction
B. Spontaneous pneumothorax with mediastinal flap
C. Pulmonary embolism

3. An 80-year-old male patient was admitted with severe bronchospasm but no history of chest pain prior to admission. The patient gave a previous history of coronary artery disease and bypass surgery. He had been a very heavy smoker. In the emergency room, pulse oximetry had indicated desaturation and the patient had been placed on 4 liters of oxygen. The patient's venous pressure had to be assessed from wrist measurement, and was noted to be 20 cmH₂O, hence elevated. He was treated with intravenous furosemide (Lasix). The bronchospasm subsided.
The diagnosis is:

A. Carcinoid syndrome
B. Bronchial asthma
C. Bronchospasm caused by congestive heart failure

4. A 90-year-old female patient was transferred from another hospital to the intensive care unit of the present hospital and had arterial lines and a pulmonary flotation catheter placed. Although the pulmonary

artery pressures were normal or slightly reduced, the nurse noted a prominent V wave in the wedge tracing. Transesophageal echocardiography enabled a diagnosis to be made.
The diagnosis is:

A.   Cardiogenic shock due to acute mitral regurgitation
B.   Ventricular septal defect
C.   Dehydration and hypovolemia with mitral regurgitation

5.   A patient who had had a temporary pacemaker placed in a teaching hospital was seen with tamponade. The patient was in shock with pulsus paradoxus. An echocardiogram showed diastolic collapse of the right atrium and right ventricle with signs of significant pericardial tamponade.
The diagnosis is:

A.   Perforated ventricle with hemopericardium
B.   Iatrogenic cardiac rupture
C.   Mediastinal pneumothorax

6.   A 24-year-old male presented after an automobile accident with blunt trauma to the chest. The collision had occurred 6 weeks prior to admission. The patient was mildly symptomatic with shortness of breath. After a complete evaluation, an echocardiogram was obtained that revealed the diagnosis.
The diagnosis is:

A.   Pseudoaneurysm
B.   Transient post-traumatic anxiety reaction
C.   Contusion of the right ventricle

7.   A 45-year-old Caucasian female patient presented with shock. Her history indicated that she had had a valve replaced about 3 years previously, and was mildly hypertensive. Examination did not reveal valve clicks. Transthoracic echocardiography was performed.
The diagnosis is:

A.   Heart failure obscuring valve clicks
B.   Valvular regurgitation due to endocarditis
C.   Clotted prosthetic valve

8.   An African-American female with a prosthetic Bjork-Shiley valve presented with hypotension. Examination of the heart revealed the absence of clicks. Thrombolytic therapy was instituted immediately while the patient underwent transesophageal echocardiography, which was required on account of inability to obtain valve visualization due to obesity. Following thrombolytic therapy, the patient's vital signs returned to normal.
The diagnosis is:

A. Clotted prosthetic valve
B. Myocardial infarction with response to thrombolytic medication
C. Pulmonary embolism

9. An 80-year-old male patient with prostate cancer was admitted with a history of a cerebrovascular accident. He had swelling of his right leg and venous thrombosis, as well as shortness of breath and desaturation. The patient had not been fully anticoagulated with coumadin. The diagnosis is:

A. Pulmonary and systemic embolism from clots in the leg
B. Acute myocardial infarction
C. Pulmonary embolism and stroke unrelated

10. A male patient age 5 years was seen in the emergency department doubled up with chest pain, clutching his knees and crying. He was unable to extend the neck or to sit without bending, making attempts to examine him almost impossible. His history indicated recurrent streptococcal infections with joint pains and an elevated antistreptolysin-O titer. A loud three-component pericardial friction rub was heard. The diagnosis is:

A. Juvenile chronic arthritis
B. Lyme disease
C. Rheumatic pericarditis

ANSWERS

True or False

1. *F;* 2. *T;* 3. *T;* 4. *F;* 5. *F;* 6. *F;* 7. *T;* 8. *T;* 9. *T;* 10. *T.*

Clinical Vignettes

1. *A. CT scan.* Clearly *A* would be the procedure of choice and would yield the diagnosis of dissecting aneurysm, probably due to cystic medial necrosis. In the absence of hypertension in a young patient, this is the most likely diagnosis. Type III dissecting aneurysms (Fig. 7-5) refer to ruptures of the aorta occurring beyond the subclavian artery and proceeding into the thorax and the abdomen.
2. *C. Pulmonary embolism.* The diagnosis is clearly that of *C,* pulmonary embolism. There are no signs of myocardial infarction, and in this case the right ventricle was palpable. Severe shortness of breath and elevated venous pressure bring to mind the possibility of pulmonary embolism, although a right ventricular infarction cannot be ruled out. Pulsus paradoxus was not mentioned. The patient's blood gases were abnormal, indicating a respiratory hypoxia with tachypnea. Spontane-

ous pneumothorax would have led to the physical findings of amphoric breathing, movement of the mediastinum and trachea, and shock.

3.   *C. Bronchospasm caused by congestive heart failure.* In this patient, the elevated venous pressure, the response to intravenous furosemide, and the previous history of bypass surgery point to *C*, bronchospasm caused by CHF rather than to bronchial asthma or to carcinoid syndrome. With respect to the latter, the patient showed none of the accompanying symptoms (e.g., flushing, skin changes, or diarrhea).

4.   *A. Cardiogenic shock due to acute mitral regurgitation.* A ventricular septal defect cannot be ruled out in the presence of a V wave in a patient in shock caused by rupture of the ventricular septum. The most likely diagnosis, however, is *A*. The presence of normal pressures even in the pulmonary capillary wedge tracing is not unusual in a patient in shock. Dehydration and hypovolemia with mitral regurgitation is unlikely in a patient in true cardiogenic shock. The TEE in this case clearly showed acute severe mitral regurgitation.

5.   *B. Iatrogenic cardiac rupture.* The absence of a mediastinal flap or movement of the mediastinum and trachea rule out *C*, and perforation of the ventricle with a hemopericardium is an unlikely event. Placement of the pacemaker associated with cardiac rupture therefore points to *B* as the diagnosis.

6.   *C. Contusion of the right ventricle.* A is unlikely, in that this patient's physical findings were not symptomatic of a pulmonary embolism with tachypnea, desaturation, shock, or pleuritic pain. *B*, post-traumatic anxiety reaction, cannot be absolutely ruled out as shortness of breath is common in anxiety disorders. Contusion of the right ventricle, however, is an important condition to rule out because of the possibility of sudden death. The answer therefore is *C*.

7.   *C. Clotted prosthetic valve.* The diagnosis is clearly *C*. In the absence of clicks, heart failure does not obscure valve clicks. Valvular regurgitation usually presents with relative murmurs.

8.   *A. Clotted prosthetic valve.* Myocardial infarction is an unlikely diagnosis in the absence of characteristic changes. Pulmonary embolism is unlikely in the absence of tachypnea, desaturation, and cyanosis. The most likely diagnosis is therefore *A*. Special types of Bjork-Shiley valves are prone to clotting and thrombolytic therapy can be immediately helpful.

9.   *A. Pulmonary and systemic embolism from clots in the leg.* In this particular case, the diagnosis is *A*, since the patient had an atrial septal defect which led to both pulmonary and systemic embolisms. *B* can be ruled out with certainty; *C* is unlikely.

10. *C. Rheumatic pericarditis.* The history of streptococcal infection and the friction rub suggest the diagnosis. Lyme disease may involve neck pain, but is caused by a spirochete rather than a streptococcus and is usually heralded by a skin rash.

BIBLIOGRAPHY

Trauma

Blalock A, Rabvith MM: A consideration of the non-operative treatment of cardiac tamponade resulting from wounds of the heart. *Surgery* 1962; 52:330.

Borch O, cited in Warburg E: *Subacute and chronic pericardial and myocardial lesions due to nonpenetrating traumatic injuries: A clinical study.* London, Oxford University Press, 1938.

Council on Scientific Affairs: Automobile-related injuries: Compounds, trends, prevention. *JAMA* 1983; 23:3216.

DeMuth WE, et al: Contusions of the heart. *J Trauma* 1967; 7:443.

Jones EW, Helmsworth J: Penetrating wounds of the heart: Thirty years' experience. *Arch Surg* 1968; 96:671.

Liedtke AJ, DeMuth WE Jr: Nonpenetrating cardiac injuries: A collective review. *Am Heart J* 1973; 86:887.

Louhimo I: Heart injury after blunt trauma. *Acta Chir Scan* 1, 1986; 380 (suppl).

Rea WJ, et al: Coronary artery laceration: An analysis of 22 patients. *Ann Thorac Surg* 1969; 71:518.

Shaikh KA, et al: Aortic rupture in blunt trauma. *Am Surg* 1986; 52:47.

Sugg WL, et al: Penetrating wounds of the heart: An analysis of 459 cases. *J Thorac Cardiovasc Surg* 1968; 56:531.

Symbas PN: *Cardiothoracic Trauma.* Philadelphia, Saunders, 1989:1–159.

Dissection

Ciggaroa JE, et al: Diagnostic imaging in evaluation of suspected aortic dissection: Old standards, new directions. *N Engl J Med* 1993; 328:35–43.

Cook JP, Safford RE: Progress in the diagnosis and management of aortic dissection. *Mayo Clin Proc* 1986; 61:147.

Duch PM, et al: Improved diagnosis of existing types II, III aortic dissection with multiplaned transesophageal echocardiography. *Am Heart J* 1994; 127:699–701.

Lindsay J Jr: Aortic dissection. *Heart Dis Stroke* 1992; 2:69.

Nienaber CA et al: Diagnosis of thoracic aortic dissection: Magnetic resonance imaging versus transesophageal echocardiography. *Circulation* 1992; 85:434.

Slater EE, DeSanctis RW: The clinical recognition of dissecting aortic aneurysm. *Am J Med* 1976; 60:625.

Vassile N, et al: Computed tomography of thoracic aortic dissection: Accuracy and pitfalls. *J Comp Asst Tom* 1986; 10:211.

Pulmonary Embolus

Bell WR, et al: The clinical features of submassive and massive pulmonary embolism. *Am J Med* 1977; 62:355.

Bomalaski JS, et al: Inferior vena cava interruption in the management of pulmonary embolism. *Chest* 1982; 87:767.

Dalen JE, et al: Pulmonary embolism, pulmonary hemorrhage, and pulmonary infarction. *N Engl J Med* 1965; 272:1278.

Douglas JG, et al: Pulmonary hypertension and fenfluramine. *Br Med J* 1981; 283:881.

Sasahara AA, et al: Clinical [word missing] of thrombolytic agents in venous thromboembolism. *Arch Intern Med* 1982; 142:684.

The Urokinase Pulmonary Embolism Trial. *Circulation* 1973; 47:1 (suppl 2).

Coronary Syndromes

Anderson JL, Gomez MA: The management of acute myocardial infarction. *Cardiology* 1995; 75:391–393.

Chatterjee K: Complications of acute myocardial infarction. *Contemp Intern Med* 1994; 6:11–26.

Lemtry R, et al: Prognosis in rupture of the ventricular septum after acute myocardial infarction and role of early surgical intervention. *Am J Cardiol* 1992; 70:147.

Marriott HJL: Ischemic heart disease. In Marriott HJL: *Bedside Cardiac Diagnosis*, Philadelphia, Lippincott, 1993:217–228.

Pepine CJ: Adjunctive therapies for acute MI became a little clearer in 1993. *J Myocard Ischemia* 1994; 6:6–7.

Radford MJ, et al: Ventricular septal rupture: A review of clinical and physiologic features and an analysis of survival. *Circulation* 1981; 64:545.

Reeder GS, Gersh BJ: Modern management of acute myocardial infarction. *Curr Prob Cardiol* 1993; 18:81–156.

Roberts R, et al: Pathophysiology, recognition and treatment of acute myocardial infarction and its complications. In Schlant RC et al(eds): *Hurst's The Heart*, 8th ed. New York, McGraw-Hill, 1994:1107–1184.

Shah PK, Swan HJC: Complications of acute myocardial infarction. In Chatterjee K, Parmley WW (eds): *Cardiology*. Philadelphia, Lippincott-Gower, 1991: 7.179–7.203.

8

CLINICAL ANTECEDENTS TO AUSCULTATION

THE CARDIAC EXAMINATION

THE HISTORY
  Basic Principles

GENERAL EXAMINATION
  Vital Signs
  Skin
  Head and Neck
  Chest/Heart
  Abdomen
  Extremities
  Musculoskeletal

CLINICAL EVALUATION OF COMMON SYMPTOMS AND SIGNS

ASSOCIATED WITH HEART DISEASE AND THEIR AUSCULTATORY

ACCOMPANIMENTS
  Angina Pectoris
  Dyspnea
  Syncope
  Cough/Hemoptysis
  Fatigue
  Palpitations
  Edema
  Cyanosis

THE CARDIAC EXAMINATION (Cardiac Pearl 42)

This chapter will begin with a "true-to-life" patient evaluation: the history and examination. It looks at specific symptoms or signs to illustrate the clinical method and prioritizes their auscultatory concomitants. The clinician cannot rely solely on auscultation, no matter how skillfully performed, as the sole means of gathering diagnostic information. This chapter is intended to acquaint the student with the basic components of a general cardiac examination as well as to guide in the evaluation of symptoms commonly associated with heart disease.

THE HISTORY

Basic Principles

Taking a good history is one of the most important segments of the initial clinical evaluation of a patient. The history allows the practitioner to establish rapport with the patient as well as gather information. Because many people feel anxious, embarrassed, or confused at the beginning of the office or clinic visit, the interviewer bears the responsibility of putting the patient at ease and encouraging open communication.

An adequate history is essential to obtain a full clinical picture and relate it to the patient's social, familial, and economic circumstances; general personality style and morale level; and occupational background and recreational habits. The history is akin to an inquiry into the "scene of the crime" in a detective story. The patient provides the details of the "scene"; the interviewer needs to interpret the information, distinguish significant "clues" from irrelevant material, and arrange the clues to form a tentative diagnosis.

An important ingredient in the patient interview is simple good manners. Conduct the interview in a private room or office in order to convey respect for the patient's confidentiality; the presence of clinical trainees or other third parties is guaranteed to hinder full and frank disclosure. Offer the patient a comfortable chair near or beside your desk so that he or she will not be distracted by feelings of physical awkwardness, or have to shout to answer your questions. Imagine yourself in the patient's place; make good eye contact and keep your vocal tone pleasant and reassuring. A bored, impatient, or irritable manner may upset or intimidate the patient and inhibit open communication. Consideration for the patient's feelings should also extend to the matter of delays in keeping scheduled appointments. "Running behind" may be misinterpreted by the patient, or significantly increase his or her anxiety, unless staff explains delays in a courteous and timely manner.

During the process of history-taking, it is best not to interrupt the patient's answers unless they wander into obvious irrelevancy. Many times significant information about the patient's symptoms will emerge in this way, and may save you additional questioning later on. Try to avoid leading questions; that is, questions that suggest a specific answer. For example, it is better to ask, "Can you point to the location of your chest pain?" than "Do you feel pain under your breastbone?" Most patients want to be cooperative and may answer a leading question in a way that inadvertently confuses the diagnosis. If a leading question is unavoidable, it can be phrased to elicit a detail that might not emerge otherwise. If a history of smoking is relevant, one can ask the patient how many cigarettes they presently smoke (as distinct from "Do you smoke?"). It is then less stressful for the patient to describe how many packs they smoke per day or per week.

It is a good idea to allow time for the patient to ask questions, particularly if tests must be ordered or test results interpreted. Many persons are annoyed or unnerved by treadmill tests, medication challenges, or similar procedures. The wise practitioner will be prepared to explain these tests to the patient's satisfaction, avoiding medical jargon or arousing fears by suggesting that the test is unusual. Table 8-1 is a list of commonly used cardiovascular tests.

General External Assessment (Spot Diagnosis)   Although cardiology is concerned with internal body structures and functioning, do not underestimate the importance of an overall external assessment of the patient. Inspection of the face, eyes, extremities, spine, and dentition are inexpensive methods of suggesting a tentative diagnosis. The specific significance of skin color and other facial features will be discussed below and illustrated by tables. The clinician should note the patient's general body habitus, gait, facial or postural expressions of pain, vocal tone, and other features of personality. Many of these spot diagnoses have eponyms, and more complete descriptions of each are supplied in Table 8-2.

Social History (Cardiac Pearl 43)   An adequate social history is necessary to determine certain aspects of the patient's prognosis as well as diagnosis. The social history supplies information about two important dimensions of the patient's lifestyle: (1) the presence or absence of social support (or social stress) derived from family and friendship networks; (2) patterns of substance use or abuse.

Social support   A patient's family and living circumstances may be relevant to the diagnosis and will affect treatment regimens. The patient's cardiac dysfunction may have been precipitated or exacerbated by family tension, marital separation, unemployment or job loss, poor housing or homelessness, recent bereavement, and other such pressures. If the patient has a history of military service, posttraumatic stress reactions or service-related injuries may be relevant to the diagnosis. If the patient lives alone, the existence of friendship networks is an important factor in recovery. In addition, the patient's illness will almost always impose major stress on the family; an important example is a work-related injury, loss of employment, and workman's compensation.

Substance use/abuse   Substance use or abuse is often implicated in cardiac syndromes, either directly (e.g., cardiotoxic substances including cocaine,

Table 8-1 Common Tests of Cardiovascular Structure and Function

Test	Description	Indications
Exercise testing Treadmill Bicycle ergometer	Patient is monitored by ECG while exercising on a motorized treadmill or bicycle ergometer. Can be combined with echocardiography or scintigraphy. Treadmill speed and elevation are increased every 3 min until patient becomes symptomatic	To confirm diagnosis of angina; determine severity of limitation of activity; assess prognosis of persons recovering from MI; evaluate responses to therapy. Use in screening asymptomatic persons is controversial
Nuclear medicine studies Scintigraphy Technetium Thallium	Radionuclide is injected; images reveal areas of ischemia or hypoperfusion	To assess extent of ischemic area; distinguish between reversible ischemia and persistent defects
Radionuclide scanning	Images left ventricle and measures its ejection fraction and wall motion	When exercise ECG is difficult to interpret, or its results differ from clinical impression; to localize ischemic area; to distinguish ischemic from infarcted myocardium
Ventilation/perfusion (V/Q) scan	Injection of radiopharmaceuticals (xenon and technetium)	To rule out suspected pulmonary embolism
Imaging modalities Computed tomography (CT) Magnetic resonance imaging (MRI)	Injection of intravenous contrast material	Main application is evaluation of pericardial disease Best noninvasive test for evaluating aortic dissection; also used to assess pericardial disease, cardiac neoplasms, chamber size, myocardial thickness, and congenital defects
Ultrafast CT	Rapid CT	Detection of coronary calcification
Positron emission tomography (PET)	Imaging by means of tagged isotopes, e.g., glucose, ammonia	To provide qualitative and quantitative information about blood flow and myocardial metabolism; can distinguish between "stunned" and infarcted myocardium as well as to determine myocardial viability

Cardiac catheterization		
Bedside flotation catheters, right heart	Insertion of balloon (Swan-Ganz) catheter in pulmonary artery or central vein	Used to diagnose shunts, pericardial disease, right-sided valvular lesions, distinguish between pulmonary and cardiac disease
Left heart		Quantitative assessment of mitral and aortic stenosis; used to confirm preoperative assessments of valvular lesions and to obtain selective coronary arteriograms
Intracardiac electrophysiologic testing	Multipolar electrode mapping/simulation	Diagnosis and treatment of severe arrhythmias in patients for whom ambulatory monitoring is unsuitable
Echocardiography		
Doppler ultrasound	Use of sound waves for imaging Doppler flow recordings, tissue Doppler imaging	Evaluation of deep venous thrombosis, patency of inferior vena cava, carotid bruits; assessment of transvalvular gradients and pulmonary artery pressure; patterns and directionality of blood flow
Transesophageal (TEE)	Information about intracardiac masses	Need for information about posterior structures and prosthetic valves, clots, mobility of valves, and dissecting aneurysm
Stress echocardiography	Dobutamine, pacing, dipyridamole Echo Doppler in esophagus	To detect ischemia, induced wall motion abnormalities
Drug injections		
Dobutamine	Infused as a form of stress testing in patients unable to exercise; used with echo and/or thallium	Used with stress echocardiography
Ergonovine	Administered per IV to induce vasospasm	Differential diagnosis of Prinzmetal's angina
Adenosine	Injected prior to scintigraphy (contrast imaging)	To induce vasodilation in patients unable to exercise
Dipyridamole		

nicotine, or alcohol) or indirectly (e.g., obesity, cardiac arrhythmias or electrolyte imbalances caused by eating disorders). In addition, substance abuse often causes or results from stressful family situations or living circumstances.

Family History (Cardiac Pearl 33)   The family history may be vital to the diagnosis, in that certain disorders (e.g., congenital cardiac disorders, cardiomyopathy, coronary artery disease, premature hypertension or stroke, and metabolic disorders) often run in families. Other cardiac syndromes are associated with abnormal genetic karyotypes such as those involved in Turner's syndrome or Down's syndrome; in addition, familial and/or environmental disorders predispose to obesity and heart disease.

In addition, the family history may assist in making the diagnosis of an obscure condition (e.g., a prolonged QT interval in which syncope may be a feature, as well as sudden death). In patients with Marfan's syndrome or hypertrophic cardiomyopathy, the risk of severe cardiac disease in the patient's blood relatives warrants the examination of other family members.

Past Medical History   This is a source of valuable information about previous illnesses (rheumatic fever, chorea, scarlet fever); past surgeries or procedures (chorea atrial bypass surgery, valve replacement, congenital heart surgery, angioplasty); previous hospitalizations (for myocardial infarction, heart failure, sudden death syndromes); medications administered, including those for treatment of heart failure and those that may cause heart failure (doxorubicin, beta blockers, digitalis). Drug interaction should not be missed in the history (use of warfarin with aspirin or pain medications or Zyloprim). Patient's previous history of heart murmurs detected at routine examination such as Army physicals are of importance, and when they occurred. If there is a history of heart murmurs it is important to inquire as to when they were heard. For example, if they were heard at birth, valvular heart disease may be suspected; shortly after birth, shunts may be suspected and, later on, degenerative or rheumatic heart disease.

Review of Systems (ROS)   It is extremely important to review the other organ systems of the body in obtaining a good history. Many cardiovascular disorders are associated with diseases in or traumatic injury to other organ systems. For example, thyroid disease is an important cause of heart disease; it may be induced by therapy with amiodarone (Cordarone), and present with atrial fibrillation, intractable heart failure, pericardial effusion, or cardiomyopathy. Similarly, a history of diabetes coupled with hypertension and hyperlipidemia suggests the possible presence of occult coronary artery disease. System review, when it is carried out in a systematic fashion, is directed toward evaluating the patient as a whole in addition to assisting with the diagnosis of a specific cardiac symptom endorsed by the patient.

GENERAL EXAMINATION

Vital Signs

The first part of most physical examinations is the measurement and recording of the patient's vital signs. The two most important of these, from the standpoint of cardiovascular assessment, are the patient's pulse and blood pressure. The third important vital sign, respiration, will be dealt with later in the chapter.

The Pulse Auscultatory findings and pulse measurements are complementary in clinical diagnosis. Pulses are felt at the wrist and elbow; the subclavian, carotid, and temporal arteries; the abdominal aorta; the femoral, popliteal, dorsalis pedis and anterior tibialis arteries. Palpation is performed with the tips of the fingers, with light application.

Analysis of pulsus The patient's pulse should be evaluated for the following features:

- Presence or absence
- Volume: small, normal, large
- Character: bounding, bisferiens, anacrotic, parvus, dicrotic, alternans, paradoxus, thready
- Rate: rapid, normal, slow
- Regularity
- Pulse deficit: presence or absence
- Effects of local pressure on blood vessel
- Tenderness
- Overlying bruits

Normal pulses (Fig. 8-1) have a (1) percussion wave; (2) dicrotic notch; and (3) tidal wave. Percussion wave is in systole; tidal wave is in diastole.

The different types of abnormal pulse and their clinical significance will be discussed in relation to auscultatory events.

Dicrotic Pulse A dicrotic pulse is most likely to be felt at the upper and lower extremes of cardiac output. The presence of a dicrotic pulse may be a similar phenomenon, accentuated in the presence of events that either markedly increase the percussion wave or markedly reduce it, as in high- or low-output states. Interposed between the percussion and tidal wave, the dicrotic notch and wave ordinarily have no special significance (Fig. 8-1).

Clinicians should note that the dicrotic wave is normally not easy to feel. It is felt, however, in high-output states (e.g., fever and high-output heart failure) and in hypotensive states with constricted vessels (e.g., myocardial infarction, pericardial tamponade, and constrictive pericarditis). The auscultatory findings that may be associated with a dicrotic pulse would include midsystolic murmurs due to flow and high-output states; the murmur

Table 8-2 Eponymous Disorders and Associated Cardiovascular

Disorder	Description	CV findings
Barlow's syndrome	Marfanoid habitus	Systolic click and murmur
Bernheim's syndrome	Right atrial outflow is obstructed by left ventricular septal thickening	Prominent A and V venous waves, exaggerated Y descent; increased jugular venous distension (JVD)
Budd-Chiari syndrome	Occlusion of the hepatic veins (from a variety of causes (clots, tumors)	May indicate right-sided heart failure or constrictive pericarditis
Cornelia de Lange syndrome	Severe mental deficiency, associated with a small mandible, bushy eyebrows, and low hairline	High risk of ventricular septal defect (VSD)
Cushing's syndrome	Truncal obesity, diabetes stria	Hypertension
Down's syndrome	Mongolism; caused by trisomy of chromosome 21	Risk of endocardial cushion defect and tetralogy of Fallot
Dressler's syndrome	Pericarditis following MI or open heart surgery	High ESR, pericardial and pleural effusions; occasional tamponade; right heart failure
Ehlers-Danlos syndrome	Bruising, cigarette paper scars, fragile skin	AI and MVP; aortic regurgitation
Eisenmenger's syndrome	Bidirectional or right-to-left shunt caused by pulmonary hypertension secondary to VSD	Single P$_2$, loud
Friedreich's ataxia	Slowly progressive disorder due to genetic defect in long arm of chromosome 19	Cardiac abnormalities, progressive weakening of cardiac (cardiomyopathy, HOCM)
Gaisbock syndrome	Polycythemia	Hypertension and primary polycythemia
Holt-Oram syndrome	Genetic syndrome marked by absent radius and "fingerized" thumbs, extra phalanx	Genetic ASD
Hurler's syndrome	Boar-like facies, hepatomegaly	Cardiomyopathy, ischemic heart disease, valvular lesions, nodules
Hutchinson's syndrome	Premature senility, marked by alopecia and dwarfism	Myocardial infarction
Jaccoud's arthritis	Variant of rheumatic arthritis; MP joints mobile but swollen	Rheumatic heart disease
Kaposi's sarcoma	Malignant indurated skin lesion associated with HIV infection	High output states
Kawasaki syndrome	Mucocutaneous lymph node syndrome; cause unknown	May produce arteritis of coronary and extremity vessels; ischemia and conduction defects, aneurysms of coronary arteries

Klinefelter's syndrome	Seminiferous tubule dysgenesis; results from abnormal genetic karyotype (47, XXY or 48, XXYY)
Klippel Feil syndrome	Webbed neck
Lentige's syndrome	VSD
Libman-Sacks endocarditis	High risk of VSD Associated with systemic lupus erythematosus
Loeffler's syndrome	May produce acute or chronic MR; may be a source of thrombotic emboli; may cause aortic valve disease Severe endocardial fibrosis, with eosinophilia; most common in Africa Restrictive cardiomyopathy
Marfan's syndrome	Systemic connective tissue disease, inherited as an autosomal dominant; long limbs; skeletal, eye disorders Anuloaortic ectasia, resulting in AR; abnormalities of aortic and mitral valves; easily ruptured chordae tendineae; dissection of aorta, MVP
Noonan's syndrome	Antimongoloid eyes, hoarseness Pectus excavatum; pulmonary stenosis in 50 percent of patients; ASDs and VSDs; HOCM
Ortner's syndrome	Hoarseness Mitral stenosis
Osler-Rendu-Weber syndrome	Capillary telangiectasia Pulmonary AV fistulae
Raynaud's phenomenon	Hands change color Scleroderma, primary pulmonary hypertension
Reiter's syndrome	Tetrad of urethritis, conjunctivitis, arthritis, mucocutaneous lesions; cause unknown; most common in young males Carditis; aortic regurgitation
Retz syndrome	Costochondritis Simulates angina
Stokes-Adams syncope	Form of cardiogenic syncope Intermittent ventricular arrest
Takayasu's disease	"Pulseless disease"; occlusive, polyarteritis of unknown cause; most common in Asians; typically affects branches of the aortic arch Cerebrovascular insufficiency with transient ischemic attacks; absent pulses in the arms and legs, bruits over arteries
Tangier's disease	Orange tonsils Low HDL cholesterol and strong family history of heart disease
Taussig-Bing syndrome	Double outlet, RV, VSD Reversed differential cyanosis, large VSD
Tietze's syndrome	Sprain or inflammation of chondrocostal junctions Mimics pain of angina
Turner's syndrome	Amenorrhea, shield chest, cubitus valgus, webbed neck Hypertension; cardiac abnormalities including CoA, AS, bicuspid aortic valve, aortic dissection, subaortic stenosis
Werner's syndrome	Premature senility Atherosclerotic heart disease, heart attacks
Whipple's disease	Malabsorption disorder caused by infection of the gut Pericarditis, AI, coronary artery disease
Williams' syndrome	Hypercalcemia, mental retardation Supravalvular aortic stenosis

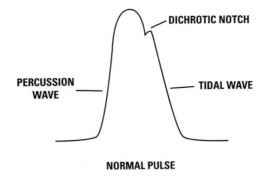

Figure 8-1   Wave pattern in a normal pulse.

of mitral regurgitation; and softening heart sounds with tachycardia in low-output states. The percussion wave is systolic; the tidal wave is diastolic and must be distinguished from the two systolic waves in pulsus bisferiens.

Anacrotic Pulse   The anacrotic pulse (Fig. 8-2) is a slow-rising pulse with a distinct shoulder on the upslope; the shoulder is followed by a wave. On occasion, the anacrotic pulse is rounded, dome-shaped and small. The visual imagery that comes to mind is the slow-relaxing tendon reflex of myxedema.

Palpate an anacrotic pulse with your thumb, with the patient's right arm extended; place your index and third finger around the patient's arm. It is important to keep the patient's arm extended and to support it with your thumb behind the elbow and your two fingers placed on the artery at the ulnar border of the elbow. This technique is easier and safer than carotid palpation, in a patient who has carotid disease or sensitivity and who may develop bradycardia. The proximity of the brachial artery to the skin makes it relatively simple to palpate. Note that an anacrotic pulse is

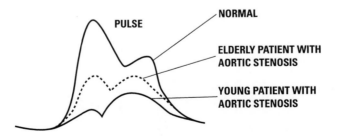

Figure 8-2   Anacrotic pulse. Comparison of pulse contour of normal, elderly, and young patient with aortic stenosis.

difficult to feel in the radial artery but is easily felt in the brachial or femoral artery.

The anacrotic pulse is characteristic of aortic stenosis. The arterial tracings previously used had elaborate timing intervals to measure the pulse upslope and correlate it with the severity of the aortic stenosis. This technique is not used at present. Clinicians should understand, however, that most patients with aortic stenosis are older, their arteries are noncompliant, and consequently the anacrotic pulse is easily obscured by the apparent large volume of the pulse ("tardus non parvus"). There is no inconsistency between a slow-rising pulse with a full volume, or an even larger apparent pulse volume. The anacrotic shoulder on the upslope in systole is extremely useful in detecting the presence of an anacrotic pulse in these patients.

The only circumstance that helps to determine the presence of an anacrotic pulse apart from other findings in the diagnosis of aortic stenosis is the simultaneous palpation of the carotid pulse and auscultation over the cardiac apex. The carotid pulse normally follows S_1 immediately. The normal time interval between these two events is very slight and representative of the period of time that it takes to open the aortic valve (approximately 30 ms). The delay in a patient with aortic stenosis is clearly much greater and the pulse is palpable close to S_2. This timing differential is valuable in diagnosing a patient in whom the pulse wave is large and the slow-rising nature of the pulse may be difficult to detect in a brachial artery.

Bounding Pulse   There are two types of bounding pulse: the large bounding pulse associated with aortic valve runoff, as in aortic regurgitation, patent ductus arteriosus, or a ruptured sinus of Valsalva opening into the right or left heart. The large bounding pulse is also seen in high-output states.

The second type of bounding pulse is the small collapsing pulse (Fig. 8-3) seen in mitral regurgitation and ventricular septal defect. Bounding pulses are empty between beats, rapidly rising and rapidly falling.

Small Volume Pulse/Thready Pulse (Cardiac Pearl 71)   Pulses fitting these descriptions are usually seen in patients in shock. They are commonly associated with tissue perfusion and narrow pulse pressure. A dicrotic notch and a "tick-tack" rhythm may be present in small-volume or thready pulses.

Pulsus Bisferiens   A bisferiens pulse (Fig. 8-4) is seen in significant aortic regurgitation and may be encountered in patients with hypertrophic obstructive cardiomyopathy (HOCM). Bisferiens pulses are rare in normal individuals and in mitral valve prolapse. The name of this pulse comes from the Latin, and means "having two peaks." Since the second peak is

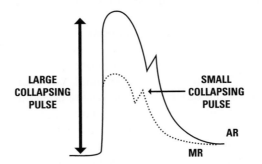

Figure 8-3 Collapsing pulses. AR, aortic regurgitation; MR, mitral regurgitation.

not related to the tidal wave. As both peaks are systolic, it is not prominent in hypertrophic obstructive cardiomyopathy, and resembles a plateau.

Bisferiens pulse is composed of a percussion wave (spike) and a second wave, referred to classically as a dome, both of which are in systole. It must be distinguished from the percussion and tidal waves of a dicrotic pulse which are systolic and diastolic, respectively; thus palpable as outward

HYPERTROPHIC CARDIOMYOPATHY
WITH OBSTRUCTION (IHSS)

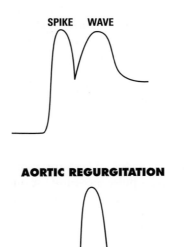

AORTIC REGURGITATION

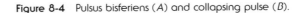

Figure 8-4 Pulsus bisferiens (A) and collapsing pulse (B).

deflections. The Valsalva maneuver increases the gradient and may accentuate a bisferiens pulse.

The waterhammer pulse is a variation of the bisferiens pulse, although
it results from a rapid percussion wave and a rapid downslope. The waterhammer pulse is characterized by a wave with a rapid upslope and rapid
downslope; it is empty between beats. It contrasts with the anacrotic pulse
of aortic stenosis, which has a slow upslope, slow downslope, and is full
between beats. The clinician can best appreciate the bounding pulse of a
pulsus bisferiens by wrapping the hand around the patient's arm just above
the wrist and elevating the wrist. Visible pulsatile impulses in the carotid
pulses may be seen in this condition (Corrigan's sign), as they are in patients
with hyperkinetic states, in coarctation of the aorta (CoA), in patent ductus
arteriosus (PDA), and in extreme bradycardia. NOTE: In acute aortic regurgitation the marked decline in stroke volume produced by the torrential
backflow across the aortic valve may obliterate the presence of a bisferiens
or a collapsing pulse.

Pulsus Paradoxus   Pulsus paradoxus (Fig. 8-5) is the most important sign
of raised intrapericardiac pressure. Pulsus paradoxus is best described with
reference to normal changes in blood pressure resulting from the breathing
cycle. Physiologically, inspiration causes an increased capacitance in the
lungs, resulting in a decrease in left ventricular filling and stroke volume;
these events tend to decrease blood pressure on inspiration. In tamponade
and constrictive pericarditis, the inspiratory decrease in blood pressure is
marked (> 10 mmHg) and is termed pulsus paradoxus. It can be detected by
palpation. The pulse may disappear at the wrist on inspiration in pericardial
tamponade; this phenomenon is easily recognized with the sphygmomanometer. Systolic pressure at expiration is noted and may be higher; slow
deflation of the cuff during inspiration will detect a lower systolic pressure.

Pulsus paradoxus is an important sign of pericardial tamponade. It may
be present in constrictive pericarditis and effusive constrictive pericarditis. It
is occasionally a confusing physical finding in chronic obstructive pulmonary
disease (COPD), hypovolemic shock, pulmonary embolism, pregnancy,
marked obesity, and obstruction of the superior vena cava and right ventricular infarction. Pulsus paradoxus is commonly seen in intensive care units
in patients with chronic obstructive pulmonary disease, or during asthma
or respiratory distress. It is evident during the examination on inspiration,
and from the blood pressure recorder in arterial lines. Pulsus paradoxus is
associated with the absence of a y descent in the venous pulse; a fall in
blood pressure on inspiration; tachycardia; tachypnea; and characteristic
echocardiographic findings with collapse of the right atrium, right ventricle,
and left atrium in diastole in pericardial tamponade.

Pulsus paradoxus is rarely seen coincidentally with Kussmaul's sign in
tamponade except in the presence of constrictive pericarditis and acute
pulmonary embolism. Thus, it is not usual to see these two signs at the

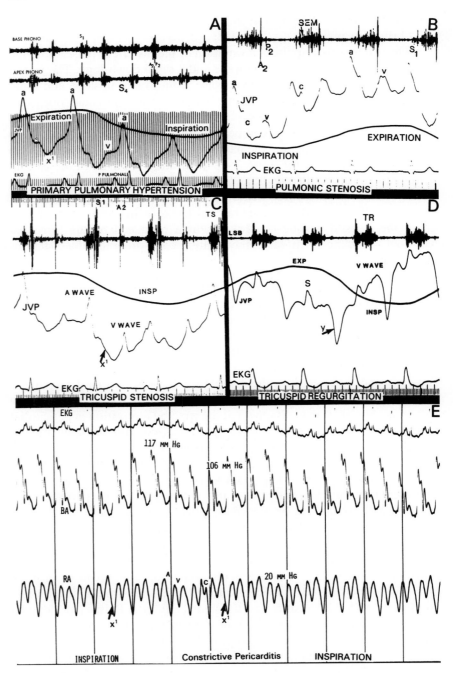

Figure 8-5   Pulsus paradoxus.

same time in patients with pericardial tamponade. In general, Kussmaul's sign occurs in a much more advanced stage of pericardial tamponade. Watching for inspiratory changes in the venous pressure while taking the blood pressure in patients with suspected tamponade is an important clinical exercise in suspected tamponade.

Reversed Pulsus Paradoxus   Reversed pulsus paradoxus is seen in hypertrophic obstructive cardiomyopathy (HOCM), in which the outflow gradient is reduced on inspiration by increasing venous return. Reversed pulsus paradoxus is difficult to elicit, and is abolished by the Valsalva maneuver or amyl nitrite.

The auscultatory findings of a patient with constrictive pericarditis have been described previously. The presence of a pericardial knock in diastole, coincident with the sudden cessation of the y descent in the venous pulse; the presence of a normal-sized heart; and the clinical presence of ascites, hepatomegaly, and engorged neck veins point to the diagnosis.

Pulsus Alternans   Pulsus alternans (Fig. 8-6) is probably the most important sign of left ventricular failure but is not often elicited at the bedside. It is characterized by fluctuation of pulse pressure with every other beat; it distinguishes true myocardial failure from other causes of heart failure due to elevated left ventricular pressure (diastolic failure). Both systolic and diastolic failure may give rise to S_3s and S_4s. Pulsus alternans is frequently noted after the presence of premature ventricular or atrial beats.

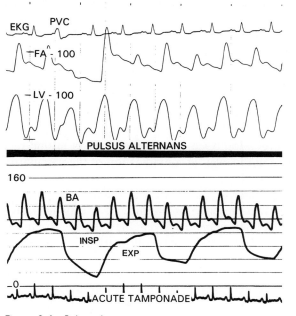

Figure 8-6   Pulsus alternans.

Pulsus alternans can be detected by light palpation of the radial pulse (Harvey), although the measurement of blood pressure by the sphygmomanometer is the most efficient means of detection. After palpation of the systolic pressure or the point at which the pulse is felt or heard on release of the pressure on the sphygmomanometer cuff will give rise to two levels of systolic pressure with alternating beats. S_2, and less commonly S_1 and S_2 together, alternate in volume in pulsus alternans.

Pulsus alternans is caused by alteration in ventricular contractility and indicates significant left ventricular myocardial failure. In HOCM significant systemic pulsus alternans is not observed, although left ventricular alternans may be present. Heart sound and loudness of the murmur will also alternate in pulsus alternans. In aortic stenosis, the loudness of the systolic murmur alternates in a fashion similar to S_2 alternation in a patient with myocardial failure.

Palpation of other arterial pulses   In some situations the palpation of other arteries may aid in differential diagnosis.

Carotid Pulses   The palpation of carotid pulses can be difficult and should always be performed with care. Palpation should never be performed over both carotid pulses at the same time. Keep in mind that carotid massage may cause changes in the following: tachycardias; atrial flutter rate (due to a breakup of the atrial flutter); and an alteration of the ratio of the flutter waves to ventricular complexes. Carotid massage will not change ventricular tachycardia but may stop reentrant supraventricular tachycardia with a pause. Pressure on the carotid sinus can also evoke or pronounce bradycardiac response and a fall in blood pressure.

Auscultation over a carotid artery may reveal the presence of carotid stenosis; pressure over the artery may induce symptoms of faintness or feelings of presyncope. The vasodepressor response is an exaggeration of the normal vagal response and may be the cause of blackout spells in patients.

Corrigan's sign (visible pulsatile impulses in the carotid arteries) is associated with aortic regurgitation. Ocular plethysmology is an indirect method of measuring pulses in the eyes, as an indication of the vascularity from the branches of the internal carotid artery. Carotid pulses are important in detecting the presence or absence of carotid lesions. They can be classified by volume or by the presence or absence of overlying bruits. Occasionally, arteriovenous fistulae may be heard in the neck due to carotid jugular communication. This phenomenon may follow traumatic injury to the neck.

Carotid pulses are extremely important to evaluate not only by palpation but also by duplex Doppler measurement and echocardiography. Recent studies have shown the importance of the carotid anatomy at the siphon and the presence or absence of obstructive plaque. The Doppler signals of the velocity, waveform, and presence or absence of thrombus or plaque are vital pieces of information in locating the focus of a stroke.

Femoral Pulses   Palpation of the femoral pulses is useful in patients with aortic regurgitation (AR). Specifically, Duroziez's murmur may be evoked by this technique. Pressure on the femoral artery proximal to the stethoscope produces a systolic murmur; distal compression elicits a diastolic murmur. The hemodynamic explanation of this phenomenon is as follows: the high velocity of flow clearly induces a systolic murmur and the retrograde flow the diastolic murmur. Occasionally, the clinician may hear a double sound over auscultation of the femoral artery in patients with a loud S_4 and pronounced atrial contraction.

In Traube's sign, a loud "booming" or "pistol shot" sound is heard when a stethoscope is placed over a patient's femoral artery in severe aortic regurgitation.

Temporal Pulses   Palpation of the superficial temporal pulses is useful in patients with temporal arteritis. This technique may evoke tenderness; aneurysms may also be palpable. Pulses in the temporal area are tortuous and may have overlying bruits.

Pulseless Disease (Idiopathic Arteritis of Takayasu)   "Pulseless disease," or Takayasu's syndrome, is a form of occlusive polyarteritis of unknown cause. Stenosis of vessels occurs with absence of pulses. Takayasu's syndrome is most common among Asians, particularly females. It has some of the features of an autoimmune disease: Patients may have features of systemic lupus erythematosus (SLE) with arthritis and fever. They may present with hypertension caused by renal artery stenosis or vascular insufficiency caused by mesenteric vessel occlusions. They may also present with symptoms of stroke and with coronary artery disease.

Takayasu's syndrome is a rare condition, usually associated with an elevated sedimentation rate (ESR). A more thready pulse is seen in shock and may be caused by cardiogenic or noncardiac shock. The patient's pulse is barely palpable; in some cases there is a "gap" between the blood pressure taken with cuff and intraarterial blood pressures. Loud systolic bruits are heard over the origins of vessels. Pulses in the femorals are smaller than brachial pulses, especially in cases involving young patients with coarctation.

Pulses and Migraine   Occasionally, auscultation over the cranial pulses may indicate the presence of a continuous murmur due to arteriovenous malformation. Patients with stereotypical unilateral migraine should be examined closely for this murmur on account of the risk of cerebral hemorrhage. Tender nodular pulses over the cranium in association with an elevated sedimentation rate suggest temporal arteritis, an important cause of blindness and headaches in the elderly.

Pulse Volume   Measurement of pulse volume is useful in intensive care units in patients with hypotension with the presence of a large volume pulse. These findings suggest sepsis; examination of the patient may reveal a septic focus. In particular, such patients should be examined for the presence of bacterial endocarditis. Changing murmurs may also be present in bacterial endocarditis.

In some instances pulse volume may be relevant to differential diagnosis. Mitral regurgitation may be characterized by a small collapsing pulse, in which the pulse volume and pressure are wide but the cardiac output is low. Pulse volume increases in high-output states; in the presence of signs of heart failure, a full-volume pulse with normal pulse pressure suggests diastolic failure with a high-output state. In myocardial failure the pulse volume is small, diastolic pressure increased, and so-called decapitate hypotension may be present as well as pulsus paradoxus.

Blood Pressure

Arterial pressure measurement   Although blood pressure is one of the basic vital signs, it is rarely measured with adequate care. In an initial cardiac examination, blood pressure should be taken in all four limbs, with the patient standing, lying, and sitting. The highest pressure measured should be correctly recorded for all four limbs. Auscultation is an important part of the procedure, in that auscultatory findings are necessary not only for the accurate measurement of blood and pulse pressures, but also for ruling out pseudohypertension.

Before the sphygmomanometer cuff is applied, systolic blood pressure should be taken first by palpating at the patient's wrist. Systolic blood pressure is always measured by palpation; it should be 5 to 10 mmHg below the auscultated pressure. The bell of the stethoscope is used to take blood pressures. Allow a pause for the return of venous blood before taking sequential blood pressure measurements (Cardiac Pearl 91). Proper palpation gives the clinician a measurement closer to the true systolic blood pressure, and allows detection of the auscultatory gap, which is the difference between the palpated pressure and the auscultated pressure.

When the sphygmomanometer is used, care must be taken to choose the right cuff size, which is proportionate to the width of the patient's arm. The ideal width of the cuff should be 20 percent wider than the arm where it is placed and should fit snugly. Recommended dimensions are 13 by 35 cm. A small cuff may produce too high a reading and a large cuff a low reading. Cuffs that are too large also tend to slip down, obscuring the appropriate position for auscultation of the brachial artery. After a cuff of the proper size has been applied in the appropriate location and inflated correctly at 3 mmHg/s, the clinician listens over the artery with the stethoscope for the Korotkoff sounds (named for a Russian military physician) as the cuff is deflated at 3 mmHg/s. The Korotkoff sounds are listed sequentially in Table 8-3. Blood pressures should be measured in both arms and legs; in the legs it may exceed that in the arms in systole by 20 mmHg to

Table 8-3 Eponymous Signs Associated with Cardiovascular Measurements or Disorders

Sign	Description	Significance
Barham's sign	Local pressure applied to pulse artery of AV fistula	Causes slowing of heart rate in AV fistula
Broadbent's sign	Rib retraction	Constrictive effusive pericarditis
Cheyne-Stokes respiration	Repeated cycle of gradual increase in depth of breathing followed by gradual decrease to apnea	
Corrigan's sign	Visible pulsatile impulses in the carotid pulses	Indicates aortic regurgitation, hyperkinetic states, CoA, PDA, and extreme bradycardia
de Musset's sign	Patient's head bobs in time with the pulse	Aortic regurgitation
Duroziez' sign	Diastolic murmur over a partially compressed peripheral artery (usually the femoral)	Aortic regurgitation
Homan's sign	Pain in calf elicited by forcible dorsiflexion of foot	Venous thrombosis
Janeway lesions	Painless erythematous lesions on palms or soles	Infective endocarditis
Korotkoff sounds	Low-pitched sounds ← vibration of artery, detected using the stethoscope bell when obtaining BP Clear tapping sound Soft murmurs Louder murmurs Muffled sounds Sounds cease	Appearance of the sounds indicates systolic pressure; complete disappearance measures diastolic pressure
Kussmaul's sign	Increase in jugular venous pressure during inspiration	Constrictive pericarditis; restrictive cardiomyopathy
Levine's sign	Patient clenches fist over chest while describing chest pain	Angina; acute myocardial infarction
Osler's nodes	Painful red raised lesions on the extremities	Subacute bacterial endocarditis
Osler's sign	Brachial or radial artery is palpable when BP cuff is inflated above systolic pressure	Noncompressible blood vessels
Quincke's sign	Alternating reddening and blanching of fingernail bed following light compression	Chronic aortic regurgitation
Roth spots	Exudative lesions in retina	Infective endocarditis
Traube's sign	"Booming" or "pistol shot" sounds heard over the femoral arteries	Chronic aortic insufficiency

palpation, but are equal in diastole. The patient is kept supine when measuring blood pressure in the legs.

The appearance of the Korotkoff sounds (or fluctuations of the needle or mercury column) indicates systole and the complete disappearance of the sounds signifies diastole. Attenuation of the sounds should not be interpreted as identifying diastole. Pulse pressure is defined as the difference between systole and diastole. It increases in (1) states of vasodilation; (2) high-output states; (3) conditions in which systolic pressure is elevated (e.g., older patients with noncompliant arteries). Diastolic hypertension in the elderly is unusual, since the diastolic blood pressure tends to fall as people age. Elevated diastolic blood pressure in an elderly patient suggests the diagnosis of renal hypertension as the cause of the hypertension. The pulse pressure $(S - D)$ exceeds D in collapsing pulses. Blood pressure in the legs in AR may exceed that in the arms by 20 to 60 mmHg. Whitecoat hypertension is avoided by reporting blood pressure measurements at the end of the examination or in the home, with a 24-h blood pressure recorder.

Blood pressure measurement in children   The measurement of blood pressure in children is similar to the procedures followed for adults, although the cuffs used are smaller. In infants, the flush technique is utilized by inflating the blood pressure cuff until the limb blanches and then letting the blood pressure decrease until the color returns.

Although pediatric cardiologists advocate attenuation phase IV of the Korotkoff sounds (Table 8-3) as representing diastolic pressure, adult cardiologists tend to use phase V, namely, the absence of the pulse.

Pseudohypotension   Pseudohypotension is a condition in which the patient's intraarterial and central blood pressures are higher than those auscultated by a cuff. When this condition pertains, the practitioner should obtain intraarterial pressure measurements with intraarterial lines. This specification is a particularly important consideration in intensive care units, in which accurate measurement of vital signs is critical. Pseudohypotension commonly results from intense vasospasm caused by low cardiac outputs. The low-output state is usually caused either by hypovolemia or by cardiogenic shock.

Doppler recording of blood pressure   Clinicians should note that Doppler recordings of blood pressure are accurate for systolic pressures but not accurate in detecting diastolic pressures. Auscultatory methods are useful in detecting mean arterial pressure. This is the point at which the maximum excursion of the column of mercury or needle is seen. Using an aneroid manometer, the clinician can measure mean arterial pressure fairly easily.

Venous pressure (Cardiac Pearl 44)

Measurement of Jugular Venous Pressure   The jugular venous pressure represents right atrial pressure, and has been likened to the manometer of the heart. The internal jugular vein has been likened to nanometers, hence the venous pressure is measured from the level of the right atrium below to the meniscus in the internal jugular vein. Measurements from the right atrium are made at the phlebocentric axis which corresponds to the middle of the right atrium with the patient lying supine or at 45 degrees. The angle of bruit which was used in the past to measure venous pressure is an inaccurate anatomical landmark for this purpose and probably hemodynamically not relevant.

External jugular veins   The anatomical entry points of the external jugular vein into the internal jugular make the external jugulars unreliable and confusing as a means of measuring venous pressure. The external jugular veins communicate with the superior vena cava after making two turns of nearly 90 degrees. It is difficult to communicate pressure accurately through two turns which are almost right angles; not infrequently the entry points of the external jugular veins are thrombosed.

Internal jugular veins   The internal jugular veins are important to examine, with one exception. During modest inspiration, partial compression of the left innominate vein is usually present. The right internal jugular veins tend to line up with the superior vena cava, allowing better transmission of pressures. Thus it is preferable to examine the right internal jugular vein in measuring venous pressure.

Identification of Venous Pulsations   It is possible to identify and measure the right internal jugular pulse as a noninvasive bedside procedure. Right atrial pressure can also be measured in this way. Place the patient in the body position that allows the top level or meniscus in the vein to be readily detected. Have the patient breathe in and out gently, without tightening the muscles of the neck. These muscles can very easily obscure venous pulsations if they tighten up from anxiety or labored breathing. Once the patient's respiration has settled into a regular pattern of gentle breaths, you should be able to measure the heights of the respective venous waves if necessary.

The height of the venous pressure is measured from the midpoint of the meniscus from the base before the v-y rise. The exception to this rule is constrictive pericarditis, in which the measurement is taken from the meniscus before the second decrease or dip in the pulse pressure. Measurement from the phlebocentric axis is more accurate than from the angle of Louis, on account of the variable distance from the mid-right atrium to the angle of Louis.

Abnormalities of Venous Pressure   During inspiration, the veins ordinarily undergo inspiratory collapse. In constrictive pericarditis and restrictive cardiomyopathy, however, the jugular venous pressure is elevated on inspiration. This phenomenon is called Kussmaul's sign, and may represent either absence of inspiratory collapse or a true elevation of venous pressure. Kussmaul's sign may be obscured by the presence of peripheral venous congestion. It is a rare sign in pericardial tamponade, occurring late.

A summary of the events and heart sounds associated with venous waves and wave segments may be found in Table 8-4.

Table 8-4   Venous Waves, Associated Events, and Heart Sounds

Venous wave	Associated event	Heart sound
A wave	Atrial systole	Precedes S_4
X or x' wave	Atrial diastole	Precedes S_1 and follows S_1
C wave	Carotid pulse transmission	Follows S_2
V wave	Atrial filling	AT tricuspid valve opening
		Follows S_2
Y descent	Rapid ventricular filling	Follows S_3
H wave	Slow-filling ventricle	Precedes S_4

A waves   A waves are characteristically described as "flicks in the neck." They are visible to the naked eye in patients with tricuspid valve stenosis. In this abnormality, the a wave is high and markedly evident, as it is in elevated venous pressure. Large a waves are seen in tricuspid obstruction caused by right atrial myxomas; in pulmonary hypertension; with atrial thrombi; and in tricuspid atresia. The "a" wave is presystolic and is not to be confused with cannon waves, which are systolic. The presence of "a" waves allows the clinician to distinguish between tetralogy of Fallot and pulmonary stenosis with intact septum; the latter condition is marked by prominent venous a waves. Auscultatory counterparts of these diagnoses are well referenced. The occurrence of a prominent "a" wave should raise the index of suspicion for tricuspid stenosis (Fig. 8-7). The clinician should look for middiastolic rumbles that increase on inspiration; tricuspid opening

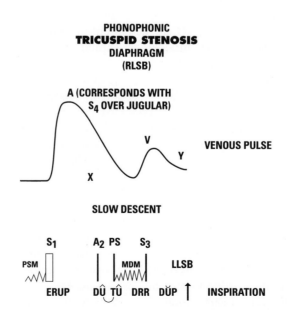

Figure 8-7   Venous pulse in tricuspid stenosis.

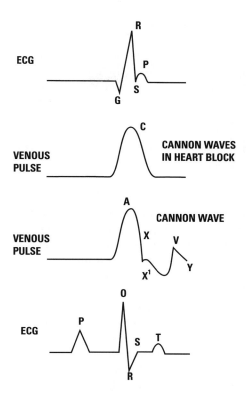

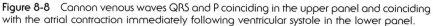

Figure 8-8 Cannon venous waves QRS and P coinciding in the upper panel and coinciding with the atrial contraction immediately following ventricular systole in the lower panel.

snaps and presystolic venous and hepatic pulsations; by signs of pulmonary valve stenosis or pulmonary hypertension.

Cannon waves (Fig. 8-8)   Cannon waves occur in ventricular diastole, represent abrupt elevation of venous pressure, and are caused by the reflux of blood when the atrium contracts against a closed atrioventricular valve. Seen regularly, cannon waves signify the presence of premature beats, which may be bigeminal; if so, alternating cannon waves may be noted. This phenomenon may be seen in pacemaker syndromes in which atrial synchrony is lost. Cannon waves are also an important indication of third-degree atrioventricular block, and are also seen in junctional rhythm.

"C" and "cv-y" waves   The c wave is a positive deflection seen at the beginning of the outward deflection which begins the x_1 descent. The c wave is observed in patients with prolonged PR intervals and soft S_1s; it precedes the carotid pulse. The c wave has little clinical significance except in the context of severe tricuspid regurgitation. In these patients cv-y pulsation occurring in right ventricular systole creates a marked positive or lateral surge of tricuspid regurgitation, reflecting right ventricular pressures, on both the upslope and the downslope of the wave. These surges corre-

spond with a lateral movement alternating with an inward movement ("rocking ear sign").

"Cv-y" pulsations are an important finding; they clearly reflect right ventricular pressures. If a patient with "cv-y" pulsations is standing upright, the pulsations may be seen in the neck and ears. When the clinician observes the patient from behind, the lateral movements of the ears will be clearly visible. The "cv-y" wave is also present in systolic abdominal pulsations in the liver. *"V" waves* "V" waves are postsystolic waves seen in atrial filling, in contrast to the presystolic "a" waves. A "v" wave may be seen as a slow lateral surge in the patient's neck, whereas the "a" wave is a rapid lateral flick. Dominant "v" waves are seen in tricuspid regurgitation, in which they are systolic events ("cv-y" waves). "V" waves are coincidental with a pansystolic murmur of tricuspid regurgitation that increases on inspiration. The "v" wave seen in atrial fibrillation is a diastolic event. A dominant "v" wave is seen in patients with atrial septal defects without significant pulmonary hypertension or tricuspid regurgitation. A prominent "cv-y" descent may occasionally be seen in mitral regurgitation in association with an atrial septal defect and in endocardial cushion defects. Prominent "a" and "v" waves may appear in Bernheim's syndrome. In this syndrome, right atrial inflow is obstructed by the septal thickening. "V" waves are delayed in mild tricuspid regurgitation.

Descending segments: X, X' and Y The wave descents represent atrial relaxation. They are reduced in tricuspid stenosis, but increase on inspiration, which allows rapid filling of the atrium to proceed. Thus, inspiration produces a reduction in venous pressure but prominent x and y descents. The x' descent disappears altogether in right ventricular hypertension but is seen in tamponade (Fig. 8-9). Note that the x' descent is a systolic event and the y descent a diastolic event. X' is referred to as "x prime" and is caused by the relaxation of the atrium during ventricular systole. The "a" wave and the x descent are absent in patients with atrial fibrillation.

The x' descent is obscured in patients with tricuspid regurgitation but increased in tricuspid stenosis. A normal or absent x descent may be seen after open heart surgery, and in cases of congenital absence of the pericardium. *Y descents* A slow "y" descent suggests tricuspid valve obstruction or right ventricular obstruction and right ventricular relaxation. In constrictive

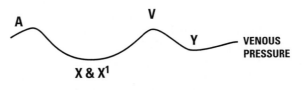

VENOUS PULSE IN TAMPONADE

Figure 8-9   Venous pulse in tamponade.

pericarditis, the "x" descent is absent and the "y" is prominent. The "y" descent in constrictive pericarditis is often interrupted by a halt in the descent attributed to impaction of the heart against the fibrous sac (Fig. 8-10). This wave corresponds with an audible pericardial knock.

An exaggerated "v" wave and "y" descent may be seen in Bernheim's syndrome. The septum of the left ventricle bulges into the opposite ventricle, creating an outflow tract gradient and interfering with filling, and producing a gradient across the aortic valve. This phenomenon is seen in slow hearts with tricuspid regurgitation.

Skin

An eminent cardiologist has noted that there is value to observing the patient before undressing the patient. With regard to the skin, a skillful clinician can make some observations relevant to differential diagnosis before asking the patient to disrobe (Marriot).

Facial Discoloration   Although facial discoloration is more noticeable in Caucasians than in darker-skinned persons, changes in a patient's complexion color may often provide useful clues for later follow-up. Specific examples include the malar icteric flush of right heart failure due to mitral stenosis; the violaceous hue of carcinoid syndrome; the pallor of pheochromocytoma; the peaches-and-cream complexion of myxedema; and the cyanotic coloration of chronic obstructive pulmonary disease or tetralogy of Fallot (Table 8-5).

Dermatologic Disorders   After the patient disrobes, the examiner should inspect the skin of the trunk and extremities for lesions associated with cardiac disease. Dermatologic lesions or other changes in the skin may be grouped into the following categories:

Rashes and eruptions   Red spots on the trunk (erythema eruptiva) may be seen in hypertriglyceridemia secondary to diabetes. A red erythematous

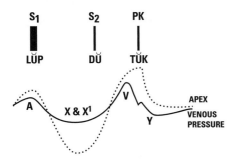

Figure 8-10   Phonocardiogram venous pressure and apex cardiogram in constrictive pericarditis.

Table 8-5   Head and Neck Abnormalities in Clinical Syndromes with Associated Cardiovascular Symptoms

Disorder	Head/neck features	Associated CV findings
"Type A" personality	Hostile, anxious, impatient, "driven"	Coronary artery disease
Alcohol abuse	Alcoholic facies (flushing, "red nose"); acne rosacea; parotid enlargement	Hypertension, esophageal varices, tachycardia ← delirium tremens (DTs)
Carcinoid syndrome	Episodic flushing, violaceous coloring, telangiectasia of the face	Tricuspid stenosis, pulmonary hypertension, tricuspid regurgitation, pulmonary valvular disease; accentuated P_2
Cornelia de Lange's syndrome	Bushy eyebrows, small mandible, tilted nose with broad tip	VSD
Down's syndrome	Mongoloid facies; prominent epicanthic folds, large tongue, mental deficiency, simian crease in hand	Endocardial cushion defect, Fallot's tetralogy
Hypothyroidism	Puffy eyes, dry skin and hair, "peaches-and-cream" coloring, absent outer third of eyebrow	Pericardial effusion, bradycardia, atherosclerotic heart disease, cardiomyopathy
Kearns-Sayre syndrome	Bilateral asymmetrical ptosis	Heart block
Klippel-Feil syndrome	Webbed neck, low ears, cleft palate, facial asymmetry, torticollis	Ventricular septal defect
Libman-Sacks		
Lupus erythematosus	"Butterfly" rash, neck rash, alopecia, Raynaud's phenomenon, photosensitive skin	Mitral regurgitation, myocarditis, hypertension, cardiac arrhythmias
Marfan's syndrome	Subluxation of the iris, ectopic lentis, long face, malpositioned ears, high-arched palate, pigmented cartilage	Atrial septal defect

Mulberry Nanism	Triangular face, low-bridged nose, bulging, forehead; small head and nose	Constrictive pericarditis
Myotonia dystrophica	Receding hairline, cataracts, wasted masklike face	Cardiomyopathy
Noonan's syndrome	Short stature, dental malocclusion, neck webbing	Valvular PS, HOCM
Obesity	Cyanotic, sleepy	Pickwickian syndrome, hypertension, angina
Osteogenesis imperfecta	Clear or blue sclera	Mitral valve prolapse
Pheochromocytoma	Episodic pallor, sweating; occasional papilledema or retinal hemorrhage	Episodic hypertension with cardiomegaly; variable A_2; palpitations, precordial pain, tachycardia, angina
Polychondritis	Destruction of cartilage in nasal bridge and edges of ears	Aortic insufficiency, aortic valve dissection, aortic regurgitation, pericarditis
Polymyositis/dermatomyositis	Dusky red rash over "butterfly area" of face and neck; periorbital edema with purplish suffusion over upper eyelids	Myocarditis
Renal disorders and failure	Dry or itching skin; cyanotic eyes	Pericarditis with or without tamponade; hypertension, CHF
Thyrotoxicosis	Stare and lid lag, fine hair, moist warm skin	Tachycardia, atrial fibrillation, palpitations, presbycardia
Turner's syndrome	Ptosis, micrognathia, low-set ears, epicanthal folds, cataracts, webbed neck	Hypertension, aortic dissection, bicuspid aortic valve, aortic stenosis, coarctation of aorta
Werner's syndrome	Balding and "old" faces in children; cataracts, small-margined eyes	Atherosclerotic heart disease, heart attacks
Williams' syndrome	Turned-up nose, broad cheeks, peg teeth, large ears	Supravalvular aortic stenosis

rash (Janeway lesions) may be present in the skin in infective endocarditis. Kaposi's sarcoma is seen in HIV-positive patients with associated cardiac problems. Circular patches of rapidly enlarging macules (erythema marginatum) are seen in acute rheumatic fever. A gradually expanding area of redness (erythema chronicum migrans) is seen in patients with Lyme disease and complete heart block. Erythema, desquamation, or a polymorphous rash in children may be associated with coronary artery disease in Kawasaki's syndrome.

Changes in the skin's texture or elasticity   Thin, fragile skin with scarring is seen in patients with Ehlers-Danlos syndrome. "Turkey skin" (hyperelasticity) is seen in pseudo-xanthoma elasticum and is associated with angina, claudication, ulcers, aortic regurgitation, and mitral valve prolapse. Crackling of the skin on palpation is seen in patients with pneumomediastinum and millwheel murmurs. Cardiogenic shock may produce peripheral cyanosis in the skin of extremities with poor perfusion. Dry and eruptive skin is seen in myxedema. Scaly feet are seen in keratoderma blennorrhagica, and aortic regurgitation associated with Reiter's syndrome.

Changes in skin pigmentation   Leopard spots (multiple pigmented areas) are seen in the Lentiges syndrome and associated with HOCM and pulmonary stenosis. Yellow-orange spots are associated with rhabdomyomas of the heart and tuberous sclerosis. Brown skin may be seen in Addison's disease and hemochromatosis. Yellow skin is seen in patients with right heart failure, hepatic failure, pulmonary hypertension, elevated venous pressure, and telangiectasia. "Café-au-lait" patches are associated with pheochromocytoma.

Head and Neck

Clinical syndromes with head and neck abnormalities associated with cardiovascular symptoms and disorders are listed in Table 8-5.

Mouth and Pharynx   Tangier's disease is associated with a low high-density lipoprotein (HDL) cholesterol count, orange tonsils and a strong family history of heart disease. A high-arched palate is seen in patients with Marfan's syndrome. A cleft palate with erupted teeth in a neonate is associated with Ellis-van Creveld syndrome and subaortic stenosis. Hoarseness and a large tongue are present in primary amyloidosis and in Ortner's syndrome in mitral stenosis.

Chest/Heart

Visual inspection, palpation, and percussion of the thoracic area are important segments of an initial cardiac examination and are carried out in sequence.

Inspection   Before proceeding to observation of the patient's chest movements during respiration, note any external abnormalities of the thoracic area. These include skin rashes and other dermatologic lesions; bloating of the chest; deformities of the rib cage or spine (Table 8-6); congenital stigmata; gynecomastia in male patients; and surgical scars. A bulging pulsatile mass in the sternum may be caused by an aneurysm. Gynecomastia may indicate the presence of liver failure or of Klinefelter's syndrome (Table 8-2), which is associated with congenital heart disease, mitral valve prolapse, and atrial septal defects.

Next, observe the patient's respiratory rate and pattern. Locate the trachea in front of the midline and watch the movements of the chest as the patient inhales and exhales. Is there indrawing of the ribs? Does the patient complain of or appear to be in pain? Watch for the presence of Levine's sign (Table 8-2), in which the patient makes a clenched fist over the chest while describing the pain. Levine's sign points to angina or myocardial infarction. Listen for wheezes and stridor. Count the rate of respiration. Is the patient hyperventilating? Are there apneic pauses? Note the presence of Cheyne-Stokes (Table 8-2) or other abnormal respirations. Look for indrawing ribs and stridor, waxing and waning respiration with pauses, "Cheyne Stokes" breathing, irregular Biot's respiration, deep sighing respiration of Kussmeul in diabetic ketoacidosis, as well as snoring in sleep apnea.

Palpation   Palpate the chest for crepitus and elicit vocal fremitus over an area of consolidation. Note any unusual findings in skin texture or elasticity. If Tietze's syndrome (Chap. 7) or other musculoskeletal disorders are suspected in the differential diagnosis of chest pain, examine the rib cage for localized tenderness and swelling.

Percussion   Percuss the chest for absolute dullness (indicating effusion or masses) and listen for bronchial breathing, egophony, rhonchi, rales, sibili,

Table 8-6   Chest Deformities, Associated Findings, and Methods of Examination

Condition	Findings
Pectus excavatum	Tilting corrugated diaphragm may be necessary to gain apposition
Blown chest	Diminished breath sounds
	Heart must be auscultated from subxiphoid area
Straight back syndrome	Signs of pulmonary hypertension simulated
	Midsystolic murmur
	Loud P_2
	Widely split S_2
	Right ventricular impulse
Kyphoscoliosis	May cause pulmonary hypertension
Pigeon chest	Small bell may be required for intercostal auscultation
Prominent left border	Enlarged right ventricle

and crepitations. Measure the vital capacity of the lungs. Listen for distant breath sounds. Elicit rib retraction in constrictive effusive pericarditis (Broadbent's sign) and dullness below the scapula (Ewart's sign). Examine the lymph nodes. In assessing rales associated with congestive heart failure (CHF), note that they occur late in its development but may persist after CHF regresses (phase lag).

Percussion is a valuable technique in a variety of circumstances:

- Delineating right atrial enlargement
- Estimating heart size (Chap. 2)
- Detecting retrosternal masses
- Detecting pleural effusions and ascites
- Detecting hepatosplenomegaly
- Detecting a pneumothorax.

Examination of Cardiac Thrills and Impulses   After the general visual and manual examination of the thoracic area, the clinician should evaluate the patient for the presence and character of thrills and cardiac impulses.

Thrills (Cardiac Pearl 79)   Cardiac thrills are palpable "purring" vibratory murmurs. They may be felt at the apex (mitral stenosis, mitral regurgitation), Erb's point (ventricular septal defect), pulmonary area (pulmonary stenosis), or aortic area (aortic stenosis). Systolic thrills may be felt in the aortic area in aortic stenosis.

Cardiac impulses   Manual examination of the chest is often valuable in the detection of chamber enlargement. One or two hands may be used to palpate the chest for evaluation of cardiac impulses. It is useful to palpate the apex and precordium with both hands.

Aortic pulsation may be felt with aneurysms, in patients with luetic (syphilitic) aneurysms, and rarely in those with Marfan's syndrome with type I dissections. Pulsations of the neck are evident in a patient with a unfolded aorta. Precordial pulsation designates or denotes long-standing right ventricular enlargement and may be seen in a variety of forms of congenital heart disease in pulmonary hypertension. A palpable diffuse apical impulse may be seen in left ventricular aneurysms. Subxiphoid pulsations are useful in detecting right ventricular enlargement.

Left ventricular impulses (Cardiac Pearl 81)   The beating heart rotates counterclockwise, impacting the thorax and giving rise to a localized impulse. The apex beat is the lowest and outermost point at which cardiac impulses are felt or seen (10 cm from the midsternal line in the fourth or fifth intercostal space). The point of maximum impulse is the point at which the maximum impulse is felt.

The left ventricular apical impulse is an outward counterclockwise thrust. Prominent impulses of the left ventricle may lead to retraction of the parasternal area (Cardiac Pearl 82), often mistaken as a parasternal lift. The cardiac impulse can be normal, hyperdynamic, or sustained at the apex with retraction in the precordial area. The left ventricular impulse may be hyperkinetic in patients with mitral regurgitation and in the presence of shunts. The impulse may be sustained, diffuse, and perceptible over a wide area in ventricular aneurysms (Cardiac Pearl 60). The initial systolic impulse is noted in isometric systole, during which the ventricle twists counterclockwise, impacting the ribs. This phenomenon coincides with the "E" wave of the apex cardiogram. In sustained ventricular impulse, the patient may have left ventricular hypertrophy. In some cases, a triple ripple (Chap. 6) may be felt at the apex in idiopathic hypertrophic subaortic stenosis, corresponding with a presystolic a wave and a double apical impulse. In systole, the left ventricular impulse is an excellent indication of good left ventricular function in a normal patient or in rocking diastolic failure. A poorly felt flattened impulse is seen in dilated cardiomyopathy, systolic failure, mitral regurgitation, and aortic regurgitation. This association may result from segmental wall motion that may be present in these conditions.

In patients with angina pectoris, a presystolic impulse and diffuse apical impulse may be seen, felt, or heard; these are relieved by nitroglycerin. In mitral valve prolapse, an outward hypokinetic impulse is interrupted by a deep notch, corresponding with a midsystolic click. Although this phenomenon is clearly visible on the apex cardiogram, it is not evident clinically. In constrictive pericarditis, the ventricle pushes against the chest wall during systole and retracts in ejection. During diastole, there is a return of a rapid impulse to the chest wall which is abruptly checked.

Right ventricular impulses (Cardiac Pearl 80)   Right ventricular impulses are heaving impulses sustained with a clockwise rotation and are felt to the left of the sternum in the fourth intercostal space. Sternal heaves are significant of pulmonary hypertension. In patients with tetralogy and trilogy of Fallot, right ventricular impulses are not felt and "a" waves are not seen, probably on account of the ventral septal defect. In severe mitral regurgitation, systolic pulsations of the precordial area may be mechanical, caused by displacement of the right ventricle by a dilated left atrium during systole. Hyperkinetic right ventricular impulses are associated with atrial septal defect; they may be felt or seen in the subxiphoid area.

If both left ventricular and right ventricular impulses are present, a null zone is present between the left and right ventricles. The use of both hands is helpful in examining patients with pulmonary hypertension or pulmonary stenosis, in that pulsations of the pulmonary artery may be evident with alternating right ventricular impulses. These impulses alternate with parasternal heaves of right ventricular dilatation. Pulmonary clicks,

P$_2$ and systolic thrills may also be felt. RV impulses may be palpable in chest deformities and straight back syndrome.

Abdomen

The abdomen should not be neglected in the initial cardiac examination. The clinician should inspect the patient's abdomen for eversion of the umbilicus, venous engorgement, and protuberance. All of these conditions have important clinical connotations. An everted umbilicus and distended abdomen suggest ascites. Truncal obesity is a predisposing factor in coronary artery disease. A protuberant abdomen with purple striae indicates Cushing's disease (Table 8-2), a condition associated with hypertension and polycythemia.

Abdominal Veins   Venous pulsations may be present in the abdomen as well as the thorax. By "milking" the abdominal veins upward, the examiner can determine whether all the veins drain upward, an indication of an inferior vena caval obstruction. An obstruction is indicated if the veins above can be milked downward toward the umbilicus, as these normally drain to the superior vena cava. In superior vena caval obstruction, superficial veins traverse the subcostal ridge and can be milked downward. Distended veins over the umbilicus may be caused by portal hypertension and often associated with liver cirrhosis and pulmonary hypertension.

Abdominal Bruits   Examination of the abdomen for tenderness, bruits, and pulsation is carried out routinely to rule out the possibility of abdominal aneurysms, renal artery stenosis, and portal hypertension. Bruits over the renal arteries may be heard in patients with hypertension in the flanks or abdomen. In general, abdominal bruits are not significant in the differential diagnosis of younger persons, but may be helpful in diagnosing patients who are hypertensive or in older patients.

Male Genitalia   In male patients, examination of the scrotum may reveal the presence of pulsatile or distended varices associated with tricuspid regurgitation. A right-sided testicle that is lower than its counterpart may be associated with situs inversus. Sacral examination may provide the first clue to edema.

Liver

Enlargement   An acutely enlarged liver is associated with tricuspid regurgitation (TR) and heart failure. The clinician palpates for hepatomegaly after percussion of the upper border, to clarify that the liver is truly enlarged and not ptosed (drooping). In tricuspid regurgitation, the liver may be tender and pulsatile with systolic pulsation (Cardiac Pearl 59). An enlarged liver is best palpated gently with the closed fist below the liver, the knuckles pointing caudad. Pain designates acute liver enlargement in patients with heart failure.

Ascites and Distension   Ascites (excessive accumulation of fluid in the abdominal cavity) can be determined by palpating the liver with rapid hand movements ("dipping"). This technique displaces the fluid and allows the liver border to be felt; the same is true for the spleen. The clinician should examine the liver for tenderness and nodules. Venous pressure can be noted during palpation of the abdomen. Hepatojugular reflux, more recently called the abdominal jugular test (Cardiac Pearl 98), should be elicited. In this test the examiner observes jugular venous pulsations to see if they rise more than 1 cm with sustained (30 s) pressure on the right upper quadrant of the abdomen. Positive findings indicate increased central blood volume.

Percussion of the abdomen may reveal the presence of fluid by demonstrating shifting dullness. The abdominal periphery is dull and the abdomen is resonant. When the patient is turned on the left side, the bowel area becomes resonant due to fluid rising upward. If ascites is suspected and cannot easily be elicited, have the patient assume the knee-elbow position (Chap. 2). The presence of ascites can then be determined by percussing over the umbilicus. The veins over the umbilicus may give rise to a venous confluence (caput medusae). There may be a continuous overlying murmur, a sign of portal hypertension.

Abdominal distension may be caused by gas in an ileal intestinal obstruction, and bowel sounds may be absent. Abdominal distension in physiological pregnancy and upper truncal obesity is related to coronary heart disease.

There are a number of serious cardiac abnormalities associated with abdominal findings. Patients with enlargement of the liver may have right heart failure, right ventricular infarction, cor pulmonale, pulmonary hypertension, or constrictive pericarditis. Ascites is not commonly seen in heart failure, although in advanced states, anasarca may be present with ascites, swelling of the legs, and pitting of the skin resembling orange peel (peau d'orange). The examiner should note such signs of liver failure as parotid enlargement and gynecomastia (in males), as well as the presence of testicular atrophy, spider nevi, and high-output states.

Extremities

Inspect the patient's extremities for pigmentation, unilateral swelling, and pallor. The skin and toenails are examined for trophic changes. Dry skin may be present in patients with hypothyroidism. Tenderness over the veins is palpated using the finger technique, in which the examiner runs the fingers serially down the patient's calf. Tenderness elicited by hyperextension of the foot is equivalent to a positive Homan's sign (Table 8-2). In either case, deep vein thrombosis is suspected. Dependent rubor of the legs and cyanosis are seen in patients with poor arterial pulses and poor circulation.

Arterial Bruits (Cardiac Pearl 63)   The patient's lower limbs should be examined for bruits, starting with the femoral, popliteal, dorsalis pedis, and posterior tibialis pulses. Palpate the brachial-femoral pulse to determine the presence of coarctation. Bruits over the femoral arteries may be systolic or continuous, depending on the degree of stenosis. There may be bruits audible over the iliac arteries.

Reflexes and Skin   The clinician should determine the patient's ankle-brachial ratios. In patients with myxedema, the deep tendon reflexes (DTRs) may be myotonic. This phenomenon is particularly evident in the ankle jerk. Lesions may be seen in the skin of the legs with patients with bacterial endocarditis. Peripheral cyanosis and clubbing should be evaluated by examining the fingers and toes. These signs may appear in patients with patent ductus arteriosus. Reversed cyanosis, in which the patient's fingers are bluish but the toes are pink, is seen with transposition of the great vessels and Taussig-Bing syndrome. Differential cyanosis, with pink fingers and blue toes, is seen in reversed ductus (Eisenmenger's syndrome). Wasting of the muscles of the body as a whole is observed in the presence of chronic heart failure and may be caused by cardiac cachexia.

Musculoskeletal

Several types of arthritis and other musculoskeletal disorders are associated with cardiovascular abnormalities.

Arthritides   Polyarthritis may be seen in Whipple's disease (a rare malabsorption disorder with wide systemic manifestations) with pericarditis, aortic regurgitation, and coronary artery disease. Rheumatoid arthritis, gonococcal arthritis, Lyme disease, and gout are associated with aortic regurgitation and right-sided endocarditis, cardiomyopathy, heart block and atherosclerotic heart disease, respectively.

Seronegative arthritis may be associated with aortic regurgitation. A buzzing or vibration systolic murmur may be heard in straight back syndrome, a condition in which the heart is compressed between the spine and the sternum. Arthritis with erythema annulare (erythema chronicum migrans) may be seen in patients with Lyme disease in association with complete heart block and cardiomyopathy.

Abnormalities of the Spine and Musculature   Friedreich's ataxia is associated with cardiomyopathy and conduction defects. Patients with this disorder often present with atactic gait and weakened legs. Marfan's syndrome may include kyphosis, scoliosis, and poker spine associated with mitral valve prolapse, aortic incompetence and dissection. Severe spinal abnormalities (e.g., in hunchbacks) may cause heart failure. They are seen in patients with pulmonary hypertension and "frozen shoulder" (scapulohumeral periarthritis), and is associated with previous myocardial infarction.

The muscles should be palpated for tenderness. The onset of polymyalgia rheumatica, a vascular syndrome of unknown origin, is often marked by arthralgia and myositis with muscle tenderness. Polyarteritis nodosa is associated with pericarditis, myocarditis, and arrhythmias; myocardial infarction may occur secondary to coronary vasculitis.

CLINICAL EVALUATION OF COMMON SYMPTOMS AND SIGNS ASSOCIATED WITH HEART DISEASE AND THEIR AUSCULTATORY ACCOMPANIMENTS

The most common symptoms of heart disease include chest pain, dyspnea, syncope, palpitations, and fatigue. None is specific to cardiac syndromes; all may have a range of other causes. Diagnostic accuracy requires careful assessment of the overall clinical picture and, in most cases, diagnostic testing.

Angina Pectoris

Differentiation of Pain   An important part of the differential diagnosis of angina pectoris is obtaining a precise description of the pain. The pain of angina is often ephemeral, mercurial in nature, and may be replaced by so-called anginal equivalents (e.g., nausea, vomiting, dyspnea, palpitations, faintness, belching, or diaphoresis). It may be helpful to ask the patient to rate the pain on a scale of 1 to 10; anginal pain is usually rated moderate to moderately severe. By contrast, the pain of aortic dissection is typically described as the worst ever experienced by the patient.

Location and radiation   The location of angina may be retrosternal or subxiphoid. In 80 to 90 percent of cases, patients describe the pain as behind or slightly to the left of the midsternum. The pain may be described as radiating into the right or left arm; the neck, teeth, or lower jaw; between the shoulders; or in the left back. On occasion it may be felt in the wrist.

Quality   Anginal pain is rarely sharply localized, and may not be described explicitly as pain. Patients may refer to sensations of "gas cramps," tightness, squeezing, burning, "having a band around my chest," "indigestion," or a vague ill-defined discomfort. NOTE: Sharp, cutting, knife-like pain is rarely caused by cardiac disorders.

Duration   Angina is typically of short duration; most episodes last between 3 and 15 m and subside completely. If the pain lasts longer than 30 m, suspect unstable angina or myocardial infarction.

Provoking factors   Angina is frequently brought on by activity or emotional excitement. Provocations mentioned most frequently include exertion (particularly lifting or other activities involving upper body muscles), walking uphill, exposure to cold, initial activity upon arising, and sexual intercourse. Angina may also be precipitated by emotional upsets, particularly anger and food, especially followed by exertion and lying down in the supine position.

Relieving factors   Relief of pain following sublingual nitroglycerin is a strong factor in the differential diagnosis of angina. Other factors that relieve angina include cessation or removal of provocations, carotid compression, or change in body posture (usually, moving from a recumbent to an upright position).

Timing   Angina pectoris is more likely to occur in the morning or during daytime exertion; Prinzmetal's angina, by comparison, is most likely to occur at night.

Auscultatory findings   Few clinicians look for auscultatory signs when examining a patient with angina, although they can be helpful in the diagnosis.
    Typical auscultatory findings include:

- An S_4
- Late systolic murmur
- An S_3
- Reverse splitting of S_2 (uncommon).

These findings may be elicited either while the patient is experiencing pain, or after the treadmill test (Table 8-1). At one time the late systolic murmur was attributed to papillary dysfunction; however, changes in ventricular shape are now thought to be the cause. Alterations in left ventricular stiffness and function will lead to reverse splitting of S_2 and filling sounds (Cardiac Pearl 85).
    In evaluating angina patients, the examiner should consider pretest probability factors. Factors that raise the pretest probability of angina include the following:

- Previous history of heart disease
- Prior bypass surgery or angioplasty
- Obesity
- "Type A" personality with hostility

- More than one of the following risk factors:
  Age
  Male gender
  Genetic predisposition
  Blood lipid abnormalities
  Arterial hypertension
  Diabetes mellitus
  Smoking.

Dyspnea

Dyspnea refers to a person's conscious awareness of discomfort in breathing; sometimes it is defined as a sensation of breathlessness that is excessive for the person's level of activity. When a patient presents with dyspnea, it is sound clinical practice to record the level of exertion that induces it as an aid in differential diagnosis.

Cardiac Dyspnea Most causes of acute dyspnea are either cardiac or pulmonary; however, dyspnea may also be associated with anemia, obesity, and some psychiatric syndromes (e.g., panic disorder and phobias). For this reason it is extremely important to obtain an accurate history in patients complaining of dyspnea. There are three types of dyspnea associated with heart disease; they result from elevated left atrial and pulmonary venous pressures or from hypoxia.

1. Nocturnal orthopnea. Nocturnal orthopnea is dyspnea that occurs at night when the patient is lying down; it is relieved by sitting up. A patient who is orthopneic has a small volume pulse with constricted peripheries and ancillary respiratory muscles. The sternocleidomastoids are hyperactive. These patients are known to sit bolt upright in bed and may sleep on several pillows. They often develop shortness of breath if they assume the supine position, which acts like an intravenous bolus, in increasing end-diastolic pressure and provoking dyspnea.
2. Paroxysmal nocturnal dyspnea. This form of dyspnea is more specific for cardiac disease; it is also relieved by sitting or standing up. It is sometimes defined as inappropriate breathlessness at night.
3. Syndrome of early pulmonary edema. This condition may result from onset or worsening of left atrial hypertension. In this syndrome, patients who develop heart failure may sit up, walk around the room, and even open a window in an effort to get air. Dyspnea in pulmonary edema is associated with diaphoresis, cyanosis, and the production of pink, frothy sputum.

Auscultatory findings The following are commonly heard on auscultation of patients with cardiac dyspnea:

- An S_3
- An S_4
- A summation gallop (may disappear in sitting position or with diuresis)
- Pulmonary ronchi or rales at the bases of the lungs

In dyspneic patients in heart failure, auscultation may indicate:

- Diastolic filling sounds
- Tricuspid regurgitation (Fig. 8-11)
- Accentuated pulmonic component of S_2
- Basal rales in the axilla and at the back of the lungs

On occasion, nocturnal chest pain causes severe dyspnea; subsequent administration of nitroglycerin may relieve both the chest pain and the dyspnea. It is also possible for patients with left-sided heart failure to present with concurrent asthma. They may wheeze, causing the rhonchi (continuous adventitious noises) to be heard throughout the chest field. These rhonchi may interfere with auscultation and obscure the diagnosis of heart failure. In general, medium rales at both bases are heard in patients with heart failure, in association with diastolic filling sounds.

Cheyne-Stokes Respirations (Cardiac Pearl 69)   Cheyne-Stokes respirations (Chap. 6; Table 8-2) are not specific to heart failure; they may be seen in uremia, in certain central nervous system (CNS) disorders, or in elderly patients with depressed CNS function under sedation. These respirations should, however, be carefully noted during a cardiac examination because of their association with acute heart failure. Cheyne-Stokes respirations may frequently be observed in patients with severe left ventricular failure with low cardiac output.

Dyspnea in patients with Cheyne-Stokes respirations differs from nocturnal dyspnea in important respects. In Cheyne-Stokes, both the rate and the volume of respiration alternates; with an apneic period following hyperpnea; there is no circadian pattern; and there are apneic intervals. Auscultation of the heart for S_3 and S_4 during an apneic period can provide the examiner with useful information. The apneic period in Cheyne-Stokes is associated with prominent pulsations over the cardiac chambers without the interference of extraneous sounds. NOTE: Inotropic drugs may abolish Cheyne-Stokes respirations by increasing cardiac output.

Episodic Dyspnea   Episodic dyspnea unrelated to changes in the patient's body position may occur as a result of arrhythmias (e.g., sudden atrial fibrillation) (Fig. 8-11) which can be detected by auscultation. Gross bradycardia can also cause episodic dyspnea (e.g., in patients with intermittent high-grade arteriovenous block).

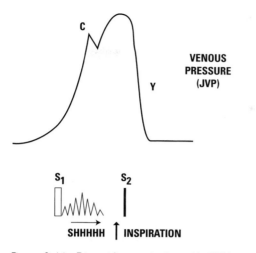

Figure 8-11 Tricuspid regurgitation with C-VY wave.

Episodic dyspnea may occur in patients with muscle abnormalities or cardiac masses, as in cases of left atrial myxoma. It may develop in patients with intermittent ischemia characterized by alteration in cardiac shape or papillary muscle dysfunction and compliance abnormalities. Clinicians should keep in mind the possible implications of episodic dyspnea, as episodes of intermittent ischemia may be clinically silent. The patient's difficulty in breathing may be the presenting symptom.

Episodic dyspnea is also seen in congenital cardiac abnormalities [e.g., tetralogy of Fallot and Eisenmenger's syndrome (Table 8-2)] in which there is a sudden alteration of shunting. An increase in a right-to-left shunt may cause dyspnea; in children, difficulty in breathing may be reduced by squatting, which decreases the right-to-left shunt. Increased right-to-left shunting may also cause hypoxia, convulsions, and syncope. Increasing episodic dyspnea is an ominous symptom in patients with aortic stenosis or aortic regurgitation, and is associated with a poor prognosis. Episodic auscultatory signs should be sought.

Mitral Stenosis and Myxomata Dyspnea associated with these conditions is discussed in Chaps. 5 and 6.

Pheochromocytoma Pheochromocytoma is a rare disorder marked by episodic or sustained hypertension secondary to a tumor of the adrenal medulla. Patients may present with dyspnea and chest pain. Dyspnea associated with pheochromocytoma, however, usually occurs as part of a symptom cluster that includes nausea, headache, visual disturbances, profuse sweating, and palpitations.

Findings typically include pallor, fluctuating blood pressure, A_2 loudness, and postural tachycardia. Facial pallor is a common finding in these patients (Table 8-5).

Carcinoid Syndrome   See Chap. 10.

Pulmonary Embolism   Dyspnea associated with pulmonary embolism is discussed in Chap. 7.

Anxiety-Induced Dyspnea   Dyspnea associated with anxiety is seen in hyperventilation syndrome. Hyperventilation is defined as an increase in alveolar ventilation leading to hypocapnia. It may be caused by a range of organic conditions, including lung diseases, fever, pain, sepsis, and liver dysfunction. Patients with dyspnea of psychogenic origin develop sighing respirations, and complain of difficulty getting their breath. This type of dyspnea is difficult to evaluate unless it is carefully differentiated from cardiac or pulmonary dyspnea. The presence of dyspnea does, however, indicate that the hyperventilation is chronic rather than acute or organic. These patients may present with associated tachycardia or bradycardia with hypotension. No specific auscultatory findings are present.

Acute hyperventilation   Acute hyperventilation is also associated with anxiety, but may be associated with carpopedal spasms, tetany, paresthesias, and stridor rather than dyspnea. Patients may develop syncope during the attacks. Treatment is usually with anxiolytic medications. As in anxiety-induced dyspnea, no systemic cardiovascular findings are present.

Inspiratory Dyspnea   Inspiratory dyspnea is associated with extreme obesity and hypercalcemia. Stridor may develop, and may also be seen in patients who hyperventilate. Stridor is an important cause of inspiratory dyspnea; it may be found in Pickwickian syndrome (obesity-hypoventilation syndrome), in that the weight of the obese person's soft tissues presses upon the ventilatory apparatus. Signs of pulmonary and systemic hypertension may also be seen in obese patients. Stridor is sometimes caused by tumors of the larynx and Kussmaul inspirations (deep rapid respirations seen in coma or diabetic ketoacidosis). It may occur in acute anaphylaxis and hypocalcemia.

Syncope

Syncope is transient loss of consciousness due to inadequate cerebral perfusion. It is not an unusual problem, particularly in the elderly. The differential diagnosis of syncope is critical, in part because of the number of conditions associated with faintness or dizzy spells that fall short of complete loss of consciousness. The examiner needs to rule out seizure disorders, hypoglycemia, epilepsy, vertigo caused by labyrinthitis or Menier's syndrome, head trauma, or hyperventilation syndrome. True syncope can also have psychogenic causes, which may require assessment.

The following factors usually characterize syncope, in contradistinction to transient neurologic deficits or other causes of dizziness:

- Patient has known heart disease
- Patient is more likely to be elderly or male
- Episode is abrupt in onset (because of this characteristic, patients with syncope should always be evaluated for possible injury caused by falling)
- Episode is transient (duration is several s to a few m)
- Patient recovers consciousness promptly without confusion or neurologic symptoms.

Causes of Syncope   The causes of syncope can be grouped into four categories. Psychogenic causes have already been mentioned. The other three are more significant in association with cardiovascular disorders.

1. Vasomotor (sometimes called vasovagal) syncope. Vasomotor syncope is usually caused by excessive stimulation of the vagus nerve or impaired reflex control of peripheral circulation. Occasionally the Jarisch-Bezold reflex following vessel reperfusion after myocardial infarction may be involved. Episodes of vasomotor syncope may be heralded by nausea, diaphoresis, or pallor, and can often be aborted by having the patient lie down or by removing the stimulus. This form of syncope may be brought on by heat, physical pain, or other stress (blood donation, closed spaces, certain types of injury).

   Vasovagal syncope may also be caused by cough, micturition (sometimes called post-micturition syndrome), or postural effects, for which a variety of autonomic disorders may be responsible. In vasodepressor syncope, hypotension occurs. On occasion, vasovagal syncope is associated with sinus bradycardia. Hypovolemia may be present in these patients and may be a precipitating factor. Bradycardia typically disappears on carotid sinus stimulation. Syncope may occur with drinking cold water (glossopharyngeal syncope).

   One specific cause of vasomotor syncope is carotid sinus syndrome (Cardiac Pearl 100). Syncope may occur in patients with carotid obstructions worsened by wearing tight collars, using electric shavers, or by other movements of the neck. In patients who have had carotid endarterectomies, touching the carotid sinus may evoke bradycardia with a feeling of faintness, which usually resolves after a brief period of time. Carefully monitored carotid sinus massage may be diagnostic of vasomotor syncope.

2. Orthostatic (or postural) hypotension. Syncope may occur in patients who develop vasodepressor syncope with bradycardia and a fall in blood pressure on assuming the upright position. Following recovery,

they are pale, diaphoretic, have slow heart rates and may have apical midsystolic murmurs. They have a history of dim vision, dizziness, and autonomic hyperactivity. Drug therapy is of limited value. Cardiac pacing may be required.

In older males, a syndrome of chronic idiopathic orthostatic hypotension may develop. Syncope caused by orthostasis in older patients may be indirectly caused by the patient's medications (especially vasodilators, tricyclic antidepressants, diuretics, and adrenergic blocking medications) or by an autonomic nervous system disorder (e.g., diabetes mellitus). Abnormalities of serotonic metabolism may be responsible (Grubb). It may occur in the Shydrager syndrome in older patients.

3. Cardiogenic syncope. This form of syncope may cause sudden death. It may be due either to mechanical causes or arrhythmias. Syncope that is brought on by exertion or that occurs while the patient is lying down is almost always cardiac in origin.

   Mechanical causes may include the following:
   - Aortic stenosis
   - Pulmonary stenosis
   - IHSS (HOCM)
   - Idiopathic pulmonary hypertension or right-to-left shunting
   - Left atrial myxoma obstructing mitral valve.

Auscultatory findings   Auscultatory findings associated with these conditions are discussed in Chaps. 5 and 6. Syncope associated with ball valve clots and myxomas may have an associated loud S_1 and a middiastolic murmur preceded by a thud. These may vary in loudness depending on the patient's posture. It is important in patients with syncope to rule out organic heart disease. Myxomas, right-to-left shunting as in tetralogy of Fallot, and aortic stenosis with syncope have a poor prognosis.

Cardiogenic syncope in congenital disorders is frequently associated with cyanosis. For example, tetralogy of Fallot may present with cyanotic attacks and syncope. In cyanotic congenital heart disease, right-to-left shunting is increased and patients lose consciousness; cyanosis of the lips may occur. Auscultatory findings pertain to the diagnosis, i.e., holosystolic murmurs due to a ventral septal defect. There are no specific auscultatory findings.

Arrhythmic causes of cardiac syncope include:

- Disorders of automaticity (sick sinus syndrome)
- Conduction disorders (atrioventricular block, sino-atrial block)
- Tachyarrhythmias [ventricular and supraventricular (regular/irregular) tachycardias; Fig. 8-7].

Auscultatory findings in ventricular and supraventricular tachycardias are discussed in Chap. 7. The recognition of these is primarily electrocardiographic.

Stokes-Adams Syncope Stokes-Adams syncope (sometimes called Stokes-Adams attacks) is a form of cardiogenic syncope caused by intermittent ventricular arrest. Atrial diastolic murmurs or sounds may be heard on auscultation. In some instances the examiner may hear only silence. Precordial thumping resumes and maintains heartbeat (Don Michael).

Miscellaneous Causes of Syncope There are a few miscellaneous causes of syncope that may need to be ruled out in the differential diagnosis. Syncope may be caused by hyponatremia (as in Addison's disease, chronic adrenocortical insufficiency), in which the PR interval is short. Syncope may also occur due to prolonged standing. This form of syncope is caused by a fall in the level of venous return; tachycardia occurs and the blood pressure falls.

Cough/Hemoptysis

Cough may occasionally be associated with vasovagal syncope; most causes of this type of coughing are relatively benign (colds, inhaled tobacco smoke, etc.). Nocturnal cough, on the other hand, should raise the index of suspicion for aspiration, occult pulmonary edema, heart failure, or sinus and postnasal drainage. Patients with early pulmonary edema may present with a nocturnal cough as the sole manifestation of their condition. Nocturnal cough is also a significant symptom of heart failure. Cough in association with hemoptysis (expectoration of blood or bloody sputum) may be due to heart failure, although pleuritic pain with hemoptysis is associated with pulmonary infarction due to pulmonary embolism. Hemoptysis, however, may occur in association with the pink-tinged frothy sputum of pulmonary edema. It may also occur due to bronchial congestion. In rare cases of massive hemoptysis, rupture occurs due to pulmonary hypertension resulting from rupture of a pulmonary artery caused by a catheter or by rupture of an aneurysm. In patients with massive hemoptysis, the classic auscultatory findings of heart failure and pulmonary embolism may be elicited.

Fatigue

Fatigue is an important cause of low-output cardiac states. There is very little emphasis in the literature concerning fatigue as a symptom of heart failure, but it is one of the most important to consider in differential diagnosis. Fatigue is common in patients who have low cardiac output (e.g., mitral regurgitation). Auscultation may reveal signs of mitral regurgitation or congestive heart failure. Auscultatory signs include a soft S_1, presence of pulsus alternans, and filling sounds with or without those of mitral regurgitation. Fatigue is also a common symptom in dilated cardiomyopathies with low cardiac output. The presence of fatigue and an impoverished sense of well-being indicate the extent of heart failure. Improvement in a sense of well-being with resolution of fatigue is concomitant with an increase in cardiac output and improvement in myocardial performance. Arrhythmias (e.g., atrial fibrillation) may induce fatigue, as may bradycardia with low cardiac outputs. On occasion, fatigue may be the patient's predominant complaint and should not be confused with dyspnea. Hypotensive states and hyponatremia may be associated with fatigue (Chap. 6).

Palpitations

Palpitations are defined as a person's conscious awareness of heart action. They may reflect normal perception of changes in heartbeat under nonproblematic circumstances (e.g., aerobic exercise, biofeedback, or some types of meditation) or a heightened awareness of changes that disturb the patient. Palpitations may be irregular, regular, rapid, or slow. In most clinical cases, they result from one of the following conditions:

- Increased cardiac output associated with noncardiac conditions
  Thyrotoxicosis
  Anemia
  Anxiety or stress reactions
- Cardiac abnormalities that increase stroke volume
  Bradycardia
  Valvular regurgitation
- Arrhythmias (Fig. 8-7)
  Premature ventricular contractions (PVCs)
  Supraventricular or ventricular tachycardia.

Physiologic palpitations associated with sinus tachycardia are often anxiety-induced. To complicate the picture, anxiety may result from palpitations caused by other factors and then exacerbate them. Palpitations due to supraventricular or junctional ventricular tachycardia, bradycardia, other arrhythmias, and premature ventricular contractions may all cause feelings of apprehension with an awareness of the heartbeats. Organic heart disease of any type is associated with palpitations, but mitral valve prolapse (MVP) in particular is commonly implicated.

Because of the "positive feedback loop" between palpitations and anxiety, changes in heartbeat require careful evaluation. Auscultation is frequently helpful in differential diagnosis. In general, the auscultatory findings of patients with palpitations are those of the causative arrhythmia, with important exceptions: S_1 in complete heart block, in ventricular tachycardias, and in atrial fibrillation is variable. Carotid sinus pressure, as previously discussed, may be a clue to the diagnosis.

Measurement of the heart rate may also be useful in evaluating palpitations. The heart rate in patients with regular tachycardias such as reentrant supraventricular tachycardia is approximately 140 to 180 beats per minute, while patients with atrial flutter may present with a heart rate that abruptly varies with carotid sinus compression. In ventricular tachycardia the heart-rate is commonly 160 to 180 beats per minute while in sinus tachycardia it is up to 140 and slows with carotid sinus compression. In atrial fibrillation, however, the apex rate is counted by auscultation of the heart and may vary from the 40s to 200; the pulse rate is lower than the apical rate, leading to a so-called "pulse deficit." The heart rate is completely irregular.

Edema

Edema is swelling of the lower extremities caused by subcutaneous fluid collection. In bedridden patients, the sacrum should be examined for pitting edema as it is the most dependent point in these patients. Facial edema is occasionally seen in superior vena caval obstruction, right heart failure, or constrictive pericarditis.

Edema is classified on a scale of 1 to 4, with 4 the highest level of severity. At level 1, indentations can be produced in the patient's skin with strong pressure; at level 4, there is obvious swelling and indentation with light pressure. This scale may be useful in categorizing the extent of the swelling.

Like other symptoms associated with heart disease, edema is not specific to cardiac abnormalities; however, cardiogenic causes of edema include:

- Elevated right atrial pressures
- Right-sided valvular abnormalities
- Cor pulmonale.
- Left heart failure

Other causes may include peripheral venous insufficiency, venous obstruction, cirrhosis, or nephrotic syndrome. On occasion edema is idiopathic. In extreme cases, anasarca results with edema of the extremities as well as of the abdominal wall, giving the skin a pitted "orange peel" appearance. Edema may be caused by heat or potentiated by calcium channel blockers [e.g., nifedipine (Adalat, Procardia)]. Pitting of the legs may be seen due to venous obstruction following vascular surgery. It is rarely seen in the edema associated with renal failure or with severe hypoalbuminemia in nephrotic syndrome. Edema confined to one leg should prompt the clinician to consider the possibility of deep venous thrombosis and examine the patient for deep vein tenderness and a positive Homan's sign (Table 8-2).

In some conditions edema is found in conjunction with ascites. Massive ascites and lower extremity edema may be seen in conditions in which the venae cavae are obstructed or in Budd-Chiari syndrome (occlusion of the hepatic veins; Table 8-2), which is associated with enlargement of the liver, jaundice, and splenomegaly. Constrictive pericarditis is an important cause of ascites with minimal edema. Edema of the lower extremities, ascites, and right heart failure in the absence of pulmonary hypertension may be seen in the presence of right ventricular infarction.

Findings in right heart failure include Kussmaul's sign (an increase of venous pressure on inspiration, Table 8-2) and the murmurs of tricuspid regurgitation. In conditions in which the inferior vena cava is obstructed, there may be dilated veins over the abdomen that drain upward into the superior vena cava from below the umbilicus. It is extremely important in all cases of edema and ascites to rule out the presence of constrictive pericarditis, as well as the presence of right ventricular infarction. It is also important to rule out conditions such as occult mitral stenosis in which S_1 is accentuated, but no other findings are obvious in which right heart failure predominates.

There are a variety of conditions in which right heart failure may predominate over left heart failure in patients with cardiomyopathy. These patients may not give a history of orthopnea or dyspnea; rather, they present predominantly with edema, anasarca, and signs of right-sided heart failure. The physical findings in these patients usually include a right ventricular S_4 heard in the subxiphoid area, a holosystolic or ejection murmur that gets louder on inspiration in the subxiphoid area, the presence of pulsatile veins in the neck, and gross edema of the lower extremities. Right ventricular infarction is a good example.

Cyanosis

Cyanosis is an important physical sign in the context of heart disease. It is defined as the presence of an absolute amount of more than 4 g/dL of reduced hemoglobin with oxygen saturation of 88%. Occasionally, methemoglobinemia (a condition in which the oxygen-carrying capacity of the blood is reduced because ferrous hemoglobin has been oxidized to methemoglobin) with concentration of 0.5 g/dL may also cause cyanosis. Methemoglobinemia may be produced by a number of chemical agents, including benzocaine, nitrobenzene, nitrites, dapsone, and pyridium. Hereditary methemoglobinemia is a rare disorder associated with bluish discoloration of the skin in infancy. Anemia is an uncommon cause of cyanosis as it is more difficult for anemic patients to develop these levels of hemoglobin reduction.

Cyanosis is divided into two categories: central and peripheral. Central cyanosis is present in the nose, tongue, mucous membranes of the face, and usually results from respiratory failure or a right-to-left shunt. In patients with chronic obstructive pulmonary disease, the central cyanosis is frequently due to a right-to-left shunt in the lungs. Central cyanosis is the hallmark of patients with congenital heart disease, such as tetralogy of Fallot, Eisenmenger's syndrome, and rare conditions such as transposition of the great vessels and truncus arteriosus. Of these abnormalities, Fallot's tetralogy is probably the most common condition seen in the pediatric population. In adults, cyanosis and syncope may be associated with the clotting of a ball valve. Central cyanosis can usually be detected by inspection of the oral mucous membranes. Peripheral cyanosis usually has nonrespiratory causes (e.g., vasoconstriction and reduced cardiac output).

Differential cyanosis occurs in patients with reversed ductus; and in the lower extremities associated with clubbing of the left upper limb and sparing of the right upper limb (Cardiac Pearl 19). Reversed cyanosis sparing the lower extremities and involving the upper extremities is seen in Taussig-Bing syndrome and transposition of the great vessels in the presence of a patent ductus (Cardiac Pearl 20). Cyanosis restricted to a single extremity suggests local vascular disease and may be due to deep venous obstruction.

TRUE OR FALSE

1. Nonpitting edema is due to lymphangitis.
2. Trunk cyanosis may be due to crowd suffocation.
3. The right ventricle, if palpated, always suggests RVH.
4. An S_4 is heard over distended veins in tricuspid stenosis and cor pulmonale but not precordially.
5. Percussion has little value in cardiology.
6. Phase lag may cause rales to persist after CHF has cleared even though rales are a late sign of CHF.

CLINICAL VIGNETTES

The following vignettes present actual cases of patients who were affected by diseases and conditions discussed in this chapter. At the end of each case, choose the *one* answer that best describes the diagnosis indicated by the vignette.

1. A 40-year-old male letter carrier complained in the course of a routine physical that his watchband became uncomfortably tight when he bicycled uphill on his route. When he got off his bicycle and took his watch off, the tightness of the band disappeared. The diagnosis is:

A. Edema
B. Angina pectoris
C. Venous obstruction

2. A diabetic male patient in his 50s presented with central chest pain that had begun 2 h earlier. The pain was moderately severe; he rated it as 5 on a scale of 1 to 10. The patient refused to lie down in bed, complaining that it made the pain worse. Allowing him to sit up and bend his head forward relieved the pain. The patient admitted to difficulty swallowing whenever he raised his neck. He denied, however, that he had previously experienced this kind of pain.

On examination, he had a pericardial friction rub; auscultation of his heart was somewhat difficult owing to his manifest pain. Nevertheless, when the patient was auscultated lying on his left side, the examiner heard a loud S_4 and an apical dyskinetic impulse. The ECG revealed the presence of Q waves. The diagnosis is:

A. Myocardial infarction underlying the pericarditis
B. Dressler's syndrome
C. Angina pectoris associated with diabetes

3. A 45-year-old female patient presented with pain in her chest worsened by inspiration, by elevating her neck, and by swallowing. Clinical examination revealed a pericardial friction rub which was present in both systole and diastole. On examination the patient had a normal venous pressure, normal pulses, and evidence of a mild left parasternal heave with an S_4 heard in the subxiphoid area. She was a nonsmoker, and examination of her chest did not reveal evidence of diminished breath sounds. A chest X-ray indicated normal heart size. The ECG showed signs of st segment elevation and PQ depression consistent with pericarditis with an ST segment depression in AVF. The patient had a temperature of 100°F with shallow but rapid respirations, attributed to chest pain. The examiner ordered a test to confirm suspicion of a diagnosis. What test did she order, and what diagnosis did she suspect?

A. Radionuclide angiography, on suspicion of left ventricular dysfunction
B. Ventilation/perfusion lung scan, on suspicion of pulmonary embolus
C. Enzyme testing, on suspicion of myocardial infarction

4. A 70-year-old woman presented with severe pain in the chest, radiating to the back. She had a blood pressure of 210/110 with a pulse rate of 110 beats per minute and a respiratory rate of 20. She was diaphoretic and looked extremely ill. There was a normal S_1 with accentuation of A_2. No diastolic murmur was evident. The patient's carotid and femoral pulses were normal. On percussion of the chest, the examiner heard dullness at the left base and an absence of breath sounds. The diagnosis is:

A. Myocardial infarction
B. Pulmonary embolism
C. Aortic dissection

5. A 30-year-old female presented with sudden attacks of shortness of breath and complained that the attacks were increasing in frequency and severity. On examination, the patient had a hyperactive appearance and a spinal deformity. Auscultation of the heart revealed the signs of classical click-and-murmur syndrome (Barlow's syndrome). While the patient was under observation, she developed an attack of dyspnea with carpopedal spasms. The diagnosis is:

A. Acute hyperventilation
B. Episodic dyspnea
C. Pheochromocytoma

6. A 50-year-old man wanted a second opinion about chest discomfort. The clinician noted that the man was overweight; a workaholic "Type A" personality; smoked heavily; was involved in a lawsuit and worried about the sale of his considerable business assets. While taking the history, the examiner noticed knuckles covered by tendon xanthomata, a red face, upper truncal obesity, and a gouty tophus in his ear. The suspected diagnosis is:

A. Prinzmetal's angina
B. Angina pectoris and Type II hyperlipidemia
C. Atherosclerosis

7. A 60-year-old female patient presented with shortness of breath and engorged neck veins, which showed absent descent. Auscultatory findings included pulsus paradoxus, a bradycardia of 55 beats per minute, and a nonpalpable cardiac impulse. The apical impulse indicated the presence of cardiomegaly, which was confirmed by chest x-ray. Echocardiography indicated the presence of pericardial effusion. Pericardial paracentesis was carried out and yielded clear fluid. The patient's pericardial effusion recurred with the same symptoms and signs. Examination of the patient revealed dry skin, myotonic (slow relaxing) tendon reflexes, and a pasty, sallow complexion. A midsystolic murmur was present with the bradycardia. The diagnosis is:

A. Hypothyroidism
B. Effusive pericarditis
C. Hypovolemic shock

8. A young man, skilled in the martial arts, presented with sudden hemiplegia. He was semi-conscious and aphasic. Examination of the patient indicated a lean, long habitus, long fingers, high-arched palate, spinal deformity and dislocated lenses. A prominent Grade IV murmur of aortic regurgitation was present early in diastole. Chest x-ray revealed a dilated aorta, confirmed by echocardiogram. A transesophageal echocardiogram then indicated presence of aortic dissection, which extended into the carotid artery. The patient was referred for urgent surgery. On the basis of these findings, the patient's cardiac abnormalities are most likely associated with:

A. Hypertension
B. Congenital tetralogy of Fallot
C. Marfan's syndrome

9. An 18-year-old female patient presented because she was concerned about her appearance. She was short in stature and had a webbed

neck. She also proved to have color blindness. The cardiac examination revealed the presence of a sharp pulse and a systolic apical murmur, and an early diastolic murmur was heard. The diagnosis is:

A. Congenital transposition of the great arteries
B. Cornelia de Lange syndrome and VSD
C. Turner's syndrome and tunnel subaortic stenosis

10. A 25-year-old male patient presented with fever and general unwellness. Examination of the heart revealed the presence of borderline cardiomegaly with clubbing of the fingers and toes, a large protuberant blue tongue and classical features of mongolism. The patient had a single S_2. A chest x-ray revealed a right-sided aorta and the ECG showed right ventricular hypertrophy. The diagnosis is:

A. Pulmonary embolism and Klinefelter's syndrome
B. Coarctation of the aorta and Marfan's syndrome
C. Tetralogy of Fallot and Down's syndrome

11. A 54-year-old man presented with chronic interstitial fibrosis. On auscultation, the principle findings were confined to the subxiphoid area and were auscultated with the diaphragm of the stethoscope. As evident to the phonocardiogram, there were five sounds present; an S_1, two components of an S_2 with P_2 heard in an atypical position, and an S_3 and S_4. On auscultation of his neck, a fourth sound was clearly heard. The diagnosis is:

A. Ebsteins' anomaly
B. Left heart failure
C. Severe pulmonary hypertension

ANSWERS

True or False

1. *T*; 2. *T*; 3. *F*; 4. *F*; 5. *F*; 6. *T*.

Clinical Vignettes

1. B. Angina pectoris. Angina may radiate to other areas (including the wrist) or be localized in these areas. In addition, the fact that uphill exertion induced the symptom raises the index of suspicion for angina.
2. A. MI underlying the pericarditis. A suspicion of the diagnosis of pericarditis was evident; the ECG showed the presence of Q-wave infarctions in this diabetic male, who had clearly developed pericarditis in association with and underlying myocardial infarction. The pericardium is involved in about 50 percent of MIs. Of patients with R-

wave infarctions, 20 percent have audible friction rubs. Although the patient's rating of the pain as moderately severe is more characteristic of angina, 20 percent to 25 percent of cases of MI present with pain of only minor or moderate severity.

3. B. V/Q lung scan, suspicion of pulmonary embolus. In view of the S_4 and parasternal heave, a lung scan was done which revealed the presence of extensive pulmonary embolism. The patient's low-grade fever also raised the index of suspicion for PE, in that about 40 percent of patients with the diagnosis present with fever. This was an example of a patient who presented with pericarditis and had an underlying pulmonary embolus causing chest pain.

4. *C. Aortic dissection.* Aortic dissection is often confused with MI. However, the presence of severe pain radiating to the back, with some signs of shock (diaphoresis) accompanied by normal or elevated blood pressure suggests the diagnosis.

   In this specific case, an immediate transesophageal echo showed a Type III dissection of the aorta with rupture of the aorta into pleural space. Surgical consultation was called and exploratory thoracentesis was done, revealing the presence of blood. Despite insistence that immediate surgery should be carried out, the patient was referred for CT scan of the aorta. The patient perished during this study. Autopsy of the ascending aorta was totally normal apart from slight ectasia and there was aortic dissection beyond the ligamentum arteriosum from the level of the subclavian down to the abdominal aorta. The patient's history was helpful in pointing out the diagnosis with severe pain in the back which got progressively worse, and the association with the pleural effusion.

   Thus, the association of chest pain, its nature and provocative features, its description by the patient, the elicitation of its nature by the physician, and the auscultatory findings, including the complete physical examination, unravel the complexities of making a diagnosis and cultivate a physician's clinical skills.

5. *A. Acute hyperventilation.* Although episodic dyspnea is associated with cardiac abnormalities, the presence of carpopedal spasms points to acute hyperventilation. The symptom cluster characteristic of dyspnea associated with pheochromocytoma is not present in this patient. Comments: The dyspnea in this case was due to hyperventilation induced by the patient's anxiety. The history of not being able to take a breath is quite characteristic in the presence of anxiety-induced hyperventilation. Treatment is by reassurance and placing a paper bag over the patient's face during an attack. Stridor is evaluated for cause and treated accordingly. In patients who have anaphylaxis with stridor, immediate epinephrine is administered; if the anaphylaxis is intractable, tracheostomy is carried out. In patients who cannot have tracheos-

tomy due to large tumors overlying the neck, femoral arteriovenous bypass may be performed.

6. *B. Angina pectoris.* The patient has a number of the classical risk factors for high pretest probability of angina: Age, gender, personality, obesity, history of smoking, evidence of hypertension. Prinzmetal's angina is more likely to occur in female patients, and to occur at night or during sleep. The patient had Type II hyperlipidemia.

7. *A. Hypothyroidism.* The diagnosis is suggested by the patient's dry skin, sallow complexion, cardiomegaly, and bradycardia.

8. *C. Marfan's syndrome.* The patient's body habitus, spinal deformity, and history of aortic regurgitation all suggest the diagnosis.

9. *C. Turner's syndrome and Tunnel subaortic stenosis.* The webbed neck, short stature, and female gender suggest Turner's syndrome which is often associated with genetic disorders, and patients typically present in early adulthood. The fact that the patient's murmur is to and fro suggests the diagnosis, although coarctation is the common associated disorder.

10. *C. Tetralogy of Fallot and Down's syndrome.* The central cyanosis evident on inspection of the oral mucosa and the mongoloid features suggest the diagnosis.

11. *C. Severe pulmonary hypertension.* A loud S_4 is not atypical to this diagnosis. The presence of five sounds, a rare occurrence, was sorted out both by phonocardiography and by acoustic spectroscopy (S_1 A_2 P_2 S_3 S_4).

BIBLIOGRAPHY

Abound FM: Neurocardiogenic syncope. N Engl J Med 1993; 328:1117–1120.

Abrams J: The precordial impulse. In Abrams J (ed): Essentials of Cardiac Physical Diagnosis. Philadelphia, Lea & Febiger, 1987.

Abrams J: Precordial motion. In Horwitz LD, Groves BM (eds): Signs and Symptoms in Cardiology. Philadelphia, Lippincott, 1985.

Abrams J: Precordial motion in health and disease. Mod Concepts Cardiovasc Dis 1980; 49:55.

Bachinsky WB et al: Usefulness of clinical characteristics in predicting the outcome of electrophysiologic studies in unexplained syncope. Am J Cardiol 1992; 69:1044–1049.

Basta LL, Bettinger JJ: The cardiac impulse: A new look at an old art. Am Heart J 1979; 97:96.

Beitman BD et al: Atypical or nonanginal chest pain. Arch Intern Med 1987; 147:1548–1552.

Bethell HJN, Nixon PCF: Examination of the heart in supine and left lateral positions. Br Heart J 1973; 9:902.

Burch GE, Ray CT: Mechanism of the hepatojugular reflux test in congestive heart failure. Am Heart J 1954; 48:373–382.

Burdine JA, Wallace JM: Pulsus paradoxus and Kussmaul's sign in massive pulmonary embolism. Am J Cardiol 1965; 15:413.

Butman SM et al: Bedside cardiovascular exam in patients with severe chronic heart failure: Importance of resting or inducible jugular venous distension. J Am Coll Cardiol 1993; 33:968–974.

Chinzer MA: Bedside diagnosis of acute myocardial infarction and its complications. Curr Probl Cardiol 1982; 7:14.

Coleman AL: *Clinical Examination of the Jugular Venous Pulse.* Springfield IL, Charles C. Thomas, 1966:11–68.

Conn RD, Cole JS: The cardiac apex impulse: Clinical and angiographic correlations. Ann Intern Med 1971; 75:185.

Constant J: Bedside Cardiology. Boston, Little, Brown, 1969.

Constant J: Clinical diagnosis of nonanginal pain: Differentiation of angina from nonanginal chest pain by history. Clin Cardiol 1983; 6:11–16.

Constant J, Lippschutz EJ: The one-minute abdominal compression test or "the hepatojugular reflux," a useful bedside test. Am Heart J 1964; 67:701.

The Criteria Committee of the New York Heart Association: Nomenclature and criteria for diagnosis of the heart and the great vessels, 9th ed. Boston, Little, Brown, 1994.

Dock W; Some paradoxes in the history of pulsus paradoxus. Am J Cardiol 1963; 11:569.

Eddleman EEJ, Langley JO: Paradoxical pulsation of the precordium in myocardial infarction and angina pectoris. Am Heart J 1962; 63:579.

Ewy GA: The abdominojugular test: Technique and hemodynamic correlates. Ann Intern Med 1988; 109:456–460.

Ewy GA: Venous and arterial pulsations. In Horwitz LD, Groves BM (eds): Signs and Symptoms in Cardiology. Philadelphia, Lippincott, 1985.

Ewy GA et al: The dicrotic arterial pulse. Circulation 1969; 39:655.

Fitzpatrick AP et al: Methodology of head-up tilt testing in patients with unexplained syncope. J Am Coll Cardiol 1991; 17:125–130.

Fowler NO: Examination of the heart, Part 2: Inspection and palpation of venous arterial pulses. New York, American Heart Association, 1965.

Fowler NO: Pericardial disease. Heart Dis Stroke 1992; 1(2):85.

Freeman AR, Levine SA: Clinical significance of systolic murmurs: Study of 1000 consecutive "non-cardiac" cases. Ann Intern Med 1993; 6:1371.

Freis ED, Kyle MC: Computer analysis of carotid and brachial pulse waves: Effect of age in normal subjects. Am J Cardiol 1968; 22:691.

Freis ED et al: Changes in carotid pulse which occur with age and hypertension. Am Heart J 1966; 71:757–765.

Friedman B: Alternation of cycle length in pulsus alternans. Am Heart J 1956; 51:701.

Hardison J, Rodgers CM: Cardiovascular manifestations of sickle-cell anemia. In Hurst JW (ed): Update I: The Heart. New York, McGraw-Hill, 1979:185.

Harvey WP: Cardiac Pearls. Newton, NJ, Laennec Publishing Co., 1994.

Hejtmanick MR et al: Acromegaly and the heart: A clinical and pathologic study. Ann Intern Med 1948; 29:22.

Heppner R et al: Aortic regurgitation and aneurysm of sinus of Valsalva associated with osteogenesis imperfecta. Am J Cardiol 1973; 31:654.

Hirschfelder AD: Variations in the form of the venous pulse: A preliminary report. Johns Hop Hosp Bull 1987; 18:265–267.

Kane FJ et al: Angina as a symptom of psychiatric illness. South Med J 1988; 81:1412–1416.

Leatham AL: An introduction to the examination of the cardiovascular system, 2nd ed. Oxford, Oxford University Press, 1978.

Lindsay J Jr: Aortic dissection. Heart Dis Stroke 1992; 1(2):69.

Manolis AS et al: Syncope: Current diagnostic evaluation and management. Ann Intern Med 1990; 112:850–863.

Massumi RA et al: Reversed pulsus paradoxus. N Engl J Med 1973; 289:1272.

Meadows WR et al: Dicrotism in heart disease. Am Heart J 1971; 82:56.

Middlekauff HR et al: Syncope in advanced heart failure: High risk of sudden death regardless of origin of syncope. J Am Coll Cardiol 1993; 21:110–116.

Mounsey JPD: Inspection and palpation of the cardiac impulse. Prog Cardiovasc Dis 1967; 10:187.

Newman JH, Ross JC: Chronic cor pulmonale. In Hurst JW (ed-in-chief): The Heart, 7th ed. New York, McGraw-Hill, 1990:1220–1229.

O'Rourke MF: The arterial pulse in health and disease. Am Heart J 1971; 82:687.

O'Rourke RA: The measurement of systolic blood pressure: Normal and abnormal pulsations of the arteries and veins. In Hurst JW (ed-in-chief): The Heart, 7th ed. New York, McGraw-Hill, 1990:157–160.

Okel BB, Hurst JW: Prolonged hyperventilation in man. Arch Intern Med 1961; 108:757.

Rebuck AS, Pengelly LD: Development of pulsus paradoxus in the presence of airway obstruction. N Engl J Med 1971; 284:1309–1311.

Reddy PS et al: Cardiac tamponade: Hemodynamic observations in man. Circ 1978; 58:265–272.

Rich LL, Tavel ME: The origin of the jugular C wave. N Engl J Med 1971; 284:1309–1311.

Roberts WC et al: Severe valvular aortic stenosis in patients over 65 years of age: A clinicopathologic study. Am J Cardiol 1971; 27:497–506.

Ryan JM et al: Experiences with pulsus alternans, ventricular alternation and the state of heart failure. Circulation 1956; 14:1099.

Sharpe DN et al: The non-invasive diagnosis of right ventricular infarction. Circ 1978; 57:483–490.

Smith D, Craige E: Mechanism of the dicrotic pulse. Br Heart J 1986; 56:531.

Sra JS et al: Comparison of cardiac pacing with drug therapy in the treatment of neurocardiogenic (vasovagal) syncope with bradycardia or asystole. N Engl J Med 1993; 328:1085–1090.

Stevenson LW, Perloff JK: The limited reliability of physical signs for estimating hemodynamics in chronic heart failure. JAMA 1989; 261:884–888.

Tavel ME et al: The jugular venous pulse in atrial septal defect. Arch Intern Med 1968; 121:594–629.

Wachtel F et al: The relation of pectus excavatum to heart disease. Am Heart J 1956; 52:121.

Wade WG: Pathogenesis of infarction of the right ventricle. Br Heart J 1959; 21:524–554.

Wood P: Diseases of the Heart and Circulation, 2nd ed. Philadelphia, Lippincott, 1956:26–32.

Wood P: Diseases of the Heart and Circulation, 3rd ed. Philadelphia, Lippincott, 1968.

9

TESTS ADJUNCTIVE
TO AUSCULTATION

ELECTROCARDIOGRAPHY
  ECG in Congenital Heart Disease
  The ECG in Differential Diagnosis
  ECG Findings in Common Clinical Conditions

RADIOGRAPHY

IMAGING
  CT And MRI
  Fast Cine MRI
  Echocardiography
  Phonocardiography

STRESS TESTING
  Treadmill Exercise
  Stress Echocardiography

This chapter discusses common techniques that are used in confirming or making a diagnosis of heart disease, as mandated by auscultatory findings. Ordering tests must be done in a logical manner justifiable by a tentative diagnosis. Today's physician must be able to arrive at the final diagnosis with a maximum of astuteness and grace—and at a minimum of cost.

ELECTROCARDIOGRAPHY (Cardiac Pearls 54 and 55)

In the past, data from electrocardiography and vectorcardiography were not evaluated separately. Both were methods of studying the electrical activity of the heart. The electrocardiogram (ECG) directly records electrical forces, representing them in two dimensions as horizontal, transverse, and sagittal. The vectorcardiogram adds the dimension of time, thus enabling physicians to study the entire shape and form of cardiac complexes.

Table 9-1   Normal ECG Complex

Wave	Description
P	Caused by atrial depolarization. In normal sinus rhythm, the P wave is upright in leads I, II, V_4, V_5, V_6, and aVF; it is inverted in aVR.
QRS	Represents ventricular depolarization.
Q	The first negative deflection of the QRS complex; not always present. May be pathologic when present.
R	The first positive deflection of the QRS complex.
S	The negative deflection following the R wave.
T	Follows the QRS complex; caused by ventricular repolarization. Usually upright in leads I, II, V_3, V_4, V_5, and V_6; inverted in aVR.

Table 9-1 lists the component waves of the normal ECG complex; Fig. 9-1 illustrates the complexes, intervals, and segments of the ECG.

ECG in Congenital Heart Disease

The ECG in congenital heart disease has relevance to both the auscultatory and clinical findings. Thus, in complete situs inversus with dextrocardia, the characteristic ECG shows an inverted P wave, and lead I has a rightward axis. This result is caused by an inversion of atrial situs and polarization originating and proceeding from rightward and interiorly from the left sinoatrial node. Thus, the P wave is inverted in lead I of the standard 12-

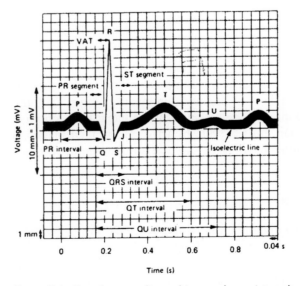

Figure 9-1   The electrocardiographic complexes, intervals, and segments. The U wave is normally not well seen. (From Gomella LG, Clinician's Pocket Reference, 7th ed. p. 327, Appleton & Lange, 1993).

lead electrocardiogram and upright in the AVR augmented lead (i.e., the right-arm augmented lead). The chest x-ray in these patients shows dextrocardia with complete situs inversus with identification of the right-sided stomach and a left-sided liver.

Auscultation over the heart reveals a normal S_1 and S_2 with the positions of the sounds identical to those seen in a normal person but heard on the right side. The heart is usually normal in complete situs inversus. In situs solitus with dextrocardia, however, or situs inversus with levocardia, cardiac anomalies are commonly present. The spleen is present and single in all these conditions.

The ECG in Differential Diagnosis

The cardiac axis represents the sum of the vectors of the electrical depolarization of the ventricles. The axis therefore locates the electrical orientation of the patient's heart within the body. In normal persons the axis points downward and to the left. Figure 9-2 depicts the normal axis and axis deviations; Table 9-2 lists the clinical conditions associated with axis deviations.

Atrial Septal Defect/Ostium Primum   The ECG is useful in distinguishing secundum atrial septal defect from ostium primum. Left-axis deviation is present in patients with ostium primum, right-axis in the presence of ostium secundum atrial septal defects. This shift in the electrical axis is thus an important electrocardiographic indication of the correct diagnosis. Occa-

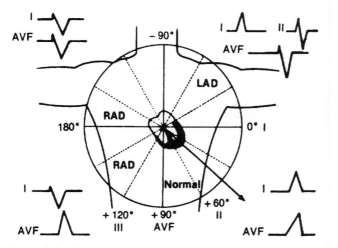

Figure 9-2   Graphic representation of axis deviation. Electrocardiographic representations of each type of axis are shown in each quadrant. The large arrow is the normal axis. (From Gomella LG, Clinician's Pocket Reference, 7th ed. p. 328, Appleton & Lange, 1993).

Table 9-2 Clinical Conditions Associated with Axis Deviations

Right Axis Deviations (RAD)	Left Axis Deviations (LAD)
Right ventricular hypertrophy	Left ventricular hypertrophy
Right bundle branch block	Left anterior hemiblock
Chronic obstructive pulmonary disease	Left bundle branch block
Acute pulmonary embolism (axis changes suddenly toward the right)	Some normal individuals
Some normal individuals	

sionally, advanced atrioventricular block may be present in the Holt-Oram syndrome, as well as prolonged QRS complexes and ectopic rhythms. Patients with atrial septal defects in the fourth decade or those who develop pulmonary hypotension frequently develop atrial tachycardias and atrial fibrillation. Complete right bundle branch block (RBBB) may be present. In sinus venosus defects, the QRS duration may be prolonged, and T waves are inverted across precordial leads. In endocardial cushion defects, the PR interval is prolonged in 50 percent of patients and the standard leads show left axis deviation. The pattern is present at birth, so that Q waves appear in leads I and aVL. The QRS axis is superior and to the left or superior and to the right. The changes seen with endocardial cushion defects and with ostium primum are also seen with a common atrium in the absence of an atrial septum.

Tetralogy of Fallot/Tricuspid Atresia Tetralogy of Fallot and tricuspid atresia are two forms of congenital cyanotic heart disease frequently encountered in clinical practice, and have many features in common. The ECG in Fallot's tetralogy, the commonest form of cyanotic congenital heart disease, is characterized by right ventricular hypertrophy with peaked T waves, a normal PR interval, and a normal QRS axis that remains vertical as the child matures. The QRS duration is normal, although right bundle branch block is seen in adult survivors. Left axis deviation arouses suspicion of tricuspid atresia. Right ventricular hypertrophy in the precordial leads is characterized by tall, monophasic R waves confined to the lead V_1; a change to a small RS pattern in V_2 is seen.

By contrast, in the ECG of a patient with tricuspid atresia, a condition sometimes mistaken for tetralogy of Fallot, P waves are biphasic in lead V_1 and positive in V_2. The QRS axis in the frontal plane is to the left, with features of left ventricular hypertrophy. Depolarization is counterclockwise, in contrast with tetralogy of Fallot, in which the axis is clockwise. Thus, in these two forms of congenital cyanotic heart disease and in atrial septal defects, the differences in ECG readings point to the correct diagnosis.

ECG Findings in Common Clinical Conditions

Systolic/Diastolic Overload Left-to-right shunts in which the ventricle is volume overloaded show signs of so-called diastolic overload with deep S waves in V_1 and tall RS in V_5 and V_6, together with deep Q waves and tall peak T waves. This is seen in ventricular septal defect as well. Right ventricular volume overload with an incomplete right bundle branch block pattern in V_1 has been described in left-to-right shunts at the atrial septal level. Auscultatory findings in these conditions are discussed in Chaps. 4, 6, and 10.

Aortic/Pulmonary Stenosis   Pulmonary stenosis and aortic stenosis display typical patterns of left and right ventricular hypertrophy with systolic overload. ST segment depression or T wave inversion also are seen. Axes are shifted to the right in pulmonary stenosis, with prominent R waves in V_1 and precordial leads with inverted T waves. In contrast, the pattern of left ventricular hypertrophy is seen in aortic stenosis, although the electrical axis may not change. ST segment depression in aortic stenosis is significant (systolic overload). Auscultatory findings are described in Chaps. 4, 6, and 10.

Acute Myocardial Infarction   Electrocardiographic features of acute myocardial infarction are present in 60 percent of cases of MI, and considered separately as they are probably the most important to recognize. S_1 is soft following acute myocardial infarction and an S_4 is commonly heard.

Ventricular Aneurysm   Ventricular aneurysm is indicated or suggested by chronic ST segment elevation, usually in precordial leads. A persistent S_3 and S_4 may be present in the absence of heart failure.

RADIOGRAPHY

One of the most common diagnostic tests is the teleradiogram of the chest taken in two projections, which produces a wealth of clinical information. All practicing physicians should become familiar with the features of this critical diagnostic tool and be able to read the chest x-ray independently without reliance on a radiologist's report. Pathognomonic appearances such as "snowman" heart in total anomalous venous drainage, rib notching in coarctation with three left-sided notches in the aorta (in the x-ray these represent the subclavian artery and pre- and poststenotic dilation of the aorta), and the coeur-en-sabot (boot-shaped) heart in tetralogy of Fallot provide examples of spot diagnoses.

IMAGING

CT and MRI

Computed tomography (CT) and magnetic resonance (MR) scans are useful to diagnose and evaluate a variety of complex congenital conditions. This is due to the clarity that these techniques bring to the anatomy of complex malformations of the heart and great vessels. The physician may need to know the position of the heart in the chest, and the relationships between the atria and ventricles and the outflow tracts with a great degree of precision prior to treatment of the condition.

CT is useful in the detection and diagnosis of mediastinal masses. In acquired heart disease in nonemergent patients, CT scans are useful in the diagnosis of dissection of the aorta, whether type I, II, or III (Table 9-3). Computed tomography may show pleural effusions associated with the dissection and evidence of an internal flap. It may reveal a dissecting hematoma, which is not seen on a transesophageal echocardiogram (TEE). CT scans are able to detect constrictive pericarditis and pericardial calcification, as well as the presence of contusions in the lungs. Thus in trauma to these structures, CT has great value. CT is also useful in the detection of prosthetic valves, as in some cases MRI cannot be used due to the interference produced in metal by the technique. CT scanning may reveal the presence of hemorrhage or air in the mediastinum, pericardium, or heart; and may be useful in detecting pulmonary disease. Spin CT, in which the CT chamber is rotated around the patient during imaging, has improved the resolution of important details in anatomy of the heart. Fast CT and contrast enhancement enable viewing of vein grafts (Fig. 9-3).

Fast Cine MRI

The cine MRI is used in the detection of many of the conditions mentioned with regard to CT, but is more specific and sensitive in evaluating complex

Table 9-3   Imaging Modalities and Associated Clinical Conditions

Imaging Modality	Clinical Conditions
CT scan	Dissecting aorta, ascending/descending
	Calcified pericardium
	Calcified myocardium
	Coronary calcifications
	Patent vein grafts
Thallium scan	Ischemic myocardium
	Non-q wave infarction
	Cardiac contusions
	Amyloid heart
PET scan	Ischemic myocardium
	Stunned myocardium
	Hibernating heart muscle
Barium swallow	Dysphagia lusoria indented by aortic muscle)
	Aberrant innominate artery
	Dextroaorta
	Hiatal hernia
	Left atrial enlargement

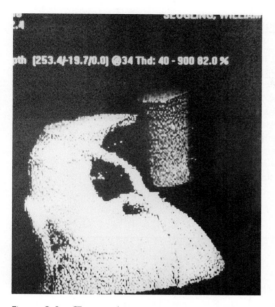

pth [253.4/-19.7/0.0] @34 Thd: 40 - 900 82.0 %

Figure 9-3 CT scan of patent vein graft. Used with permission of Bruce Brundage, M.D.

congenital heart disease, in detecting ventricular anatomy and function, as well as in measuring coronary calcification. Coronary arteries have been successfully analyzed using rapid cine MRI. Cine MRI is very useful in identifying the possible presence of shunts.

Echocardiography

Echocardiography, or cardiac ultrasound, employs high-frequency sound waves to form images of cardiac structures. This technology can document intravascular blood flow as well as tissue movement. In mitral valve disease, echocardiography is particularly valuable in the diagnosis of mitral stenosis as it relates to therapy (Table 9-4).

Three types of echocardiograms have been used in cardiac imaging: (1) M-mode (single-plane); (2) two-dimensional echocardiography; and (3) Doppler imaging, which uses reflected ultrasound to detect the direction of blood flow and tissue movement.

Historically, M-mode was the first form of cardiac ultrasound to be used. It opened a new chapter in the diagnosis of heart size, contractility, valve mobility, and septal size. Despite the limited view it provides, M-mode echocardiography was vital in the accurate diagnosis of mitral stenosis, hypertrophic obstructive cardiomyopathy and other cardiomyopathies, as well as of pericardial effusion and vegetations. M-mode also helped in detecting pulmonary hypertension and valvular diseases of the heart. M/

Table 9-4   Diagnostic Indications for Echocardiography

Not Absolutely Indicated	Desirable	Essential
Innocent systolic murmurs	Atrial septal defects	Bicuspid aortic valves
Patent ductus arteriosus	Ventricular septal defects	Complex cyanotic heart disease
Small VSD	Aortic stenosis	Suspected shunt
Pulmonary AV fistula	Pulmonary stenosis	Pseudoaneurysm
Cranial bruits	Coarctation of aorta	
Renal artery bruits	Constrictive pericarditis	
Mitral valve prolapse	Hypertension	
Idiopathic dilatation of pulmonary artery	Initial evaluation of mitral valve prolapse	
Anomalous pulmonary veins		
Coronary artery disease		

Q scans are useful today in showing aortic and mitral regurgitation, and M-mode echocardiograms may be used to provide accurate quantitative information. They are useful in detecting systolic anterior motion in HOCM.

The refinement of two-dimensional echocardiography enhanced clinicians' ability to diagnose a variety of conditions more accurately. Thus, a number of congenital disorders that could not be diagnosed previously without exploratory surgery (e.g., atrial septal defect or ventricular septal defect) could be readily visualized with two-dimensional echocardiography.

With the advent of Doppler technology it is now possible to determine the size of septal defects and the patterns of blood flow through them, as well as valve sizes and blood pressure gradients. Color Doppler imaging enables rapid visualization of shunts as well. Table 9-5 summarizes the clinical conditions that can be diagnosed or assessed with Doppler imaging.

Echocardiography in Acquired Heart Disease   With respect to acquired heart disease, two-dimensional echocardiography and Doppler imaging have enabled more precise diagnosis of tamponade and pericardial effusion.

Table 9-5   Heart Diseases That Can Be Diagnosed with the Use of Echo and Doppler Technology

Disease/Disorder Category	Condition
Congenital cyanotic	Tetralogy of Fallot
Acyanotic	Coarctation of the aorta
	Pulmonary stenosis
	Ebstein's anomaly
	Still's murmur
Complex congenital	Transposition [of the major vessels] [Truncus arteriosus]

Cardiac tumors and vegetations may be visualized with two-dimensional echocardiography.

Doppler technology permits echo-guided paracentesis of cardiomyopathies in their dilated, hypertrophic, and restrictive forms. Doppler imaging is also useful in determining the presence of cor pulmonale, right ventricular hypertrophy, and pulmonary hypertension. In addition, this technology allows superior delineation of valvular disorders. Doppler imaging has also facilitated the development of formulae for establishing the presence of gradients and diagnosing valvular dysfunction. Tamponade is recognized by diastolic collapse of the right ventricle during left ventricular relaxation.

Transesophageal Echocardiography   Transesophageal echocardiography (TEE) further extends the scope of echocardiographic diagnostic modalities. Using transesophageal echocardiography, a very precise diagnosis can often be made of cardiogenic causes of stroke. TEE enables examination and interrogation of the atrial septum for aneurysms and shunts. These defects can be demonstrated by contrast media (e.g., agitated saline or Albuminex). In addition, contrast enhancement has also improved diagnosis of dissection of the aorta and of intracardiac clots, thrombi, vegetations, and tumors. Transesophageal echocardiography has made it possible to evaluate prosthetic valves and pinpoint malfunction, especially in the aortic valve and tricuspid valve. Prosthetic valve stenosis, however, is best detected by a combination of transthoracic and transesophageal echocardiography, using Doppler quantitative technology. The use of Albuminex and agitated saline permits the diagnosis of occult foramen ovale in the atrial septum. TEE also allows assessment of the presence of pulmonary atrioventricular fistulae. Recently, although technically difficult, transesophageal echocardiography has been shown to enable the visualization of coronary artery grafts and flow reserve.

Tissue Doppler Imaging   Tissue Doppler imaging is a new technique that can evaluate myocardial and valvular movement in terms of a Doppler velocity profile. Myocardial and valvular motion that occurs at slower speeds but higher amplitudes than blood flow can be detected (Fig. 9-4). These movements are captured as images at a high frame rate (340 frames/s) and measured. These measurements provide accurate representation of cardiac tissue motion with minimal delay in image acquisition. Although these images are mostly of research value at the present time, they provide a range of data about cardiac tissue motion and correlative phenomena such as heart sounds that have been previously inaccessible to echocardiography.

Directed Echocardiography   Echocardiography has an extensive role in the diagnosis of heart disease and the evaluation of murmurs and heart sounds. The term *directed echocardiography* reflects the fact that clinical assessment of the probable diagnosis is necessary before an echocardiogram

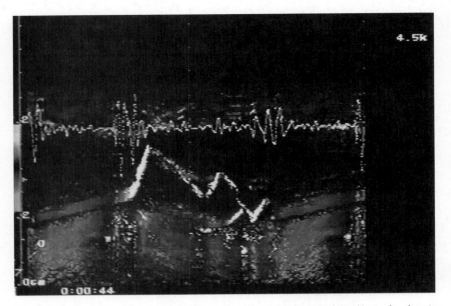

Figure 9-4 Tissue Doppler imaging of mitral valve and left ventricle in M mode, showing phonocardiographic correlates of mitral valve closure (S_1). The mitral valve closure point corresponds with S_1 and the beginning of systole.

is ordered. In other words, performing an adequate echocardiogram depends on a provisional clinical diagnosis; hence, an echocardiogram should never be ordered without a provisional diagnosis having first been made. An echocardiogram does not substitute for auscultation. Table 9-6 summarizes the forms of echocardiography associated with different probable diagnoses.

Phonocardiography

Recent years have witnessed a renewed interest in phonocardiography. This technique is particularly useful when combined with echocardiography in showing heart sounds, murmurs, and valves with Doppler imaging together with the timing of heart sounds (Fig. 9-5). As was noted in Chap. 6, auscultation does not always mirror the shape of the phonocardiogram. This observation applies to the diamond-shaped murmur in systole which is an acoustic artifact.

STRESS TESTING

Treadmill Exercise

Having a cardiac patient walk a treadmill is a useful and commonly employed investigatory procedure. The test is carried out using standard proto-

Table 9-6   Clinical Conditions and Cardiac Tissues Associated with Directed Echocardiography

Condition/Tissue	M-Mode	Newer Modes
Aortic regurgitation	M-mode	2D + Doppler
	M/Q scan	Suprasternal notch evaluation
		TEE
Mitral regurgitation	M/Q scan	PISA calculation
Mitral stenosis	M-mode slope	1/2 time
		PISA calculation
Aortic stenosis	M-mode echo	TEE gradient continuation equation
Tricuspid regurgitation	—	TTE for Doppler calculation of PAP
Myocardium	M-mode values	Appearance EF
Pericardium	M-mode	Look for tamponade
Endocardium	M-mode	TEE TN masses
Aorta	M-mode	TEE
Pulmonary artery	M-mode	2D + TEE

cols. Treadmill testing is of value in detecting cardiac ischemia, in determining maximum oxygen consumption at peak exertion and anaerobic threshold, and in evaluating patients prior to cardiac rehabilitation. Treadmill testing may help in detecting occult arrhythmias and hypotension during exercise.

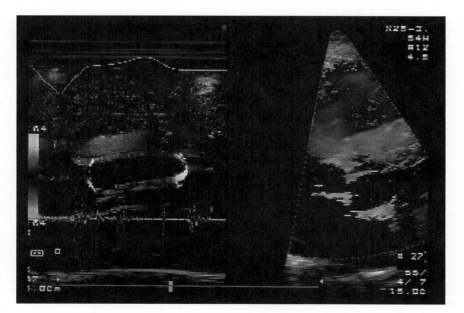

Figure 9-5 Tissue Doppler images of aortic valve closure and S_2 on the phonocardiogram. S_2 corresponds to aortic valve closure.

Although this test has a moderate degree of sensitivity and specificity, it elicits certain important signs (Fig. 9-6) which point to ischemia in patients with intermediate pretest probabilities of ischemic heart disease:

1. An S₄ and apical systolic murmur which appear after exercise.
2. An apical systolic murmur that appears immediately after exercise.
3. Disappearance of *1* and *2* as the patient rests.
4. Hypotension during exercise, indicating immobilization of cardiac muscle by ischemia, corresponding to ischemic dilatation seen on stress echocardiography.
5. Hypertension in the recovery period that is thought to be due to ischemia.

Stress Echocardiography

A stress echocardiogram allows the physician to view the motion of the patient's ventricular wall after he or she has exercised on a stationary bicycle or has been administered the pharmacological stressors dobutamine (Dobutrex), dipyridamole (Persantine), or the two drugs in combination (Table 9-7). Recently, atrial pacing and obtaining paced and resting echocardiograms have been shown to be safe, rapid methods to be used in association with stress testing (Don Michael). Auscultation of the heart using an esophageal stethoscope with atrial pacing is useful in detecting S₄s that

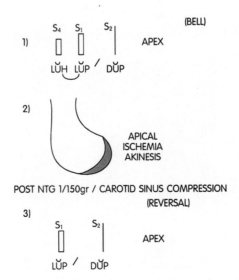

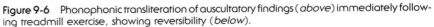

Figure 9-6 Phonophonic transliteration of auscultatory findings (*above*) immediately following treadmill exercise, showing reversibility (*below*).

Table 9-7 Forms of Stress Testing and Auscultatory Results

Condition	Treadmill Exercise	Atrial Pacing Esophageal	Dobutamine
Coronary artery disease	S_3, S_4 Apical late systolic murmur	S_4 at peak rates	S_4
Valvular heart disease	Murmur louder in stenosis, softer in regurgitation	As in TM	MSM may increase stenosis
HOCM	Systolic murmur grows louder	Systolic murmur grows louder	Systolic murmur grows louder

indicate ischemia and in evaluating the effects of pacing on stenotic and regurgitant murmurs (Don Michael).

BIBLIOGRAPHY

ECG

Romhilt DW, Estes EH Jr: A point-score system for the ECG diagnosis of left ventricular hypertrophy. *Am Heart J* 1968; 75:752.

Echo

Adhar GC, Nanda NC: Doppler echocardiography: Part II: Adult valvular heart disease. *Echocardiography* 1984; 1:219–241.

Burstow DJ et al: Cardiac tamponade: Characteristic Doppler observations. *Mayo Clin Proc* 1989; 64:312–324.

Houston AB: Doppler ultrasound and the apparently normal heart. *Br Heart J* 1993; 69:99–100.

Klein AL et al: Two-dimensional and Doppler echocardiographic assessment of infiltrative cardiomyopathy. *J Am Soc Echo* 1988; 1:48–59.

Leon DF, Shaver JA: Physiologic principles of heart sounds and murmurs. New York, American Heart Association, 1975.

Louie EK et al: Transesophageal echocardiographic diagnosis of patent foramen ovale in adults without prior stroke. *Circulation* 1991; 84(4):II-451.

Oh JK et al: Prediction of the severity of aortic stenosis by Doppler aortic valve area determination: Prospective Doppler-catheterization correlation in 100 patients. *J Am Coll Cardiol* 1988; 11:1227.

Rokey R et al: Determination of regurgitant fraction in isolated mitral or aortic regurgitation by pulsed Doppler two-dimensional echocardiography. *J Am Coll Cardiol* 1986; 7:1273–1278.

Smith MD et al: Observer variability in the quantification of Doppler color flow jet areas for mitral and aortic regurgitation. *J Am Coll Cardiol* 1988; 11:579.

Stevenson JG: Two-dimensional color Doppler estimation of the severity of atrioventricular valve regurgitation: Important effects of instrument gain setting, pulse repetition frequency, and carrier frequency. *J Am Soc Echo* 1989; 2:1.

Talano JV, Gradin JM: *Two-Dimensional Echocardiography*. New York, Grune & Stratton, 1983.

Thomas JD, Weyman AE: Doppler mitral pressure half-time: A clinical tool in search of theoretical justification. *J Am Coll Cardiol* 1987; 10:923.

Wayne HH: Syncope: Physiologic considerations and an analysis of the clinical characteristics in 510 patients. *Am J Med* 1961; 31:418–438.

Exercise Testing

Chaitman BR: Exercise testing in heart disease. In Braunwald E (ed): 4th ed. Philadelphia, Saunders, 1992:161–179.

MRI

Fulkerson PK et al: Calcification of the mitral annulus: Etiology, clinical associations, and therapy. *Am J Med* 1979; 66:967–977.

Margolis JR et al: The diagnostic and prognostic significance of coronary artery calcification: A report of 800 cases. *Radiology* 1980; 137:609–616.

Rehr RB: Cardiovascular nuclear magnetic resonance imaging and spectroscopy. *Current Problems in Cardiology,* Mosby/Year Book 1991; 16:131–215.

TEE

Seward JB et al: Multiplane transesophageal echocardiography: Image orientation, examination technique, anatomic correlations, and clinical applications. *Mayo Clin Proc* 1993; 68:523–551.

Sheikh K et al: Intraoperative transesophageal Doppler color flow imaging used to guide patient selection and operative treatment of ischemic mitral regurgitation. *Circulation* 1991; 84:594–604.

Other

ACP/ACC/AHA Task Force Statement, Clinical Competence in Electrocardiography. *J Am Coll Cardiol* 1995; 25:1465–1469.

Chen JTT: Technique of cardiac fluoroscopy. In Hurst JW (ed-in-chief): *The Heart,* 7th ed. New York, McGraw-Hill, 1990:1853.

Daffner RH: *Clinical Radiology: The Essentials.* Baltimore, Williams & Wilkins, 1993.

Dinsmore RE, Miller SW: The plain chest roentgenogram. In Eagle KA et al (eds): *The Practice of Cardiology,* 2nd ed. Boston, Little, Brown, 1989, 1445–1464.

Kerley PJ: Radiology in heart disease. *Br Med J* 1933; 2:594.

Klein RC et al: Electrocardiographic diagnosis of left ventricular hypertrophy in the presence of left bundle branch block. *Am Heart J* 1984; 108:502–506.

Maddahi J et al: Improved noninvasive assessment of coronary artery disease by quantitative analysis of regional stress myocardial distribution and washout of thallium-201. *Circulation* 1981; 64:927.

10

AUSCULTATION IN THE CARE OF SPECIAL POPULATIONS

ISSUES IN ADULT PEDIATRIC CARDIOLOGY
  Atrial Septal Defects
  Ventricular Septal Defects
  Atrioventricular Septal Defects
  Patent Ductus Arteriosus
  Coarctation of the Aorta
  Aortic Valve Stenosis
  Tetralogy of Fallot and "Tet" Syndromes
  Ebstein's Anomaly
  Corrected TGA
  Congenital TGA
  Tricuspid Atresia
  Congenital Heart Block

SPECIAL PROCEDURES IN ADULT PEDIATRIC CARDIOLOGY
  Nonsurgical Treatments
  Balloon Valvuloplasty
  Electrophysiological Abnormalities

SURGICAL TREATMENT OF PATIENTS WITH CONGENITAL HEART DISEASE
  Atrial Septal Defect
  Ventricular Septal Defect
  Atrioventricular Septal Defect
  Patent Ductus Arteriosus
  Coarctation of the Aorta
  Pulmonary Valve Stenosis
  Tetralogy of Fallot
  Ebstein's Anomaly
  Transposition of the Great Arteries
  Congenital Corrected Transposition
  Eisenmenger's Syndrome
  Tricuspid Atresia
  Electrophysiological Issues

PREGNANCY
 Reproductive Issues
 Auscultatory Findings
 Management of Heart Disease in Pregnant Patients

ISSUES IN ADULT PEDIATRIC CARDIOLOGY

Much of this chapter will be devoted to the care of patients who were born after 1950 and have survived into adult life with problems related to congenital heart defects. These patients are often seen by physicians whose adult practice leaves them without the appropriate background in pediatric cardiology. This patient subpopulation has survived into adulthood because of major advances in pediatric cardiac surgery. Paradoxically, the group's extended life span also has been accompanied by such problems as postsurgical complications; growth and nutritional abnormalities; and the combined effects of congenital heart disease, corrected congenital heart disease, created defects, and adult heart disease superimposed on congenital heart disease. Such factors complicate the management of these patients, and tax the abilities of even the specialists involved in their care.

In this chapter we will discuss some of the common conditions that are encountered and their associated auscultatory findings, both pristine and those that pertain to changes after intervention. Gender ratios in certain conditions are noted (Cardiac Pearl 32). Table 10-1 summarizes the signs and symptoms that the clinician should look for in this patient population.

Atrial Septal Defects

Patients with adult congenital atrial septal defects (ASDs) may present with added changes caused by the development of pulmonary hypertension,

Table 10-1   Congenital Heart Disease

Category	Disease
Acyanotic	ASD-pulmonary
	Bicuspid valves
	Subvalvular stenosis
	Vascular stenosis
	Pulmonary stenosis
	Infundibular stenosis
	Branch PA stenosis
	Cushion defect (ASD, VSD, PDA)
	Aortic stenosis
	Coarctation of the aorta
Cyanotic	Tetralogy of Fallot
	Truncus arteriosus
	Transposition of great arteries
	Tricuspid atresia
	Total anomalous venous drainage

abnormalities of cardiac rhythm, or auscultatory findings that have altered (e.g., a loud early P_2). Infrequently, patients may present with paradoxical embolism. This condition may be caused either by the atrial septal defect per se, by a patent foramen ovale, or by a partially closed defect. Anomalous venous connections, mitral valve prolapse, and cleft mitral valves are commonly encountered. The finger changes in the Holt-Oram syndrome (Chap. 8) may be easily observed. If closure occurs spontaneously, it does so in children younger than 30 months.

Auscultatory findings   Findings in these patients are outlined in Chaps. 5 and 6. Although in most cases these defects are left-to-right and are closed, they have been overlooked or have reopened with shunts with ratios higher than 1.5:1. Atrial fibrillation, right heart failure, and pulmonary hypertension complicate the physical findings in these adults. Thus, a typical older patient with an atrial septal defect may present with wide splitting of S_2; apparent physiological splitting of S_2; or mitral regurgitation, ventricular septal defect, or complete right bundle branch block (RBBB). In these patients, the index of suspicion should point to the diagnosis of atrial septal defect. An accentuated pulmonic valve closure sound is heard in the pulmonary area and at the apex due to an enlarged right ventricle. In adults P_2 is widely transmitted to other areas and may be closer to A_2 with fixed narrow splitting of S_2 in pulmonary hypertension.

Older patients with an atrial septal defect may manifest with diastolic tricuspid flow murmurs that grow louder on inspiration if there is a left-to-right shunt. In patients with severe pulmonary hypertension, right heart failure dominates the picture: There is a loud P_2, a palpable right ventricle, an S_4 with a Graham Steell murmur and some degree of central cyanosis. Leg edema, ascites, hepatomegaly, or venous engorgement may occur. In patients with atrial septal defect and severe pulmonary hypotension, A_2 and P_2 are narrowly split with a fixed interval between them. After atrial septal defect closure, the split narrows in children but may widen or stay wide in adults with dilated pulmonary arteries. In Lutembacher's syndrome, the signs of mitral stenosis and atrial septal defect are present. In cor triatrium, the physical signs are those of mitral stenosis (i.e., middiastolic murmurs are caused by a membrane overlying the valve and dividing the left atrium into parts). These conditions are rare.

Treatment and evaluation   Pulmonary vascular resistance is an important prognostic factor; if it is below 15 Wood units/m² (1 Wood unit = 80°C/ cm²), repair is indicated at any age. Over 15 units/m², surgery is probably contraindicated. Shunt evaluation is done by echo, magnetic resonance imaging (MRI), or cardiac catheterization. In patients with atrial fibrillation, the risk of embolic stroke may indicate the need for anticoagulant therapy. The reversibility of pulmonary hypertension is determined with Prostacyclin and high-flow oxygen used in right heart catheterization. Closure before age 24 years is associated with lower morbidity.

Ventricular Septal Defects

Ventricular septal defects are found in a variety of locations within the septum.

1. Supracristal outflow tract defects are often associated with early diastolic murmurs caused by proximity to outflow tracts and by prolapse of the aortic or pulmonic valves into the defect. These patients do not ordinarily live long if the defects are uncorrected.
2. A small Roger-type defect may be present in the perimembranous area.
3. Muscular defects may be present—trabecular in the outflow tract or adjacent to the tricuspid valve.
4. Multiple ventricular ("Swiss cheese") septal defects may also occur.
5. Septal defects may transgress the tricuspid valve ring.

Auscultatory findings   Patients present with a loud holosystolic murmur and thrill (Roger murmur), described in Chap. 6. They may over a period of time lose the murmur in the presence of pulmonary hypertension. This loss may result from spontaneous closure of the ventricular septal defect, or attenuation of flow through it. A windsock sound may appear (Chap. 5) and the murmur may attenuate (Chap. 6). With a ratio of flow higher than 1.5:1, surgical closure is warranted; if not performed in childhood, it may be required in later life. The patient's treatment is determined by the degree of pulmonary hypertension. Physical findings in patients with ventricular septal defects are fairly typical; however, they may present with pulmonary hypertension and develop Eisenmenger's syndrome, in which the holosystolic murmur is attenuated and may disappear. A single S_2 is heard. Patients with Eisenmenger's syndrome have systemic pressures that preclude surgery.

Atrioventricular Septal Defects

Atrioventricular septal defects are associated with Down's syndrome (Chap. 8). These patients may survive into adulthood whether or not surgery was performed. The chest x-ray is classical, indicating the presence of the "swan neck" deformity seen on angiography in ostium primum defects. The echocardiogram (ECG) shows characteristic floating mitral and tricuspid valves through endocardial cushion defects.

Auscultatory findings   The auscultatory findings in atrioventricular septal defects include the presence of mitral regurgitation, tricuspid regurgitation, splitting of S_2, and atrioventricular conduction abnormalities. Complete heart block, however, is rare. Primary repair is required to maximize the odds for long-term survival.

Patent Ductus Arteriosus

This condition is associated with a continuous murmur as described previously. Patients with patent ductus arteriosus may have a small shunt and need only antibiotic prophylaxis. The risk of operative mortality in adults is somewhat greater than in children. Closure in patients with a significant ductus is appropriate unless contraindicated by the presence of irreversible pulmonary hypertension; if a reversed ductal flow occurs, cyanosis and clubbing of the toes and the fingers of the left hand and pink fingers on the right side are pathognomonic. Coil devices may be used in surgery in closing ductus; they do not involve thoracotomy. With a right-sided aorta, the murmur is heard in the second right intercostal space.

Coarctation of the Aorta (Cardiac Pearl 64)

Coarctation of the aorta (CoA) is frequently misdiagnosed or missed; only 20 percent of CoAs are diagnosed in childhood or adolescence. Patients present with hypertension and other clinical findings that may include the following:

- Bicuspid valve
- Ejection sound
- "Blubbering" systolic murmur
- Splitting of S_2
- Early diastolic murmur
- Loud systolic murmur heard over the back and continuing into diastole
- Suzman's sign (pulsating axillary collaterals).

Left sternal and infraclavicular murmurs as well as periclavicular murmurs with pulsating intercostals may be heard. In CoA there is brachiofemoral peak pulse lag and hypertension. ECG allows the diagnosis to be made with Doppler imaging. The clinician should look for bicuspid valves. Treatment is usually surgical (angioplasty). The coarctation murmur may be midsystolic, late systolic, or continuous, depending on the degree of narrowing (Cardiac Pearl 21). Postoperative complications may occur.

Aortic Valve Stenosis

This condition may occur secondary to congenital bicuspid aortic valves or unicuspid valves. It may develop into critical aortic stenosis (Fig. 10-1). Patients are generally symptomatic when surgery becomes necessary. The area of the aortic valve is then calculated by the *continuation equation,* which relies on flow being equal to product of area and mean velocity on

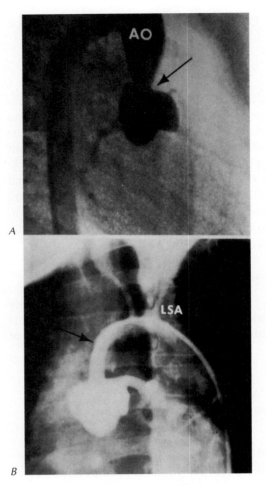

Figure 10-1 A. Lateral aortogram from a seven-year-old boy with severe supravalvular aortic stenosis; arrow points to a localized zone of obstruction just above the sinuses of Valsalva. B. Aortogram from an eight-year-old boy with tubular hypoplasia of the aorta (arrow) beginning just above the aortic sinuses and extending beyond the left subclavian artery (LSA).

both sides of a stenotic valve. Severe stenosis is indicated by a cross-sectional area of 0.6 to 0.7 cm². It is also characterized by:

- Delay of the aortic ejection sound
- Muffled S_1
- Presence of S_4
- Long and prominent systolic murmur
- Gradient of 70 mmHg or higher across the aortic valve
- Aortic valvotomy may be performed in children and young adults; however, aortic valve replacement is required in adults

- Pulmonary Valve Stenosis
- In pulmonary valve stenosis the classic signs of pulmonary stenosis are present:
  a. Enhanced inspiration
  b. Rough midsystolic murmur (RŔR)
  c. Crescendo/decrescendo thrill over the pulmonary artery (*Lu͘rrr'/dup*)
  d. Possible loud ejection click (*lu͜ trr/dup*)

As the pulmonary stenosis becomes more severe, the click occurs early; S_2 splits; and P_2 softens. In severe cases, the patient may develop a presystolic click, fatigue, dyspnea, cyanosis, epistaxis, and right heart failure. On the other hand, 25 percent of patients with pulmonary valve stenosis are asymptomatic.

Tetralogy of Fallot and "Tet" Syndromes

The tetralogy of Fallot is a congenital condition that, together with the trilogy and pentalogy of Fallot, comprise the so-called "tet" syndromes. These syndromes share the following features:

- A right-to-left shunt at atrial level, ventricular level, or both
- A right-sided aorta
- Anomalous origin of the coronary arteries

Other coronary artery anomalies are common in these patients (Chaps. 6, 8). A right-sided aorta is seen in 25 percent of tet syndromes (Cardiac Pearl 22).

Physical findings Patients may present with the classic physical findings of Fallot's tetralogy:

- Normal neck veins
- Central cyanosis and clubbing
- Long systolic murmur preceded by a click (either ejection or holosystolic)
- Single S_2 at apex

In most instances patients with this syndrome will have undergone total correction. Palliative surgery may be a feasible alternative in patients whose defects cannot be totally corrected. When examining a patient who has undergone palliative procedures, the clinician should note both the procedure in question and the findings. The more common palliative procedures include (Fig. 10-2):

1. *Blalock-Taussig,* placing a shunt from the pulmonary to the subclavian artery, associated with continuous bruit

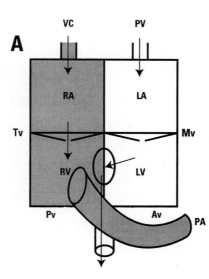

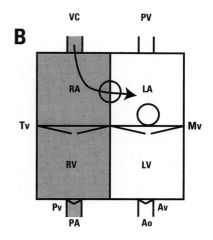

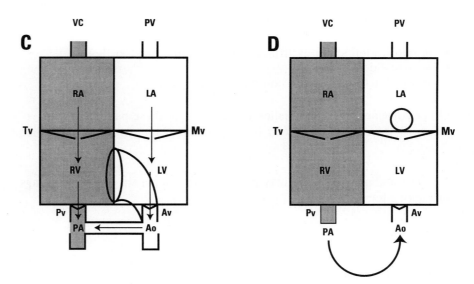

Figure 10-2 Common surgical procedures for Fallot's tetralogy and congenital TGA. A. Rastelli procedure. B. Rashkind balloon septostomy. C. Potts or Waterston shunt procedure. D. Switch procedure. VC, venacava; RA, right atrium; RV, right ventricle; PA, pulmonary artery; PV, pulmonary veins; LV, left ventricle; LA, left atrium; A, aorta; Tv, tricuspid valve; Mv, mitral valve; Pv, pulmonary valve; Av, aortic valve.

2. *Waterston:* Placing a shunt between the ascending aorta and the pulmonary artery
3. *Potts:* Placing a shunt between the descending aorta and left pulmonary artery

"Tet" patients with continuous murmurs may develop later complications: (1) pulmonary hypertension caused by flow into hypoplastic pulmonary arteries; and (2) left heart failure with pulmonary edema.

Treatment   In total corrections of tetralogy of Fallot, patients often present with pulmonary regurgitation, which may require replacement of the pulmonary valve. Left ventricular failure and dilatation may develop. Arrhythmias are common. Patients with "tet" syndromes will require antibiotic chemoprophylaxis.

Ebstein's Anomaly

Patients with Ebstein's anomaly present with arrhythmias in adult life caused by Wolff-Parkinson-White syndrome (accessory conduction between the atria and ventricle through Kent bundles) and by a variety of supraventricular arrhythmias. Atrial fibrillation is common in these patients as they age. Patients may be cyanotic at birth, although the cyanosis may be variable and is usually mild. Sudden death is a common occurrence in these patients.

Physical findings   The physical findings are complicated in patients with Ebstein's anomaly. In spite of the presence of tricuspid regurgitation, these patients have nearly normal neck veins because the enlarged right atrium dampens venous pulsation. Findings include a quiet heart with no right ventricular impulse. The enlarged right atrium can be detected by percussion to the right of the sternum. Auscultation reveals:

- Widely split S_1, occasionally split into three components (second component is high-pitched and loud; sail sound)
- Holosystolic murmur
- Splitting of S_2 caused by an RBBB configuration
- Diastolic murmur
- Diastolic sound

S_2 in Ebstein's anomaly may also be widely split because of an atrial septal defect. Wolff-Parkinson-White syndrome may be present, with signs evident in the left chest. The conglomeration of heart sounds may produce a quintuple or sextuple rhythm.

Treatment   The arrhythmias in this syndrome should be treated if hemody-namic problems are present, with ablation of bypass tracts if warranted.

Transposition of the Great Arteries (TGA)

There are two types of TGA, corrected and congenital. A comparison of normal circulatory anatomy with TGA may be found in Fig. 10-3.

Corrected TGA   In the *corrected* form of TGA, the outflow tracts, atrio-ventricular valves, and ventricles are inverted (Fig. 10-4). As a result, the systemic ventricle has the morphology of a right ventricle; it receives pulmonary venous blood and pumps it into the aorta. The venous ventricle has the morphology of a left ventricle; it receives blood from the venae cavae and ejects blood into the pulmonary artery. The systemic ventricle carries the tricuspid valve, while the pulmonary ventricle carries the mitral valve. This arrangement places stress on the systemic ventricle and leads to systemic heart failure. Patients with corrected transposition have a poor prognosis.

Physical findings   In corrected transposition, a loud A_2 can be heard over the pulmonic area and a loud P_2 over the pulmonary area (Cardiac Pearl

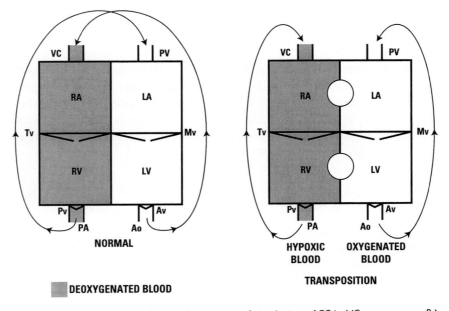

Figure 10-3 Comparison of normal anatomy of circulation of TGA. VC, vena cava; RA, right atrium; RV, right ventricle; PA, pulmonary artery; PV, pulmonary veins; LV, left ventricle; LA, left atrium; Ao, aorta; TV, tricuspid valve; Mv, mitral valve; Pv, pulmonary valve; Av, aortic valve.

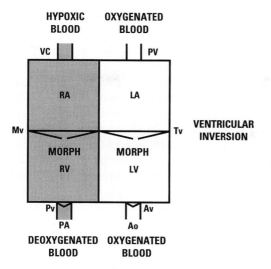

Figure 10-4 Schematic diagram of ventricular inversion in the corrected form of TGA. VC, vena cava; RA, right atrium; RV, right ventricle; PA, pulmonary artery; PV, pulmonary veins; LV, left ventricle; LA, left atrium; Ao, aorta; Tv, tricuspid valve; Mv, mitral valve; Pv, pulmonary valve; Av, aortic valve.

25). These sounds are caused by the displacement of the two outflow tracts—the pulmonary artery lying posteriorly and to the right of the aorta, which is anterior and left. Other defects may be present in cases of corrected transposition:

- Ventricular septal defects
- Tricuspid valve abnormalities
- Ebstein's anomaly between the left atrium and the systemic ventricle (the morphological right ventricle)
- Atrial septal defects
- Congenital heart block

Ebstein's anomaly in the systemic atrioventricular valve may add other physical signs to the clinical picture. Patients with corrected transposition are vulnerable to sudden death from atrial or ventricular tachyarrhythmias, and to left sided heart failure.

Treatment   Heart failure may develop acutely if the systemic ventricle with right ventricular morphology should fail. Patients may require cardiac transplantation.

Congenital TGA   Patients with the congenital form of TGA are cyanotic. One of two procedures is usually carried out shortly after birth. The patient may require an immediate Rashkind balloon septostomy (Fig. 10-2*B*) to reduce cyanosis, followed by a Mustard-Senning or switch procedure (Fig. 10-5). The Rashkind septostomy consists of baffle placement for redirection of the circulations; the venous circulation is redirected to the venous outflow tract and the arterial circulation to the aorta.

In patients with ventricular septal defect, the procedure is carried out to connect the respective ventricles with the correct outflow tracts. The ventricular septal defect itself is patched, the left ventricle connected to the aorta, and the right ventricle attached by a conduit to the pulmonary artery (Rastelli procedure; Fig. 10-2A). Specialists in adult cardiology who see patients with the Mustard procedure may encounter problems similar to those connected with corrected transposition. Patients who have had

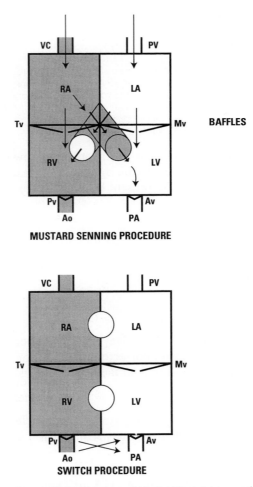

Figure 10-5 Diagram of Mustard-Senning procedure. VC, vena cava; RA, right atrium; RV, right ventricle; PA, pulmonary artery; PV, pulmonary veins; LV, left ventricle; LA, left atrium; Ao, aorta; Tv, tricuspid valve; Mv, mitral valve; Pv, pulmonary valve; Av, aortic valve.

the Mustard procedure may develop sick sinus syndrome or left-sided heart failure caused by systemic overload of the morphological right ventricle.

Treatment   Patients with congenital TGA often develop heart block and may require permanent pacemakers. Arrhythmias are common.

Tricuspid Atresia

Tricuspid atresia closely resembles tetralogy of Fallot. The physical findings in tricuspid atresia are similar:

- Cyanosis
- Left axis deviation
- Left ventricular hypertrophy (LVH)
- Other defects (pulmonary stenosis and ventricular septal defect)

Congenital Heart Block

In congenital heart block, the heart rate is usually 60 to 70 beats per minute, associated with total atrioventricular dissociation with narrow QRS complexes. The following conditions also obtain:

- Variable S_1
- Cannon sounds
- Multiple atrial sounds
- Cannon waves visible in the neck

Complete heart block in a young adult mandates a search for Lyme disease.

SPECIAL PROCEDURES IN ADULT PEDIATRIC CARDIOLOGY
Nonsurgical Treatments

New approaches have been developed for closure of patent ductus arteriosus (PDA) by (vascular) insertion of special devices that obviate the need for more invasive procedures, such as thoracic surgery. These devices include:

- Double umbrella occlusions
- Siders buttons
- Gianturco coils

Atrial septal defects can be repaired by the Rashkind double umbrella device, or by the Siders button, or by wing tip devices.

Balloon Valvuloplasty

Balloon valvuloplasty has been used in the treatment of patients with adult rheumatic mitral stenosis using the Inouye balloon, which may be single or double. Mitral valvuloplasty is then performed. Pulmonary valvuloplasty is a common procedure, while angioplasty of coarctation is being performed more frequently. Patients with subclavian steal syndrome (transient vertebrobasilar ischemia caused by localized stenosis or occlusion of a subclavian artery proximal to the vertebral artery) have been successfully treated with angioplasty. Other interventional procedures in congenital heart disease include the embolization of pulmonary atrioventricular fistulae.

Transplantation may be necessary in patients with congenital heart disease. Heart alone or heart and lung transplants may be required in these patients. Single lung transplants have the associated problems of obliterative bronchiolitis and long-term management. They also have a higher mortality than heart transplants, as well as being more difficult to perform. Lung transplants may, however, be necessary in patients with corrected TGA, atrial transposition, Ebstein's anomaly (less commonly), and other congenital cardiomyopathies. Single lung transplants are useful in idiopathic pulmonary hypertension.

Electrophysiological Abnormalities

Electrophysiological abnormalities are common in most congenital heart disease or in adult congenital heart disease. Arrhythmias, frequent in affected patients, may have serious consequences and may require pacemakers to resolve. Patients undergoing surgery for corrections of "tet" syndromes are at risk for pulmonary regurgitation, right ventricular failure, and cardiac arrhythmias. As in Epstein's anomaly, sudden death is not uncommon. Atrial arrhythmias are common following the baffle procedure in TGA.

SURGICAL TREATMENT OF PATIENTS WITH CONGENITAL HEART DISEASE

Surgical treatments of defects discussed in this section are summarized in Table 10-2.

Atrial Septal Defect

In atrial septal defect, surgical closure is recommended if the defect is larger than 1.5 cm, and the shunt greater than 1.5:1. Even after closure, these patients continue to be at risk for atrial fibrillation. With pulmonary vascular resistance less than 10 units/m^2, there is a good outcome post

Table 10-2   Complications of Surgical Procedures

Procedure	Complication(s)
Tetralogy of Fallot, correction	Progressive pulmonary regurgitation
Tetralogy of Fallot, palliative	Pulmonary hypertension
	Cyanosis ← failure of conduction
TGA, Mustard-Senning procedure	Loss of sinus function
	Atrial fibrillation
	Obstruction of venous return, CHF or edema
Tricuspid atresia, Fontan procedure	Heart failure of morphological RV to aortic valve regurgitation
	Conduit obstruction
	Thromboembolic events
	Protein-losing enteropathy

surgery. Resistance between 10 and 15 units indicates a possible need for repair; over 15 units, surgery is contraindicated. Patients over the age of 24 years with pulmonary artery pressures over 40 mmHg have a higher mortality rate. Residual ejection systolic murmurs with split but mobile S_2 (A_2, P_2) are present. The A_2P_2 split may persist in dilated pulmonary arteries. In ostium primum defects, residual mitral regurgitation may be present.

Ventricular Septal Defect

In ventricular septal defects, the palliative operation consists of banding for infants, closure for adults if the shunt ratio is higher than 1.5:1. For ventricular septal defects, the same considerations pertain with respect to surgery as it applies to the presence of pulmonary hypertension. In some cases lung biopsy may be necessary to assess the reversibility of pulmonary vascular disease. Prostacycline may be given to determine the reversibility of pulmonary hypertension. A residual systolic ejection murmur may persist, as may pulmonary hypertension and a loud P_2. If aortic regurgitation is present, this may worsen. Bundle branch and atrioventricular blocks may complicate these procedures.

Atrioventricular Septal Defect

For atrioventricular septal defects, primary repair only is undertaken whenever possible. Management guidelines are the same as those for other septal defects.

Patent Ductus Arteriosus

Closure is indicated for a hemodynamically significant ductus; in adults, the ductus is more friable. Guidelines for vascular resistance and shunt ratios are adhered to. Surgical ligation has been the standard method of management. In addition, catheterization techniques have been developed for ductus closure that do not involve surgery. Hemorrhage may occur after closure in adults.

Coarctation of the Aorta

Intervention is undertaken in the presence of proximal hypertension. Without treatment, the mean survival of patients with CoA is 35 years; fewer than 25 percent of patients live to age 50. Coarctation repairs are carried out by balloon angioplasty or by surgery. Repair is indicated by a resting systolic blood pressure gradient less than 10 mmHg. Possible complications include:

- Sudden death
- Coronary artery disease
- Heart failure
- Need to reoperate
- Aortic valve replacement
- Aortic stenosis caused by bicuspid valves
- Restenosis of the coarctation
- Formation of aneurysms at repair site

In young patients with pressure gradients greater than 50 mmHg, a positive exercise ECG, and valve areas of less than 0.6 to 0.7 cm^2, replacement can be done with bioprosthetic valves using the Ross procedure to place a homograft or bioprosthetic valve in the pulmonary position. Angioplasty also has an important role in treatment of coarctation of the aorta.

Pulmonary Valve Stenosis

This condition is usually treated with balloon valvotomy or traditional surgical correction. Possible complications include right ventricular and atrial enlargement due to pulmonary or tricuspid regurgitation.

Tetralogy of Fallot

Complications regarding such palliative procedures as the Blalock-Taussig, Waterston, and Potts may involve either insufficient shunting, causing cyanosis, or massive shunting, causing pulmonary hypertension.

Following total repair of a "tet" syndrome, possible complications include pulmonary regurgitation, left ventricular failure, and bacterial endocarditis. Prosthetic pulmonary valve replacement may be carried out. Complications include the risk of sudden death. Right bundle branch block may also develop postoperatively. Ventricular arrhythmias may develop in the presence of residual pressure gradients. Anomalous coronary arteries mandate surgical caution (Cardiac Pearl 23).

Ebstein's Anomaly

Surgery is undertaken if the cardiothoracic ratio is greater than 65 percent and systemic saturation less than 90 percent. Ablation of abnormal pathways is carried out. Mortality for the procedure is between 5 and 10 percent.

Transposition of the Great Arteries

Later complications may include systemic ventricular dysfunction in patients who have undergone the Senning or Mustard procedure, owing to the strain on the morphological right ventricle; loss of sinus function; junctional rhythm; and atrial arrhythmias. The Jayene (switch) procedure has a higher mortality rate but fewer residual complications. Atrial arrhythmias and sinus node dysfunction complicate the Senning procedure.

Congenital Corrected Transposition

Prior to organ transplantation, the double switch procedure involving atrial and arterial switching may be carried out; however, it has a higher mortality rate than transplantation.

Eisenmenger's Syndrome

There is no current surgical treatment for this abnormality.

Tricuspid Atresia

The Fontan procedure (Fig. 10-6) may be carried out as a palliative measure. It may involve:

1. A conduit from the right atrium to the pulmonary artery
2. A conduit from the right atrium to a valve or nonvalvular subpulmonary ventricle
3. A connection between the superior vena cava and the right pulmonary artery (classic Glenn procedure; Fig. 10-6) or between the superior vena cava and both pulmonary arteries (bi-directional Glenn procedure)

The Fontan procedure provides good palliative results; however, patients may develop arrhythmias, thromboembolism, or protein-losing enteropathy during the postoperative period. Complications of the Fontan procedure include:

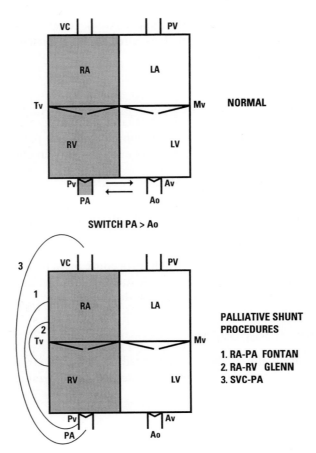

Figure 10-6 Diagram of Fontan and Glenn procedures for treatment of tricuspid atresia. VC, vena cava; RA, right atrium; RV, right ventricle; PA, pulmonary artery; PV, pulmonary veins; LV, left ventricle; LA, left atrium; Ao, aorta; Tv, tricuspid valve; Mv, mitral valve; Pv, pulmonary valve; Av, aortic valve.

- Conduit obstruction
- Pulmonary artery obstruction
- Residual left-to-right shunts
- Left ventricular dysfunction
- Mitral regurgitation

Electrophysiological Issues

Atrial septal defect is commonly associated with atrial fibrillation and Ebstein's anomaly as well as with anomalous conduction pathways that may cause sudden death. Patients who have undergone the Mustard-Senning procedure may develop sinus node disease and require pacemakers. Atrial arrhythmias may occur in congenital corrected transpositions.

In tetralogy of Fallot, ventricular ectopic rhythms may respond to phenytoin (Dilantin); these conditions too are associated with sudden death.

PREGNANCY

There is no situation in cardiovascular medicine in which evaluation of the patient is as critical as in pregnancy, especially in pregnant patients with known or suspected cardiac abnormalities.

Reproductive Issues

When a pregnant woman has adult congenital heart disease, the risks to both mother and fetus may be quite serious. In Marfan's syndrome with aortic involvement, the aorta is typically dilated (> 40 mm), and surgery is not recommended. In uncorrected coarctation of the aorta, there is a risk of aortic dissection during pregnancy. The mother's blood pressure should be controlled and activity limited.

In patients with Eisenmenger's syndrome, the mortality for both mother and fetus is extremely high. Endocarditis may occur in any of these conditions except atrial septal defect (ostium secundum), and requires careful assessment. Paradoxic emboli caused by septal defects (in particular atrial septal defects and patent foramina ovales) also require anticipatory care.

Auscultatory Findings

In Normal Pregnancy   Auscultatory findings in normal pregnancy include the following:

- Apparent cardiomegaly
- Venous waves in the neck
- Accentuated S_1 and S_2 with an ejection sound
- S_3
- Systolic murmurs heard at the left sternal edge
- Mammary soufflé
- Uterine soufflé or bruit
- Fetal heart sounds
- Exertional dyspnea, particularly in the third trimester
- Basal rales dispersed by coughing
- Left axis deviation on ECG.

In Pregnancy with Heart Disease

- Dyspnea or orthopnea
- Central or peripheral cyanosis

- Clubbing of the fingers
- Marked neck wave distention with elevated venous pressure
- Systolic murmurs greater than III/VI in intensity
- Loud, high-pitched S_4
- Other diastolic murmurs
- Localized cardiomegaly, with documented abnormal heaves or thrusts, or sustained arrhythmias
- Splitting of S_2
- Criteria for pulmonary hypertension
  a. Loud parasternal click
  b. Left parasternal lift
  c. Palpable, loud P_2.

Management of Heart Disease in Pregnant Patients

Heart disease in pregnancy usually falls into one of the following categories:
1. *Congestive failure,* as in peripartum cardiomyopathy.
2. *Acyanotic congenital heart disease* (Table 10-3). These conditions include coarctation of the aorta, Marfan's syndrome, mitral valve prolapse, shunts, Ebstein's anomaly, and hypertrophic obstructive cardiomyopathy, or HOCM.
3. *Cyanotic congenital heart disease* (Table 10-3). These conditions are less common in pregnancy, because patients with them are less likely to become pregnant. They include: tetralogy of Fallot, tricuspid atresia, Eisenmenger's syndrome, transposition of the great arteries, and truncus arteriosus.
4. *Changes in established murmurs due to vasodilatation.* Murmurs due to regurgitation tend to become softer during pregnancy, while murmurs due to stenotic valves grow louder. These murmurs may get louder or softer as described after pregnancy. Symptoms relate to these murmurs.
5. *Heart disease of adult onset* (Cardiac Pearl 90). These conditions include acute myocardial infarction, aortic dissection, endocarditis, pulmonary or systemic hypertension, valvular heart disease, rheumatic fever, chorea gravidarum, and prosthetic valvular heart diseases with their complications.

   Patients with any of the following conditions should be advised to avoid pregnancy:

- Primary pulmonary hypertension
- Grade III heart failure
- Angina pectoris
- Previous peripartum cardio
- Myopathy (PPCM).

Eight percent of cardiac patients with pulmonary hypertension develop syncope, 30 percent dyspnea, 75 percent palpitations, and 8 percent Raynaud's phenomenon (Chap. 8). These symptoms may derive from plexiform changes of the lungs or thromboembolic changes of occlusive disease. Other conditions with known high mortality in pregnancy include class III or IV heart failure from any cause, as well as severe pulmonary hypertension.

Conditions associated with increased risk of heart failure in pregnancy include the following:

- Hyperthyroidism
- Anemia
- Pulmonary embolism
- Arrhythmias
- Infection
- History of PPCM.

Failure is aggravated in the second trimester but may improve somewhat in the third trimester. In childbirth, heart failure may occur during second-stage labor (with straining) or immediately postpartum.

Toxemia in pregnancy is an important cause of hypertension and heart failure. Hemodynamic changes in pregnant patients with pulmonary hypertension, HOCM, or cyanotic congenital heart lesions with right-to-left shunts must be monitored with special care for signs of shock.

CLINICAL VIGNETTES

1. A 30-year-old female patient presented with dyspnea, central cyanosis, minimal clubbing and a grade II systolic murmur with a loud P_2. A transesophageal echo was done and Albuminex injected into the peripheral vein. A large ventricular septal defect was visible. The diagnosis is:

A. Eisenmenger's syndrome
B. COPD
C. Pulmonary edema

2. A 39-year-old female patient presented with an episode of amaurosis fugax (fleeting visual loss caused by retinal emboli). She had a history of atrial septal defect closure. S_2 was widely split. There was a tear in the septal defect between the patch and the wall of the defect. The diagnosis is:

A. Torn patch of atrial septum
B. Neck carotid clot embolus
C. Ventricular clot

3. A 25-year-old male patient was seen with a continuous murmur over the pulmonic area. The patient had clubbed fingers and toes, minimally

cyanosed, and on examination had signs of pulmonary hypertension with cor pulmonale with right ventricular enlargement and accentuated pulmonary S_2. A continuous murmur over the pulmonary artery was prominent in systole and attenuated in diastole. The physical findings suggested right ventricular hypertrophy, which the ECG confirmed, and the chest x-ray showed a large pulmonary artery with peripheral vessel oligemia. The patient had a long-standing Blalock-Taussig shunt. The diagnosis is:

A.　Eisenmenger patent ductus arteriosus
B.　Truncus arteriosus
C.　Tetralogy of Fallot

4.　A 12-year-old female patient presented with tachycardia of 180 beats per minute due to atrial fibrillation. She had a rapid heartbeat with hypotension (60 mmHg/90 mmHg) and her perfusion was impaired. The ECG showed wide QRS tachycardia with a normal axis. The QRS axis pointed anteriorly into leads V_1–V_6. Cardioversion was carried out. After the patient achieved a sinus rhythm, auscultation indicated a sail sound, tricuspid regurgitation, and diastolic sounds and murmurs. This patient had:

A.　Tetralogy of Fallot
B.　Ebstein's anomaly
C.　Coarctation of the aorta

5.　A 35-year-old female patient presented with severe congestive failure and tricuspid regurgitation. Appropriate treatment to consider would be:

A.　Valve replacement of the left sided tricuspid valve
B.　Cardiac transplant
C.　Either, depending on LV function

6.　A 30-year-old female patient presented with blackout spells. A Holter monitor recording indicated intermittent second degree type 2 AV block. A previous mustard Senning procedure has been carried out. Appropriate treatment would be:

A.　Atropine
B.　Pacemaker implant
C.　Isuprel

7.　A 58-year-old female patient was referred with a large pericardial effusion of unexplained origin, present for at least 6 weeks and increasing in size. She had complained of slight shortness of breath. Clinical evaluation was unremarkable, apart from pallor. Tendon reflexes were myotonic. What test did the examiner order, and what diagnosis did it confirm?

A. A CBC, to confirm diagnosis of anemia
B. Thyroid function tests, confirming diagnosis of myxedema
C. Pericardiocentesis, to confirm diagnosis of infectious pericarditis

ANSWERS

Clinical Vignettes

1. *A. Eisenmenger's syndrome.* The central cyanosis, clubbing, and ventricular septal defect point to the diagnosis.
2. The tear in the septal defect between the patch and the wall of the defect is not infrequently seen due to patch traction.
3. *C. Tetralogy of Fallot and pulmonary hypertension.* Pulmonary hypertension was due to the Blalock-Taussig shunt. Normally, in Fallot's tetralogy, the pulmonary artery is small, indicated by a "bay" in the left border of the chest x-ray.
4. *B. Ebstein's anomaly.* The tricuspid regurgitation, sail sound, and presence of atrial fibrillation suggest the diagnosis.
5. *A. Takayasu's syndrome.* The diagnosis is suggested by the absence of pulses, joint pains, and elevated ESR. Polyarteritis nodosa is more often characterized by hypertension. Giant cell arteritis is characterized by an elevated ESR, but is usually associated with severe headache and visual disturbances.
6. *Obstruction of the main mesenteric arteries.* Angiogram confirmed the diagnosis. This condition was surgically corrected and the patient improved.
7. *B. Thyroid function tests, confirming diagnosis of myxedema.* The patient's thyroid function tests indicated elevated TSH levels and a low T_4. She was placed on replacement thyroid medication and made a complete recovery, including the resorption of the pericardial effusion. The diagnosis is suggested by the patient's pallor, the delayed tendon reflexes, and the presence of the pericardial effusion.

BIBLIOGRAPHY

Ainger LE, Pate JW: Ostium secundum atrial septal defects and congestive heart failure in infancy. *Am J Cardiol* 1965; 15:380.

Ali Khan MA et al: Experience with 205 procedures of transcatheter closure of ductus arteriosus in 1982 patients, with special reference to residual shunts and long-term follow-up. *J Thorac Cardiovasc Surg* 1992; 104:1721–1727.

Alpert BS et al: Spontaneous closure of small ventricular septal defects: Ten-year follow-up. *Pediatrics* 1979; 63:204–206.

Alpert MA et al: Cardiovascular manifestations of mixed connective tissue disease in adults. *Circulation* 1983; 68:1182–1193.

Appelbe AF et al: Libman-Sacks endocarditis mimicking intracardiac tumor. *Am J Cardiol* 1991; 68:817–818.

Backer CL et al: Transposition of the great arteries: A comparison of results of the Mustard procedure versus the arterial switch. *Ann Thorac Surg* 1989; 48:10–14.

Baltaze HA, Wixon D: The incidence of congenital anomalies of the coronary arteries in the adult population. *Radiology* 1977; 122:47.

Barash PG et al: Management of coarctation of the aorta during pregnancy. *J Thorac Cardiovasc Surg* 1975; 69:781.

Barritt DW et al: Heart sounds and pressures in atrial septal defect. *Br Heart J* 1965; 27:90.

Basson CT et al: The clinical and genetic spectrum of the Holt-Oram syndrome (heart-hand syndrome). *N Engl J Med* 1994; 330:885–891.

Becker RM: Intracardiac surgery in pregnant women. *Ann Thorac Surg* 1983; 36:453.

Bauerlein EJ et al: Reversible dilated cardiomyopathy due to thyrotoxicosis. *Am J Cardiol* 1992; 70:132.

Beary JF et al: Postpartum acute myocardial infarction: A rare occurrence of uncertain etiology. *Am J Cardiol* 1979; 43:158.

Becker RM: Intracardiac surgery in pregnant women. *Ann Thorac Surg* 1983; 36:453.

Bedford DE: The anatomical types of atrial septal defect: Their incidence and clinical diagnosis. *Am J Cardiol* 1960; 6:568.

Besterman E: Atrial septal defect with pulmonary hypertension. *Br Heart J* 1961; 23:587.

Bialostozky D et al: Ebstein's malformation of the tricuspid valve: A review of 65 cases. *Am J Cardiol* 1972; 29:826–836.

Blake HA et al: Coronary artery anomalies. *Circulation* 1964; 30:927.

Blalock A, Taussig HB: The surgical treatment of malformations of the heart in which there is pulmonary stenosis or pulmonary atresia. *JAMA* 1945; 128:189.

Bonchek LI et al: Natural history of tetralogy of Fallot in infancy: Clinical classification and therapeutic implications. *Circulation* 1973; 48:392.

Boon AR: Tetralogy of Fallot: Effect on the family. *Br J Prev Soc Med* 1972; 26:263–268.

Borenstein DG et al: The myocarditis of systemic lupus erythematosus: Association with myositis. *Ann Intern Med* 1978; 89:619–624.

Braunwald E: The physical examination in heart disease. In Braunwald E (ed): *Heart Disease: A Textbook of Cardiovascular Medicine* 2d ed. Philadelphia, Saunders, 1984.

Brenner LD et al: Quantification of left-to-right atrial shunts with velocity-encoded cinenuclear magnetic resonance imaging. *J Am Coll Cardiol* 1992; 20:1246–1250.

Brock RC: Pulmonary valvulotomy for the relief of congenital pulmonary stenosis: Report of three cases. *Br Med J* 1948; 1:1121.

Burnard ED: A murmur from the ductus arteriosus in the newborn baby. *Br Med J* 1958; 1:806.

Campbell M: Natural history of coarctation of the aorta. *Br Heart J* 1970; 32:633–640.

Campbell M: Natural history of persistent ductus arteriosus. *Br Heart J* 1968; 39:4.

Campbell M, Baylis JH: The course and prognosis of coarctation of the aorta. *Br Heart J* 1956; 18:475.

Carruth JE et al: The electrocardiogram in normal pregnancy. *Am Heart J* 1981; 102:1075–1078.

Chatterjee K: Bedside hemodynamic monitoring. In Boolooki H (ed): *Clinical Applications of Intra-Aortic Balloon Pumps.* Mt. Kisco, NY, Futura Publishing, 1977:197.

Cheitlin MD: Congenital heart disease in the adult: Modern concepts of cardiovascular disease. 1986; 55:20.

Cheitlin MD et al: Sudden death as a complication of anomalous left coronary origin from the anterior sinus of Valsalva. *Circulation* 1974; 50:780.

Chesebro JH et al: Antithrombotic therapy in patients with valvular heart disease and prosthetic heart valves. *J Am Coll Cardiol* 1986; 8:41–56B.

Clapp S et al: Down's syndrome, complete atrioventricular canal, and pulmonary vascular obstructive disease. *J Thorac Cardiovasc Surg* 1990; 100:115–121.

Clark SL et al: Labor and delivery in the presence of mitral stenosis: Central hemodynamic observations. *Am J Obstet Gynecol* 1985; 152:984.

Clarkson PM et al: Prosthetic repair of coarctation of the aorta with particular reference to Dacron onlay patch grafts and late aneurysm formation. *Am J Cardiol* 1985; 56:342.

Clements PJ et al: The relationship of arrhythmias and conduction disturbances to other manifestations of cardiopulmonary disease in progressive systemic sclerosis (PSS). *Am J Med* 1981; 71:38–46.

Cohen M et al: Coarctation of the aorta: Long-term follow-up and prediction of outcome after surgical correction. *Circulation* 1989; 80:840.

Connelly MS et al: Congenitally corrected transposition in the adult: Functional status and complications. *J Am Coll Cardiol* 1996; 27:1238–1243.

Cumming GR: Congenital corrected transposition of the great vessels without associated intracardiac abnormalities. *Am J Cardiol* 1962; 10:605.

Cutforth R, MacDonald C: Heart sounds and murmurs in pregnancy. *Am Heart J* 1966; 71:741.

Dalen JE et al: Life expectancy with atrial septal defect. *JAMA* 1967; 100:442.

Danielson GK: Correction of atrioventricular canal. In Anderson RH, Shinebourne ES (eds): *Paediatric Cardiology* 1977. Edinburgh, Churchill Livingstone, 1978:470.

Dave KS et al: Atrial septal defects in adults. *Am J Cardiol* 1973; 31:7.

Davia JE et al: Anomalous left coronary artery origin from the right coronary sinus. *Am Heart J* 1984; 108:165.

Davis PJ, Davis FB: Hyperthyroidism in patients over the age of 60 years: Clinical features in 85 patients. *Medicine* 1974; 53:161–181.

Deal K, Wooley CF: Coarctation of aorta and pregnancy. *Ann Intern Med* 1973; 78:706.

Dines DE et al: Pulmonary arteriovenous fistulas. *Mayo Clin Proc* 1974; 49:460.

Doherty NE, Siegal RJ: Cardiovascular manifestations of systematic lupus erythematosus. *Am Heart J* 1985; 110:1257–1265.

Edwards JE: The congenital bicuspid valve. *Circulation* 1961; 23:485.

Engle MA: Ventricular septal defect in infancy. *Pediatrics* 1954; 14:16.

Fisher RG et al: Patent ductus arteriosus in adults—long-term follow-up: Nonsurgical versus surgical treatment. *J Am Coll Cardiol* 1986; 8:280–284.

Fontan F, Baudet E: Surgical repair of tricuspid atresia. *Thorax* 1971; 26:240–248.

Fontan F et al: Outcome after a "perfect" Fontan operation. *Circulation* 1990; 81:1520–1536.

Freed MD et al: Prostaglandin E1 in infants with ductus arteriosus-dependent congenital heart disease. *Circulation* 1981; 64:899–905.

Friedberg DZ, Nadas AS: Clinical profile of patients with congenital corrected transposition of the great arteries: A study of 60 cases. *N Engl J Med* 1970; 282:1053–1059.

Gault JH et al: Atrial septal defect in patients over the age of 40 years: Clinical and hemodynamic studies and the effects of operation. *Circulation* 1968; 37:261.

Gersony WM, Krongrad E: Evaluation and management of patients after surgical repair of congenital heart disease. *Prog Cardiovasc Dis* 1975; 18:39.

Gewillig M et al: Early and late arrhythmias after the Fontan operation: Predisposing factors and clinical consequences. *Br Heart J* 1992; 67:62–70.

Ghisla RP et al: Spontaneous closure of isolated secundum atrial septal defects in infants: An echocardiographic study. *Am Heart J* 1985; 109:1327–1333.

Glancy DL et al: Juxtaductal coarctation. *Am J Cardiol* 1983; 51:537.

Gleicher N et al: Eisenmenger's syndrome and pregnancy. *Obstet Gynecol Surv* 1979; 34:721–741.

Gray DT et al, for the Patent Ductus Arteriosus Closure Comparative Study Group: Clinical outcomes and costs of transcatheter as compared with surgical closure of patent ductus arteriosus. *N Engl J Med* 1993; 329:1517–1523.

Gross RE, Hubbard JP: Surgical ligation of a patent ductus arteriosus. *JAMA* 1964; 212:729–731.

Habib A, McCarthy JS: Effects on the neonate of propranolol administered during pregnancy. *J Pediatr* 1977; 91:808.

Harley HRS: What is Fallot's tetralogy? *Am Heart J* 1961; 62:729.

Hawkins JA et al: Total anomalous pulmonary venous connection. *Ann Thorac Surg* 1983; 36:548.

Heiner DC, Nadas AS: Patent ductus arteriosus in association with pulmonic stenosis: A report of six cases with additional noncardiac congenital anomalies. *Circulation* 1958; 17:232.

Henion WA et al: Postpartum myocardial infarction. *N Y State J Med* 1982; 82:57.

Hijazi ZM et al: Balloon angioplasty for recurrent coarctation of aorta: Immediate and long-term results. *Circulation* 1991; 84:1150–1156.

Holt M, Oram S: Familial heart disease with skeletal malformations. *Br Heart J* 1960; 22:236.

Homcy CJ et al: Ischemic heart disease in systemic lupus erythematosus in the young patient: Report of six cases. *Am J Cardiol* 1982; 49:478–484.

Honey M: The diagnosis of corrected transposition of the great vessels. *Br Heart J* 1963; 25:313.

Hughes CV et al: Total intracardiac repair for tetralogy of Fallot in adults. *Ann Thorac Surg* 1987; 43:634–638.

Ishikawa T, Brandt PWT: Anomalous origin of the left main coronary artery from the right anterior aortic sinus: Angiographic definition of anomalous course. *Am J Cardiol* 1985; 55:770.

Iskandrian AS et al: Cardiac performance in thyrotoxicosis: Analysis of 10 untreated patients. *Am J Cardiol* 1983; 51:349–352.

James KB, Healy BP: Heart disease arising during or secondary to pregnancy. In Douglas PS, Brest AN (eds.): *Heart Disease in Women.* Philadelphia, F. A. Davis, 1989:81–96.

Jarmakani JM et al: Left heart function in children with tetralogy of Fallot before and after palliative or corrective surgery. *Circulation* 1972; 46:478.

John S et al: The adult ductus: Review of surgical experience with 131 patients. *J Thorac Cardiovasc Surg* 1981; 82:314–319.

Kabadi UM, Kumar SP: Pericardial effusion in primary hypothyroidism. *Am Heart J* 1990; 120:1393–1395.

Keith JD et al: Transposition of the great vessels. *Circulation* 1953; 7:830.

Kitterman JA et al: Patent ductus arteriosus in premature infants: Incidence, relation to pulmonary disease, and management. *N Engl J Med* 1972; 287:473–477.

Klotz TA: Thrombophlebitis and pulmonary embolism. In Gleicher N (ed): *Principles of Medical Therapy in Pregnancy.* New York, Plenum, 1985:721.

Konishi IY et al: Dissecting aneurysm during pregnancy and the puerperium. *Jpn Circ J* 1980; 44:726.

Kramer HH et al: Cardiac rhythm after Mustard repair and after arterial switch operation for complete transposition. *Int J Cardiol* 1991; 32:5–12.

Ladenson PW et al: Complications of surgery in hypothyroid patients. *Am J Med* 1984; 77:261–266.

Landzberg MJ, Lock JR: Interventional catheter procedures used in congenital heart disease. *Cardiol Clin* 1993; 11:569–587.

Leatham AL: *Auscultation of the Heart and Phonocardiography,* 2d ed. Edinburgh, London, and New York: Churchill Livingstone, 1975.

Leatham AL: *An Introduction to the Examination of the Cardiovascular System.* Oxford, Oxford University Press, 1977.

Leatham AL, Gray I: Auscultatory and phonocardiographic signs of atrial septal defect. *Br Heart J* 1956; 18:193.

Lee RT et al: Depressed left ventricular systolic ejection force in hypothyroidism. *Am J Cardiol* 1990; 65:526–527.

Lee RV et al: Cardiopulmonary resuscitation of pregnant women. *Am J Med* 1986; 81:311.

Lewis BV, Parsons M: Chorea gravidarum. *Lancet* 1966; 1:284.

Libersthson RR et al: Coarctation of the aorta: Review of 234 patients and clarification of management problems. *Am J Cardiol* 1979; 43:835.

Liebman J et al: Natural history of transposition of great arteries: Anatomy and birth and death characteristics. *Circulation* 1969; 40:237.

Limet R, Grondin CM: Cardiac valve prostheses, anticoagulation, and pregnancy. *Ann Thorac Surg* 1977; 23:337.

Lin CC et al: Fetal outcome in hypertensive disorders of pregnancy. *Am J Obstet Gynecol* 1982; 142:255.

Lin SL et al: Transesophageal echocardiographic detection of atrial septal defect in adults. *Am J Cardiol* 1992; 69:280–282.

Lindsay J Jr: Coarctation of the aorta, bicuspid aortic valve, and abnormal ascending aortic wall (review). *Am J Cardiol* 1988; 61:182–184.

Lloyd TR et al: Transcatheter occlusion of patent ductus arteriosus with Gianturco coils. *Circulation* 1993; 88:1412–1420.

McGoon D: Long-term effects of prosthetic materials. In Engle MA, Perloff JK (eds): *Congenital Heart Disease After Surgery.* New York, Yourke Medical Books, 1983:177–201.

McWhorter JE, LeRoy EC: Pericardial disease in scleroderma (systemic sclerosis). *Am J Med* 1974; 57:566–575.

Mehta AV, Chidambaram B: Ventricular septal defect in the first year of life. *Am J Cardiol* 1992; 70:364–366.

Midei MG et al: Peripartum myocarditis and cardiomyopathy. *Circulation* 1990; 81:922–928.

Mitchell SC et al: Congenital heart disease in 56,109 births: Incidence and natural history. *Circulation* 1971; 43:323.

Moe DG, Guntheroth WG: Spontaneous closure of uncomplicated ventricular septal defect. *Am J Cardiol* 1987; 60:674–678.

Moller JH et al: Late results (30–35 years) after operative closure of isolated ventricular septal defect from 1954 to 1960. *Am J Cardiol* 1991; 68:1491–1497.

Morgan BC et al: Ventricular septal defect: I. Congestive heart failure in infancy. *Pediatrics* 1960; 25:54.

Murdoch JL et al: Life expectancy and causes of death in the Marfan's syndrome. *N Engl J Med* 1972; 286:804.

Nadas AS et al: Spontaneous functional closing of ventricular septal defects. *N Engl J Med* 1961; 264:309.

Nasser WK et al: Atrial myxoma: I. Clinical and pathologic features in nine cases. *Am Heart J* 1972; 83:694.

Nielson NC, Fabricius J: Primary pulmonary hypertension with special reference to prognosis. *Acta Med Scand* 1961; 170:731.

O'Fallon WM et al: Second natural history study of congenital heart defects: Material and methods. *Circulation* 1993; 87:4–15.

Paulus HE et al: Aortic insufficiency in five patients with Reiter's syndrome: A detailed clinical-pathologic study. *Am J Med* 1972; 53:464.

Perloff JK: Auscultatory and phonocardiographic manifestations of pulmonary hypertension. *Prog Cardiovasc Dis* 1967; 9:303.

Perloff JK: *The Clinical Recognition of Congenital Heart Disease,* 3rd ed. Philadelphia, Saunders, 1987:404.

Perloff JK: Congenital heart disease and pregnancy. In Gleicher N (ed): *Principles of Medical Therapy in Pregnancy.* New York, Plenum, 1985:665–671.

Perloff JK: Late postoperative concerns in adults with congenital heart disease. In Perloff JK (ed): *Pediatric Cardiovascular Disease.* Philadelphia, F. A. Davis, 1981.

Perloff JK: Pregnancy and cardiovascular disease. In Braunwald E (ed): *Heart Disease: A Textbook of Cardiovascular Medicine,* 3d ed. Philadelphia, Saunders, 1988.

Perloff JK: Pregnancy in congenital heart disease: The mother and the fetus. In Perloff JK, Child JS (eds): *Congenital Heart Disease in Adults.* Philadelphia, Saunders, 1991:124–140.

Perry SB et al: Interventional catheterization in pediatric congenital and acquired heart disease (review). *Am J Cardiol* 1988; 61:109G–117G.

Polikar R et al: The thyroid and the heart. *Circulation* 1993; 87:1435–1441.

Pyertiz RE: Maternal and fetal complications of pregnancy in the Marfan syndrome. *Am J Med* 1981; 71:784.

Rashkind WJ, Miller WW: Creation of an atrial septal defect without thoracotomy: A palliative approach to transposition of the great arteries. *JAMA* 1966; 196:991–992.

Redington AN et al: Right ventricular function 10 years after the Mustard operation for transposition of the great arteries: Analysis of size, shape, and wall motion. *Br Heart J* 1989; 62:455–461.

Reid MM, Murdoch R: Polymyositis and complete heart block. *Br Heart J* 1979; 41:628.

Ridolfi RL et al: The cardiac conduction system in progressive systemic sclerosis: Clinical and pathologic features of 35 patients. *Am J Med* 1976; 61:361–366.

Roberts WC et al: The congenitally bicuspid aortic valve: A study of 85 autopsy cases. *Am J Cardiol* 1970; 26:72.

Roberts WC et al: Origin of the right coronary from the left sinus of Valsalva and its functional consequences: Analysis of necropsy patients. *Am J Cardiol* 1982; 49:863.

Rodstein M et al: Atrial septal defect in the aged. *Circulation* 1961; 23:665–674.

Rome JJ et al: Double-umbrella closure of atrial defects: Initial clinical applications. *Circulation* 1990; 82:751–758.

Rosenthal A et al: Long-term prognosis (15–26 years) after repair of tetralogy of Fallot: I. Survival and symptomatic status. *Ann Thorac Surg* 1984; 38:151–156.

Rosenthal L: Coarctation of the aorta and pregnancy: Report of five cases. *Br Med J* 1955; 1:16.

Rowe RD et al: Atypical tetralogy of Fallot: A noncyanotic form with increased lung vascularity. *Circulation* 1955; 12:230.

Rowley KM et al: Right-sided infective endocarditis as a consequence of flow-directed pulmonary artery catheterization: A clinico-pathological study of 55 autopsied patients. *N Engl J Med* 1984; 311:1152.

Ruben PC: Treatment of hypertension in pregnancy. *Clin Obstet Gynecol* 1986; 13:307.

Rudolph AM et al: Patent ductus arteriosus: A clinical and hemodynamic study of 23 patients in the first year of life. *Pediatrics* 1958; 22:892.

Schrader ML et al: The heart in polyarteritis nodosa: A clinicopathologic study. *Am Heart J* 1985; 109:1353–1359.

Sciscione AC, Callan NA: Congenital heart disease in adolescents and adults: Pregnancy and contraception (review). *Cardiol Clin* 1993; 11:701–709.

Sehested J: Coarctation of the aorta in monozygotic twins. *Br Heart J* 1982; 47:619–620.

Shah D et al: Natural history of secundum atrial septal defect in adults after medical or surgical treatment: A historical prospective study. *Br Heart J* 1994; 71:224–228.

Shub C et al: Sensitivity of two-dimensional echocardiography in the direct visualization of atrial septal defect utilizing the subcostal approach: Experience with 154 patients. *J Am Coll Cardiol* 1983; 2:127–135.

Siegel RJ et al: Percutaneous ultrasonic angioplasty: Initial clinical experience. *Lancet* 1989; 2:272–274.

Soto B et al: Classification of ventricular septal defects. *Br Heart J* 1980; 43:332–343.

Spinnato JA et al: Eisenmenger's syndrome in pregnancy. *N Engl J Med* 1981; 304:1215.

St. John Sutton MG et al: Atrial septal defect in patients aged 60 years or older: Operative results and long-term postoperative follow-up. *Circulation* 1981; 64:402–409.

Steinfeld L et al: Clinical diagnosis of isolated subpulmonic (supracristal) ventricular septal defect. *Am J Cardiol* 1972; 30:19.

Sullivan JM, Ramanathan KB: Management of medical problems in pregnancy—severe cardiac disease. *N Engl J Med* 1985; 313:304.

Suwa M et al: Late diastolic whoop in severe aortic regurgitation. *Am J Cardiol* 1986; 57:699.

Swan HJC et al: Catheterization of the heart in man with the use of a flow-directed balloon-tipped catheter. *N Engl J Med* 1970; 283:447.

Tabaznik B et al: The mammary souffle of pregnancy and lactation. *Circulation* 1960; 22:1069.

Taylor GW et al: Peripartum myocardial infarction. *Am Heart J* 1993; 126:1462–1463.

Turina MI et al: Late functional deterioration after atrial correction for transposition of the great arteries. *Circulation* 1989; 80(I):162–167.

Ueland K: Cardiac surgery and pregnancy. *Am J Obstet Gynecol* 1965; 92:148.

Uretzky G et al: Reoperation after correction of tetralogy of Fallot. *Circulation* 1982; 66:202–208.

Veille JC: Peripartum cardiomyopathy: A review. *Am J Obstet Gynecol* 1984; 148:805.

Wessel HU et al: Prognostic significance of arrhythmia in tetralogy of Fallot after intracardiac repair. *Am J Cardiol* 1980; 46:843–848.

Whittemore R et al: Pregnancy and its outcome in women with and without surgical treatment of congenital heart disease. *Am J Cardiol* 1982; 50:641.

Wood P: The chief symptoms of heart disease. In Wood P (ed): *Diseases of the Heart and Circulation.* London, Eyre & Spottiswoode, 1956.

Wood P: The Eisenmenger syndrome or pulmonary hypertension with reversed central shunt. *Br Med J* 1958; 2:755–762.

Yale SH et al: Dermatomyositis with pericardial tamponade and polymyositis with pericardial effusion. *Am Heart J* 1993; 126:997–999.

APPENDIXES

APPENDIX I

Cardiac Pearls

1. A good standard stethoscope correctly used is fundamental to auscultation. It supersedes electronic devices that are currently available.

2. Loud heart sounds and high-pitched murmurs mask soft sounds and lower-pitched murmurs. Listen in the direction opposite to sources of obvious sounds or murmurs which cause acoustic obliteration.

3. Amyl nitrite softens mitral regurgitation and increases the murmur of IHSS; it thus enables clinicians to distinguish these two conditions. S_2 is physiologically split in mitral regurgitation and VSD; and paradoxically split in IHSS (HOCM).

4. If environmental noise is a problem, using a special electronic stethoscope (being developed), having a sound blocking system, or using an esophageal stethoscope may aid auscultation.

5. Triple impulses are heard or felt in IHSS; triple rubs in uremic pericarditis; triples at the base in mitral stenosis; A_2, P_2-OS triple rhythm in gallop rhythms. Triple first sounds are heard in Ebstein's anomaly; as a result, this anomaly has a quintuple rhythm of heart sounds.

6. When a patient is asked to change position, prompt standing will soften S_4; move nonejection clicks close to S_1; and will not appreciably change S_1 to ejection click duration.

7. In older patients, physiologically split S_2s in the absence of RBBB should suggest atrial septal defect, VSD, mitral regurgitation, or RV enlargement. In ASD, the split S_2 may be fixed, wide, or narrow.

8. A tapping apical impulse strongly suggests mitral stenosis. A triple impulse (triple ripple) is felt in IHSS; a double apical impulse in gallop rhythm; a diffuse impulse in ventricular aneurysms.

9. S_2 is split in ASDs and VSDs; often the split is reversed in patent ductus arteriosus (PDA).

10. An S_4 sound over the jugular veins, but not over the heart, is heard in tricuspid stenosis, but is heard over veins and heart in pulmonary hypertension.

11. A tambour-quality A_2 with an early diastolic murmur to the right side of the sternum suggests a dilated aorta, as in Marfan's syndrome or ascending aortic aneurysm (Harvey's sign).

12. Heart sounds and murmurs are softened in the presence of emphysema. In these patients, listen below the xiphoid.

13. Diastolic "cooing" or "wood saw" musical murmurs are heard in patients with retroverted aortic cusps. They are lower in pitch than "sea gull" murmurs.

14. Systolic murmurs are innocent if they keep innocent company. Innocent murmurs are rare after the second decade of life.

15. An S_3 in mitral regurgitation does not suggest failure, but implies significance.

16. A pseudo-right ventricular impulse may be caused by mitral regurgitation, which pushes the right ventricle against the chest wall during systole. This phenomenon also occurs in straight back syndrome.

17. Tilting the patient's bed upward may increase the loudness of the murmur in IHSS. Prompt squatting decreases this murmur.

18. Atrial fibrillation in a patient with IHSS is a medical emergency. In aortic stenosis, it suggests mitral valve disease.

19. Differential cyanosis (pink fingers, blue toes) with a loud P_2 suggests Eisenmenger's ductus.

20. Reversed cyanosis (pink toes, blue fingers) is seen in double outlet syndrome and transposition in the presence of ductus arteriosus.

21. Aortic coarctation is frequently missed; it is associated with bicuspid valve and subarachnoid hemorrhage.

22. Right-sided aorta is present in 25 percent of patients with tetralogy of Fallot. Right-sided aorta is also seen in Eisenmenger's syndrome and ductus arteriosus.

23. Patients with tetralogy of Fallot may have anomalous coronary arteries.

24. A child with apparent aortic stenosis may actually have type II homozygous hyperlipidemia. The murmur is caused by a xanthoma (Fogelman).

25. A_2 and P_2 switch places in TGA and dextrocardia.

26. A cyanotic patient with telangiectasia suggests the presence of pulmonary AV fistula with capillary telangiectasia.

27. Left-sided pleural effusions complicate pericarditis; right-sided pleural effusions complicate congestive failure.

28. A two-component rub becomes a three-component rub with Valsalva's maneuver. A one-component rub is rarely heard.

29. Complete heart block in a younger patient should bring to mind the possibility of Lyme disease or congenital heart block.

30. Embolism in a young patient should bring to mind the possibility of left atrial myxoma, endocarditis, patent foramen ovale, and/or atrial septal aneurysm.

31. See Table AI-1.

32. Gender preponderance: Pulmonary artery disease and CoA are more common in males; PDA and rheumatic tricuspid regurgitation in females. There is no gender preponderance for pulmonary stenosis, tetralogy of Fallot, tricuspid atresia, truncus arteriosus, Ebstein's anomaly, and TGA.

33. Disorders associated with familial transmission include IHSS, Marfan's syndrome, familial cardiomyopathy, accelerated atherosclerosis, hyperlipidemia, and sickle cell disease.

34. Disorders associated with racial origin include supracristal VSDs with prolapsed aortic cusps (Asians); sickle cell anemia and cardiomyopathy (African Americans); Chagas' disease, a form of myocarditis caused by an insect-borne protozoan (South Americans); and Takayasu's syndrome (Japanese).

35. Pulmonary branch stenosis is seen with rubella syndrome. The long murmur is heard anywhere in the chest, but often in the axilla.

36. See Table AI-2.

37. See Table AI-3.

38. See Table AI-4.

39. Bicuspid valves are the most common cause of congenital heart disease and may occur in 2 percent of persons. Coarctation of the

Table AI-1. Summary of Heart Sounds

Sound Name	Features
Train wheel quadruple rhythm	S_1-S_2-S_3-S_2
Summation gallop	S_1, S_2, (S_3 S_4) combined
Wind sock sound	Flail septum
Sigh in diastole	Aortic regurgitation
Plop in diastole	Suggests myxoma
Sail sound	Triple component in Ebstein's anomaly
Machinery or water wheel sound	Patient ductus arteriosus
Systolic buzzing murmur	Innocent Still murmur
Crunch	Pneumomediastinum
Millwheel murmur	Air embolism
Honks/whoops	Mitral valve prolapse
Seagull sound	Mitral or tricuspid valve disease
"Blubbering" murmur	Atrial regurgitation
Wood saw murmur	Atrial regurgitation

Table AI-2.   Names of Common Murmurs

Name	Description
Carey Coombs	Murmur in mitral valvulitis
Duroziez'	Double femoral murmur in aortic regurgitation
Cecil Cole	Conducted to the axilla in aortic regurgitation
Austin Flint	Apical diastolic murmur in aortic regurgitation
Graham Steell	Murmur of pulmonary regurgitation ← pulmonary hypertension
Roger	Murmur in ventricular septal defect
Means Lerman	Scratch in thyrotoxicosis
Still's	Innocent systolic murmur in a normal heart
Gibson	Machinery murmur in patent ductus arteriosus
Hamman's	Crunch murmur in pneumomediastinum
Millwheel	Murmur in air embolism
Libman-Sacks	Endocarditis in lupus erythematosus

aorta may occur in 17 percent of persons with congenital heart disease. VSD is the commonest congenital heart disease in infancy.

40. Maneuvers used during cardiac examinations: Carvallo, Valsalva, Müller, abdominal jugular test (hepatojugular reflux), Brockenborough, Braunwald, and Morrow.

41. Hangout can be compared to the workings of door hinges (Dr. James Shaver). The aortic "door" has a tight hinge, the pulmonic "door" a loose one. This differential impedance causes physiological splitting of A_2, P_2 on inspiration.

42. Observing a patient prior to formal examination yields a great deal of information. Time spent with the patient getting to know him or her is invaluable to the examination (Marriott).

43. Take the time to dicuss and evaluate the patient's financial and domestic situation. In severely ill patients, ask them to make "living wills" or trusts prior to initiating aggressive treatment. Inquire about the patient's religious affiliation or preference; some groups (e.g.,

Table AI-3.   Eponymous Signs and Their Associated Disorders

Sign(s)	Disorder
Suzman's	Coarctation of the aorta
Branham's	Arteriovenous fistulae
Corrigan's	Aortic regurgitation
Traube's	
de Musset's	
Quincke's	
Duroziez'	
Hills'	
Kussmaul's	Constrictive pericarditis
Ewart's	Pericardial effusion
Broadbent's	Constrictive effusive pericarditis
Harvey's	Loud A_2 and early diastolic murmur in aortic area

Table AI-4. Syndromes and Anomalies and Associated Disorders

Syndrome	Disorder
Eisenmenger's	Pulmonary hypertension, right-left shunt
Tetralogy of Fallot	Overriding aorta, right ventricular hypertrophy, pulmonary stenosis, ventricular septal defect
Pentalogy of Fallot	Tetralogy and atrial septal defect
Taussig-Bing	Double outlet right ventricular syndrome
Marfan's	Connective tissue disorders with cystic medial necrosis of the aorta
Ehlers-Danlos	Blue sclerae, elastic thin skin, connective tissue disorder
Down's	AV canal defect and/or tetralogy of Fallot
Heyde's	Aortic stenosis, angioma of the ascending colon
Bernheim's	Venous inflow tract obstruction due to ventricular hypertrophy and septal hypertrophy

Anomaly	Disorder
Ebstein's	Displaced tricuspid valve (usually downwards), atrial septal defect, atrialization or right ventricle
Uhl's	Right ventricular dysplasia

Jehovah's Witnesses) have beliefs that may affect the patient's attitude toward certain treatments or procedures.

44. A useful technique for measuring central venous pressure above the baseline of the phlebocentric axis is as follows: Have the patient elevate the hand supine, palms up, extended. Then watch the veins until they collapse (TDM).

45. Splitting of S_2 is best heard when the patient is in the sitting position; occasionally, however, it can be heard in the left lateral position when it suggests mitral valve prolapse with a late click (Don Michael).

46. Find S_2 before looking for S_1; that is, find S_1 in tachycardic states by finding S_2 (Leon).

47. Q waves without infarction are seen in myocarditis, left ventricular hypertrophy, cerebrovascular accidents, and pulmonary fibrosis.

48. Inability to extend the neck is common in pericarditis, especially when caused by rheumatic fever. Patients lie on their pillows in pain and do not extend their heads (Shaver).

49. Changing the position of the patient from supine to upright gradually may help to locate the upper level of the venous pressure called the meniscus.

50. Examine the patient's earlobes from behind as well as from the front for pulsations in tricuspid regurgitation. If the patient's blood pressures are low, ask them to lie down and elevate their legs. Then look for the neck veins. If the neck veins pulsate, palpate the patient's liver.

51. Café-au-lait patches and hypertension suggest pheochromocytoma.

52. Cyanosis and syncope on movement suggest ball valve clot or myxoma. Changing the patient's position may be life-saving. Facial suffusion in the supine position suggests tricuspid stenosis.

53. In a cerebrovascular accident, look for the following ten items:

- Bicuspid valves
- Atrial fibrillation
- Atrial septal aneurysm
- Contrast enhancement of the atria
- Patent foramen ovale
- Intramural clots
- Native and prosthetic valves
- Dissection
- Calcification in the distal aorta
- Neck bruits

54. Low-voltage ECG with bradycardia suggests myxedema.

55. Low-voltage ECG with conduction disturbances with bradycardia and thickened myocardium suggests amyloid heart (Carvallo).

56. Thyroid function should always be checked in patients with atrial fibrillation and in those on amiodarone (Cordarone) therapy.

57. A small collapsing pulse is seen in mitral regurgitation and VSD.

58. Nonpulsatile neck veins thrombosis of the superior vena cava. Facial edema may be present.

59. A pulsatile liver is seen in tricuspid regurgitation and tricuspid stenosis. Systolic and presystolic pulsation is best elicited by a fist below the liver to feel the impulse (Ewy).

60. A pseudo-S_3 is heard in acute AR due to mitral valve preclosure.

61. Aortic regurgitation in acute myocardial infarction suggests dissection. TEE may indicate which coronary artery is involved.

62. Listen for prosthetic valve clicks with your unaided ears prior to auscultating with a stethoscope. Clicks can be better detected in this manner.

63. In older patients, listen selectively for abdominal, femoral, and carotid bruits; these are invaluable in diagnosing stenosis in this subpopulation. These bruits may have little significance in younger patients.

64. In CoA, brachiofemoral lag is present only at the peak of the pulse, not at its onset. This phenomenon is difficult to elicit clinically, although it is more prominent in younger patients.

65. In air embolism, imminently have the patient lie on the left side to displace air into the right atrium.

66. Manometric pressures are useful in chest trauma in judging the presence of tamponade or shock.

67. In emphysema, listen over the xiphoid or below for a gallop rhythm from the right ventricle.

68. Xanthopsia suggests digitalis toxicity.

69. In Cheyne-Stokes respirations, auscultate the patient during the apneic phase.

70. Gallop rhythms may be:

- Seen and not felt
- Felt and not heard
- Heard and not seen

71. In tic-tac rhythm associated with shock, systole is longer than diastole.

72. In acute mitral regurgitation, listen over the scapula in anterior papillary muscle disease. Listen at the base of the heart for "top-of-the-head" murmur, and in posterior papillary muscle disease.

73. A systolic thrill may be felt in aortic regurgitation; it does not imply aortic stenosis.

74. A soft TR murmur which gets louder on inspiration is heard in carcinoid syndrome.

75. In severe pulmonary stenosis, pulmonary clicks are presystolic and disappear on inspiration.

76. Papillary muscle dysfunction produces late systolic murmurs which are louder on inspiration.

77. Absent M_1 in acute aortic regurgitation is due to diastolic preclosure of the mitral valve. An Austin Flint presystolic murmur is not present in this condition. A middiastolic murmur may precede a pseudo-S_3.

78. An opening snap sounds like a rattle at the apex. An S_2 snap sounds like a trill in the pulmonary area (A_2P_2OS), and is best heard at the left sternal edge.

79. Locations of cardiac thrills in different valvular disorders.

Condition	Location of Thrill
Aortic stenosis	Below the clavicle on the right side of the neck
Pulmonary stenosis	Over the pulmonary artery
Ventricular septal defect	At the left sternal edge
Mitral regurgitation	At the apex or axilla
Mitral stenosis	At the apex

80. When two hands are used to palpate the right ventricle and pulmonary artery, a rocking motion occurs in sequence at the left sternal edge.

81. In simultaneous palpation of left and right ventricular hypertrophy, a null zone can be found between the two impulses.

82. Retraction over the left sternal area may be due to left ventricular hypertrophy.

83. An isolated loud apical musical systolic murmur suggests aortic stenosis (Gallavardin).

84. If aortic valve disease is associated with atrial fibrillation, rule out rheumatic mitral valve disease (Hurst).

85. If you suspect angina, listen for an S_4, press on the carotid artery, and administer nitroglycerin. S_4 may disappear, as may late systolic murmurs.

86. In female patients with large breasts or prostheses, auscultate below them, or turn the patient to the right side prior to auscultation.

87. Musical murmurs are produced by:

- Aortic stenosis (Gallavardin phenomenon)
- Everted aortic valve cusps
- Pacemakers across the aortic valve

88. Honks and whoops are heard in mitral valve prolapse (MVP), sea gull murmurs in mitral regurgitation.

89. The development of PR prolongation in bundle branch block in the presence of infective endocarditis suggests septal abscess.

90. Pregnant women may develop life-threatening myocardial infarction, peripartum cardiomyopathy, aortic dissection, or pulmonary embolism.

91. Palpate for systolic blood pressures on account of the gap phenomenon (the difference between palpated and auscultated blood pressures). Pseudohypertension is found in incompressible arteries; pseudohypotension is caused by vasospasm in shock.

92. If a low gradient is present in aortic stenosis, auscultate and perform dobutamine, echo, and Doppler tests before deciding on surgery.

93. When you ask patients about their symptoms, phrase your questions to elicit the opposite response. For example, if you suspect angina, ask the patient, "Do you feel chest pain when you walk downhill?"

94. Cannon veins and cannon sounds are heard in complete heart block.

95. S_1 is soft in dilated cardiomyopathy but loud in hypertrophic cardiomyopathy.

96. TR and MR with elevated venous pressures, small hearts, and enlarged atria with S_3s suggest restrictive cardiomyopathy.

97. Whereas Kussmaul's sign is seen late in cardiac tamponade and pulsus paradoxus is seen early, both phenomena are encountered in patients with constrictive pericarditis and right ventricular infarction.

98. The abdominal jugular test may be useful in excluding elevated wedge pressure and right atrial pressure, as in unexplained pedal edema.

99. Pigmented cartilage in ochronosis, xanthomata, and the diagonal crease sign can be readily observed during your initial conversation with the patient.

100. Suspect carotid sinus syncope in male patients wearing tight starched collars who pass out while turning their necks.

APPENDIX II

Abbreviations for Cardiac Terminology

Abbreviation	Term
A	Aortic value closure
P	Pulmonic valve closure
M	Mitral valve closure
T	Tricuspid
S_1	First sound
S_2	Second sound
S_3	Third sound
ES	Ejection sound
NEC	Nonejection sound
RBBB	Right bundle branch block
LBBB	Left bundle branch block
PR	Short, long intervals
VSD	Ventricular septal defect
PS	Pulmonary stenosis
PDA	Patent ductus arteriosus
PH	Pulmonary hypertension
MR	Mitral regurgitation
MS	Mitral stenosis
AS	Aortic stenosis
AR	Aortic regurgitation
TR	Tricuspid regurgitation
TS	Tricuspid stenosis
PR	Pulmonary regurgitation
PS	Pulmonary stenosis
LA	Left atrium
RA	Right atrium
LV	Left ventricle
RV	Right ventricle
Ao	Aorta
PA	Pulmonary artery
JUG.VEINS	Jugular veins
APEX	Apex
LSE	Left sternal edge
RSE	Right sternal edge
PA	Pulmonic area
AA	Aortic area
HSM	Holosystolic murmur
LSM	Late systolic murmur
MDM	Middiastolic murmur
EDM	Early diastolic murmur
PSM	Presystolic murmur
OS	Opening snap
CHF	Congestive heart failure
ECG	Electrocardiogram
CXR	Chest x-ray

APPENDIX III

Heart Sounds: Overview

S_1

Apical low-pitched sound (apex)
LUP

S_1	Loud	— PR interval—mitral stenosis—mitral valve prolapse
S_1	Soft	— PR
S_1	Variable	— AV Block—Wenckebach—Type I, Grade 2, or Grade 3
S_1	Absent	— Acute aortic regurgitation

S_2 — (second intercostal space)
Basal sounds A_2 P_2 (PA)
Sharp higher pitch–*dup*
Physiologically split–*drup*

S_3 — Apex; LV subxiphoid-RV
Apical low-pitched sound in early diastole
lup' du dup (from LV) (apex)
Xiphoid or below (RV) follows S_2

S_4 — Apex; LV subxiphoid-RV
Apical low-pitched sound precedes S_1 (apex)
luh lup' dup

Systolic Sounds

S_1 to S_2

Ejection sound—left sternal border
Sharp sound heard at left sternal border *lu tuk' dup*
Heard in dilatation of aorta pulmonary or systemic hypertension
(vascular or root sounds) heard in aortic and pulmonic stenosis
(valvular sound) S_1-ES has fixed time relationship

Nonejection sound—left sternal border
Sharp sound or sounds heard between S_1 and S_2 moves to left occurring
early if patient is standing or sitting (small heart), moves to right
occurring late if patient is lying down (larger heart). May be musical
(honk, whoop), systolic, or diastolic.

Opening snap—apex; left sternal border
High-pitched sound follows A_2, note A_2-OS interval heard at LLSB, in PA may be three sounds A_2P_2OS. Heard in mitral stenosis at apex with loud S_1. Middiastolic and presystolic murmurs. Indicates mobile valve.

Pericardial knock—left sternal edge,
Sharp, low-pitched sound after S_2 heard in constrictive pericarditis.

Tumor plop—apex, left atrial, left lower sternal border, right atrial
Low-pitched sound after S_2 associated with middiastolic murmur heard with atrial tumors (i.e., myxomas).

Sail sound—apex
Heard at apex and left sternal edge in patients with Ebstein's anomaly.

S_2

Fixed wide	— ASD
Fixed narrow	— ASD with pulmonary hypertension
Single	— Eisenmenger syndrome
	Severe as PS with immobile valves and low PA pressure
Paradoxic	— Hypertension occasionally
	LBBB
	LVH
	Aortic stenosis
Soft	— A_2 (aortic stenosis)
	P_2 (pulmonic stenosis)
Physiological	— VSD, MR, RBBB, MS, RVE

Diastolic Sounds

S_3	— Protodiastolic
S_4	— Presystolic
PK	— Pericardial knock
OS	— Opening snap or click
PLOP	— Tumor

Acoustic Protracted Events (120 to 250 ms)

Timing (Tune in and determine if)

Systolic	Between S_1 and S_2
Diastolic	Between S_2 and S_1
Continuous	Between S_1 and S_1

Detection

(S_1)	Do you hear the first heart sound?
(S_2)	Do you hear the second heart sound?
S_1-S_2	Do you hear any sounds or murmurs between S_1 and S_2? If yes, this is systolic.
S_2-S_1	Do you hear any sounds or murmurs between S_2 and S_1? If yes, this is diastolic.

Classification

Systolic Murmurs

Early (ESM)	*RRR*
Midsystolic (MSM)	*Lu' RRR*
Holosystolic (HSM)	*SHHH*
Late systolic (LSM)	*Luh' SHHH*

Diastolic Murmurs

Early or immediate diastolic (EDM)	*Lup' DHH*
Middiastolic (MDM)	*Erup' Du DRR*
Presystolic (PSM)	*RRRR*

Continuous

Peaks at S_2
Starts after S_1

Character

Rough *RRR*
Blowing *SHHH*
Musical *HMM*

Pitch

High
Medium
Low

Loudness

    1 to 3 Soft to loud, no thrill (felt as a purring, vibrating series of impulses)

    3 to 6 Loud, to being loud enough to be heard without a stethoscope (6) (thrill +)

Radiation

| To axilla | Mitral regurgitation, aortic regurgitation (Cecil Cole), pulmonary branch stenosis |
| To neck | Aortic midsystolic murmurs |

Significance

    1. Innocent
    2. Vascular/root—hypertension, ectasia, aneurysm, increased flow
    3. Pathological

Location Best Heard

    1. Mitral area
    2. Left lower sternal border
    3. Aortic area
    4. Pulmonic area
    5. Erb's point 3 LICS
    6. Other areas, 3 RICS, neck, axilla, xiphoid, scapula

Features

    Innocent murmurs
    MSM
    No click
    No abnormal signs

Continuous Murmurs

Left Sided	Physiological	Right-Sided
Patent ductus arteriosus (PA)	Jugular venous (neck) (R)	Pulmonary branch stenosis
Aortopulmonary window (LLSB)	Abolished by turning neck	Pulmonary AV\fistula
Coronary AV fistula (apex)	Mammary soufflé over breast in pregnancy	Patent ductus R-L
Intercostal (axillary) in coarctation	Uterine soufflé over uterus	In pulmonary atresia

Pericardial Rubs

One-, two-, or three-component rub, LLSB, supine, sitting
Two in diastolic, one in systolic (usually two to three)
Scratchy, leathery
Chest pain on breathing or swallowing or extending neck
CG–ST elevation, PQ depression

APPENDIX IV

Cardiophonetics

Instructions on Using the Cardiophonetics Appendix, the Disc, and the Cardiophonetic Card

1. Deploy disc on computer (Macintosh or PC)
2. Click on sound file and select sound or murmur
3. Open cardiophonetic appendix to corresponding page
4. Study left upper page *how to* auscultate;
   left lower page for where to listen;
   right page for phonocardiogram, sound, and acoustic spectrogram
5. Click on phonetic and listen to sound at slow speed, read sound out of appendix
6. Click on actual sound; read sound out of appendix
7. Listen to "5" or "6" until the sound or murmur is learned
8. Use cardiophonetic card
9. Correlate card, disc, and appendix
10. Repeat process until all sounds and murmurs are learned, then read other sections

Sounds and Murmurs: A Cardiophonetic Approach   The next few pages will outline to the beginning student the sounds and murmurs of the heart. These will be described not only as systolic, diastolic, loud, soft, harsh, rough or musical, but also will be described in cardiophonetic terminology. The reason for using cardiophonetics is to develop a currency or a language that represents heart sounds which will enable the student to carry around the sounds he heard, to translate the sounds he/she hears into cardiophonetics, to express these sounds out loud, and to repeat this procedure until he/she understands and learns them. It is also intended that he/she follows the illustration shown in the endless loop of learning, which correlates heart sounds, bedside sound, computer sound, cardiophonetics on the computer, and the portable card.

Abbreviations

A_2	Aortic valve closure sound
S_1	First sound
S_2	Second sound
S_3	Third sound
S_4	Fourth sound
AP	Aortopulmonary
AR	Aortic regurgitation
AV	Arteriovenous
EDM	Early diastolic murmur
ES	Ejection sound
ESM	Early systolic murmur
HSM	Holosystolic murmur

LBBB	Left bundle branch block
LICS	Left intercostal space
LLSB	Left lower sternal border
LSM	Late systolic murmur
LV	Left ventricle
LVH	Left ventricular hypertrophy
MDM	Mid diastolic murmur
MR	Mitral regurgitation
MSM	Mid systolic murmur
NEC	Nonejection click
OS	Opening snap
P_2	Pulmonary valve closure sound
PA	Pulmonary area
PDA	Patent ductus arteriosus
PSM	Presystolic murmur
RICS	Right intercostal space
RV	Right ventricle
TR	Tricuspid regurgitation
TS	Tricuspid stenosis

Phonics Stepwise

1. All primary phonics for sounds and murmurs are taught in this lesson.

2. / mark denotes pause accent, preceding syllable.

3. ‿ indicates joined syllables, e.g., Du‿D̄R̄R̄→

4. ŭ as in up
   Û as in HER
   ↑ ↓ pitch increases or decreases
   → no change in pitch
   ↗ increasing pitch
   ↘ decreasing pitch

5. Audio notations or "phono" and "phonics" (phonophonics are shown).

6. (S₁) Denotes absence of sound or soft sound

Pronunciation Key
Pronunciations have been converted for reader friendliness.

SPELLINGS	AHD	IPA
ship, dish	sh	ʃ
cut	ŭ	ʌ
urge, term, firm	û	ɜ˞ ɜr

Heart Sounds S$_1$ and S$_2$

With physiological splitting of S$_2$
How to Listen (p. 115)

1. Listen at the apex of the heart using both the bell and the diaphragm. Examine the patient in the left lateral supine position. S$_1$ corresponds with the apical impulse and the carotid pulse. To confirm, move to the second intercostal space and listen for S$_2$. S$_1$ is soft or absent in this space. Identify S$_2$ first, then S$_1$.
2. When listening for S$_2$, sit the patient up.

Physiological Splitting of S$_2$ (p. 132)   Listen with the patient sitting up. Use the diaphragm, placing it in the second intercostal space on the left side. Have the patient breathe in and out and take a deep breath in. Listen for physiological splitting of S$_2$(drup). Do not instruct the patient to hold his respiration.

WHERE TO LISTEN

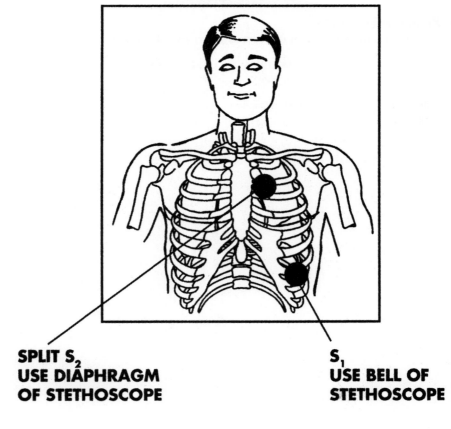

**SPLIT S$_2$
USE DIAPHRAGM
OF STETHOSCOPE**

**S$_1$
USE BELL OF
STETHOSCOPE**

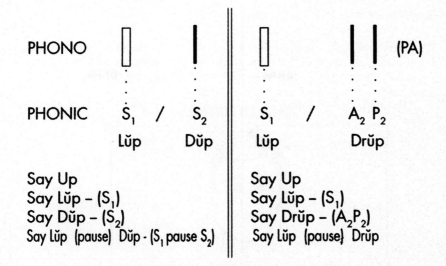

PHONO

PHONIC S_1 / S_2 S_1 / $A_2 P_2$

    Lŭp   Dŭp   Lŭp   Drŭp

Say Up   Say Up
Say Lŭp – (S_1)   Say Lŭp – (S_1)
Say Dŭp – (S_2)   Say Drŭp – ($A_2 P_2$)
Say Lŭp (pause) Dŭp - (S_1 pause S_2)   Say Lŭp (pause) Drŭp

This is Lŭp (S_1)/Drŭp (S_2) Note the accent on the Lup followed by the pause. This is the phonic for S_1 and S_2 at the apex.

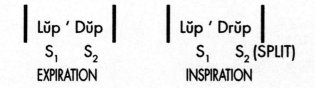

Lŭp ' Dŭp   Lŭp ' Drŭp
S_1 S_2 S_1 S_2 (SPLIT)
EXPIRATION   INSPIRATION

Lŭp sounds like a baseball hitting a mitt.
Dŭp sounds like a stone falling into water.

Heart Sounds S$_4$

1. Carry out light auscultation with bell, with patient in the left lateral supine position with full expiration. A lightly clenched fist will accentuate these sounds, heard below xiphoid process (RV origin).

WHERE TO LISTEN

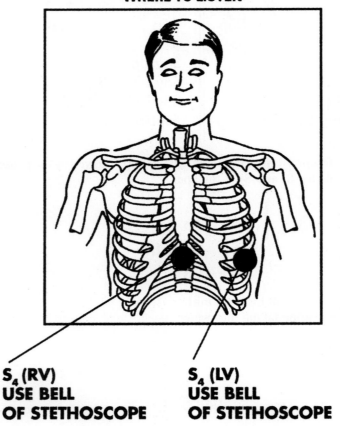

**S$_4$ (RV)
USE BELL
OF STETHOSCOPE**

**S$_4$ (LV)
USE BELL
OF STETHOSCOPE**

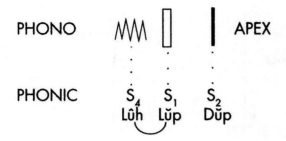

PHONO   MMM   [ ] | APEX

PHONIC $\dot{S}_4$ $\dot{S}_1$ $\dot{S}_2$
              Lûh   Lŭp   Dŭp

Say Up
Say Lŭp—(S_1)
Now say Dŭp—(S_2)
Say Lûh—(S_4) (Like Her)
Now say Lûh Lŭp / Dŭp Pause accent

This is the phonic for a presystolic gallop (S_4).
Lûh is the phonic for S_4.

| Lûh   Lŭp ' Dŭp |
     S_4 S_1 S_2

NOTE: Pause after Lŭp, accent on Lŭp.

Heart Sounds S₃

1. Conduct light auscultation with the patient heard in the left lateral supine position with full expiration. A lightly clenched fist will accentuate sounds that are of left-ventricular origin. These are heard below xiphoid process in supine position. Sounds of right-ventricular origin are accentuated on inspiration.

WHERE TO LISTEN

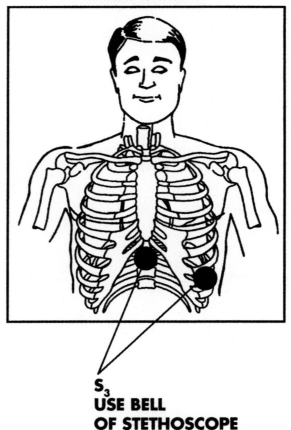

**S₃
USE BELL
OF STETHOSCOPE**

PHONO 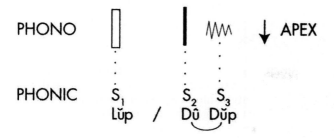 APEX

PHONIC S_1 S_2 S_3
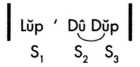
Lŭp / Dû Dŭp

Say Up
Say Lŭp Dŭp—(S_1 and S_3)
Say HER, Say DER, Say Dû (Her)
Say Dû (like Her)—(S_2)
Now say Lŭp / Dû Dŭp—(S_1, S_2 and S_3)

Note Dŭp decreases in pitch in heart failure it increases
in children.
This is the phonic for a protodiastolic gallop. (S_3)

| Lŭp ' Dû Dŭp |
   S_1 S_2 S_3

NOTE: Pause after Lŭp, accent on Lŭp.

Ejection Sound

Nonejection click or ejection click

1. Best heard using the diaphragm at the second or third left intercostal space with the patient sitting up. The sounds are high-pitched. The ejection sound has a fixed relationship to S_1; a nonejection click moves away from S_1, when the heart is large; this occurs when the patient is lying flat or with the legs elevated. ES is closer to S_1 when the patient is in the sitting or standing position and with Valsalva.

WHERE TO LISTEN

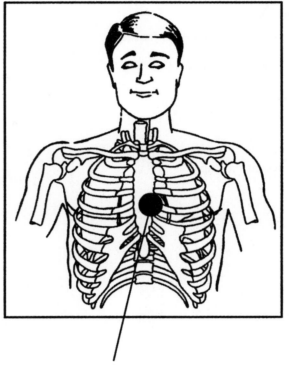

**NEC
USE DIAPHRAGM
OF STETHOSCOPE**

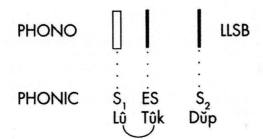

PHONO   LLSB

PHONIC   Ṡ₁ ES   Ṡ₂
          Lû Tûk Dŭp

Say Lup—As in Up
Say Lû (Like Her) S₁
Say Ter (Like Her)
Say Tû (Her)—(3)
Say Tûk (Her)—(ES)
Now say Lû Tûk Dŭp

This is the phonic for an ejection sound or a click
preceded by S₁ followed by S₂.

Lû Tûk ' Dŭp
S₁ ES   S₂

NOTE: Pause after Tûk accent on Tûk. Ejection clicks move with position
unlike ejection sounds.

Holosystolic Murmur

1. Listen at the apex or in the scapula with the diaphragm. The murmur is almost always blowing in character. The holosystolic murmur due to VSD is heard at the left sternal edge, associated with a thrill and usually blowing or musical. Listen for holosystolic murmur, associated with tricuspid regurgitation, at the right or left sternal edge; on deep inspiration, the murmur grows louder.

WHERE TO LISTEN

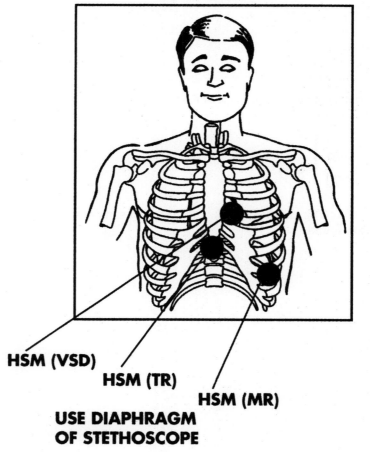

HSM (VSD)

HSM (TR)

HSM (MR)

USE DIAPHRAGM OF STETHOSCOPE

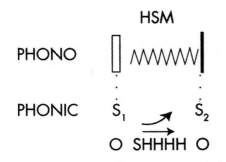

Say SHHHH Like "Shush" without the terminal "sh"
Protract the SHHH Sounding the "H"
This the phonic for a holosystolic murmur.

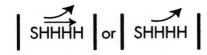

NOTE: The pitch *is* even *or* may increase at the end, occasionally giving a musical quality.

SHHHH sounds like shush without the terminal "sh."

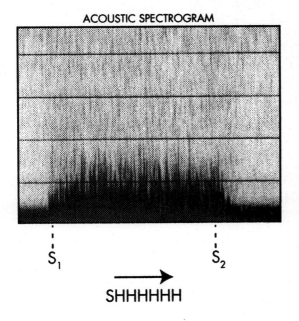

Late Systolic Murmur

1. Listen at the apex of the heart with the diaphragm. The murmur is best heard on expiration, and is accentuated by the patient clenching a fist. In click murmur syndrome, a click is heard before the murmur.

WHERE TO LISTEN

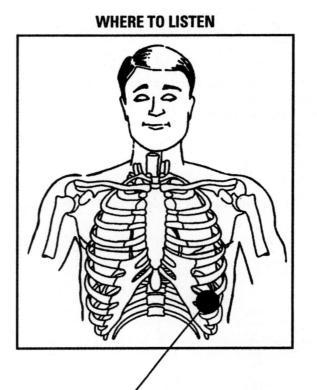

LSM (MR)
USE DIAPHRAGM
OF STETHOSCOPE

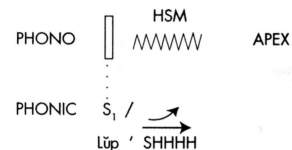

PHONO

HSM

APEX

PHONIC S_1 /

Lŭp ' SHHHH

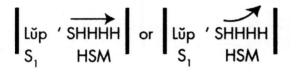

Say Lŭp (Up, S_1)
This is S_1
Now say SHHHH (HSM)
This is a holosystolic murmur.

Say Lŭp—pause—$\overrightarrow{\text{SHHHH}}$ (HSM)
This is a late systolic murmur following S_1.

| Lŭp ' $\overrightarrow{\text{SHHHH}}$ | or | Lŭp ' SHHHH |
| S_1 HSM | | S_1 HSM |

NOTE: The pitch is flat or elevated with a terminal musical character. Pause after Lŭp

ACOUSTIC SPECTROGRAM

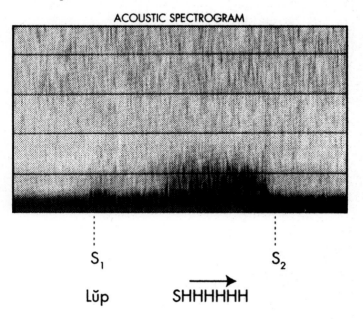

S_1 S_2

Lŭp SHHHHHH

Early Systolic Murmur

1. Use the diaphragm of the stethoscope at the left sternal edge in the second intercostal space or below the scapula. For an early systolic murmur to be heard, the patient should be in a semi-recumbent or reclining position. The patient is usually extremely sick. The murmur is heard in association with an S_3. **An S_1 may be muffled or absent. May be heard below the scapula or in the second intercostal space.**

WHERE TO LISTEN

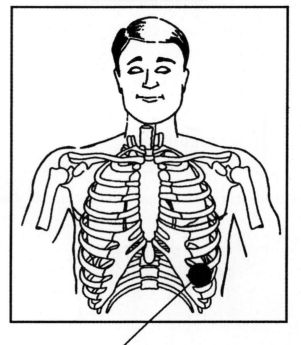

**ESM
USE DIAPHRAGM
OF STETHOSCOPE**

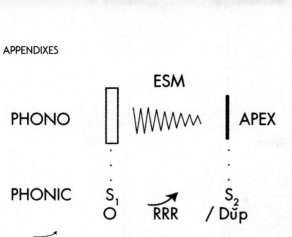

PHONO

ESM

APEX

PHONIC S_1 S_2

O ↗ RRR / Dŭp

Say ‾RR͡R—rolling R's Note pitch increasing and decreasing.

Say ‾RR͡R / Dŭp ‾RR͡R pause Dŭp (ESM + 2nd Sounds)

This is the phonic for an early systolic murmur.

RRR / Dŭp

ESM S_2

NOTE: Diamond-shaped murmurs only sound crescendo

NOTE: Pause between ‾RR͡R and Dŭp.

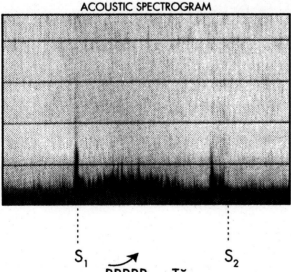

ACOUSTIC SPECTROGRAM

S_1 ↗ S_2

RRRRR Tŭp

Midsystolic Murmur

1. Listen at the left sternal edge with the diaphragm for S_1, murmur, and S_2. This is listened for at the left sternal edge. S_1 may not be heard at the base.

WHERE TO LISTEN

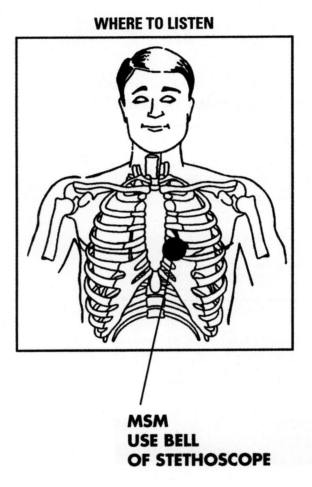

**MSM
USE BELL
OF STETHOSCOPE**

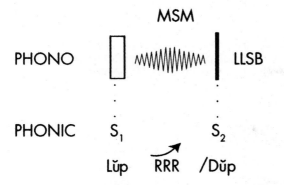

MSM

PHONO   LLSB

PHONIC S_1 S_2

Lŭp   RRR   /Dŭp

NOTE: Diamond–shaped murmurs only sound crescendo.

Say Lŭp (Up–S_2)
Now say RRR (as in ERR) Roll RRR Note Pitch (MSM)
Now say Dŭp (S_2)
This is a mid systolic murmur.
Say Lûp—RRR—pause—Dŭp
This is the phonic for a mid systolic murmur following S_1.

Lŭp RRR ' Dŭp

S_1 MSM S_2

NOTE: Pause after RRR and SHHH

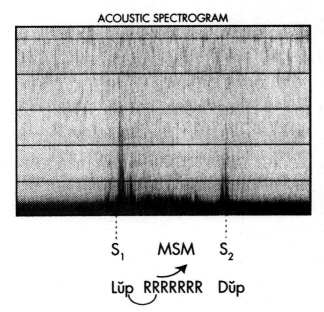

ACOUSTIC SPECTROGRAM

S_1 MSM S_2

Lŭp RRRRRR Dŭp

Early Diastolic Murmur

1. An early diastolic murmur, due to aortic regurgitation, is heard with the patient sitting up with the diaphragm of the stethoscope applied over the fifth intercostal space and at the apex. It occasionally is heard in the axilla. The pulmonary regurgitation murmur is heard in the pulmonary area.

WHERE TO LISTEN

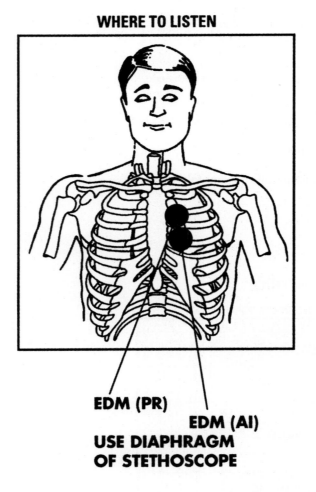

EDM (PR)

EDM (AI)
USE DIAPHRAGM
OF STETHOSCOPE

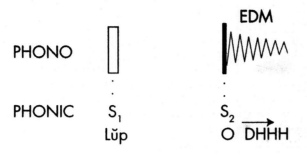

PHONO

PHONIC   S₁
           Lŭp

EDM

S₂ →
O DHHH

Say up
Now say Lŭp (S₁)

Say DHHH (blow out H) sigh, decreasing pitch.

Now say Lŭp ´ DHHH (expel air from your lips with tongue hard against palate).
This is the phonic for an early diastolic murmur.

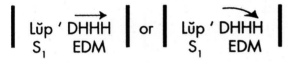

| Lŭp ´ DHHH → | or | Lŭp ´ DHHH ↘ |
| S₁   EDM | | S₁   EDM |

NOTE: DHHH often goes down in pitch. Pause after Lŭp.

DHHH sounds like the end of an aerobic session.

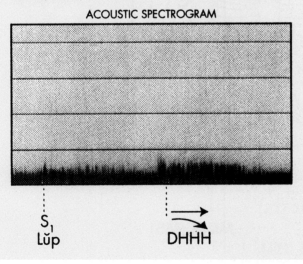

ACOUSTIC SPECTROGRAM

S₁
Lŭp

DHHH

Late Diastolic Murmur

1. Osler commented that this murmur is heard within the area of a quarter at the apex, with the patient in the left lateral position. It is accentuated by the patient clenching a fist and by expiration. Listen with the bell of the stethoscope with very light auscultation. The murmur will be missed unless the stethoscope is placed on the tapping impulse in a patient with mitral stenosis. In tricuspid stenosis, a middiastolic murmur is heard in the midclavicular line on the left sternal edge and gets louder on inspiration. In mitral stenosis, the murmur is best heard on expiration. Thrills may be present with both murmurs.

WHERE TO LISTEN

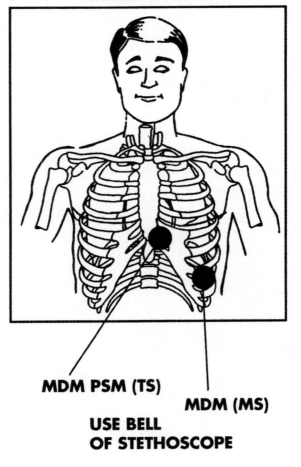

MDM PSM (TS)

MDM (MS)

USE BELL OF STETHOSCOPE

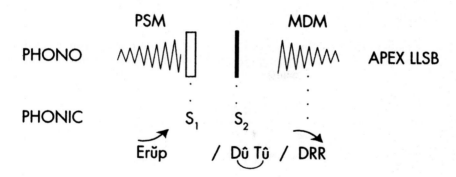

Say Err
Say ŭp

Say Erŭp (roll R)—Note pitch mark. (PSM)
Say Der (to rhyme with Her)
Say Dû (to rhyme with Her—no R)—(S₂)

Say Erŭp´ Dû Note pause (PSM) (S₂) Say Dû Tû (Der–Ter)

Now say DRR—(roll R)—(3) Note pitch mark. (MDM)

Now say Erŭp / Dû / DRR Note pitch marks.
This is the phonic for a presystolic and delayed diastolic murmur.

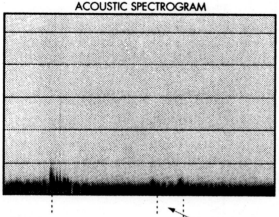

ACOUSTIC SPECTROGRAM

Continuous Murmur

1. Listen over the pulmonary artery for patent ductus arteriosus; over the apex for coronary AV fistula; left sternal edge for AP windows above the clavicle in jugular venous hums.

WHERE TO LISTEN

PDA

AP WINDOW

CORONARY AV FISTULA

USE DIAPHRAGM OF STETHOSCOPE

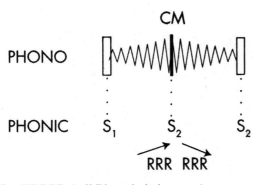

PHONO

CM

PHONIC S_1 S_2 S_2

RRR RRR

Say ERRRR (roll R's and pitch waxes)

Now say RRRR

This is the phonic for a continuous murmur.

RRRRR

RRRR sounds like a car engine being revved.

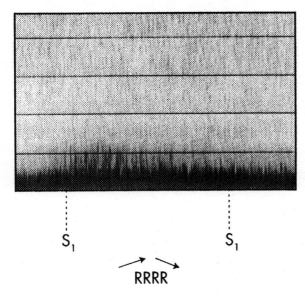

S_1 S_1

RRRR

INDEX

Page numbers followed by *t* or *f* indicate tables or figures, respectively.

A wave, 267–268
A₂. *See* Aortic valve closure (A₂)
Abbreviations, standard cardiology,
        19t
Abdomen
  distended, 279
  examination of, 278–279
Abdominal aneurysm, rupture of, 239
Abdominal bruits, 278
Abdominal veins, examination of, 278
Achilles tendon, xanthoma of, 87f
Acoustic obliteration, 6
Acoustic spectrography, 14
Adult pediatric cardiology
  issues in, 316–327
  nonsurgical treatments in, 327
  special procedures in, 327–328
AF. *See* Atrial fibrillation
Age, changes related to, auscultation
        and, 22–23
Air embolism, acute, chest pain in, 227
Alcohol abuse, head/neck
        abnormalities in, 272t
Amyl nitrite, 37–40
Anacrotic pulse, 256–257
Aneurysm
  abdominal, rupture of, 239
  aortic, phonophonic representation
        of, 130f
  dissecting, 238
    auscultatory findings in,
        phonophonic representation of,
        224f
    chest pain in, 224
    types of, 238f
  systolic ejection murmur and, 168

ventricular
  ECG in, 305
  S₃ and S₄ in, 140
ventricular septal, 189
Angina pectoris, 281–283
  auscultatory findings in, 282
  chronic stable, 74
  in differential diagnosis of chest pain,
        223
  Prinzmetal's, 75–76
  unstable, 75
Anxiety-induced dyspnea, 286
Aorta
  coarctation of, 176–177, 319
    2-D and Doppler echocardiograms
        of, 176f
    surgical treatment of, 330
  rupture of, post-traumatic, 236–237
Aortic aneurysm, phonophonic
        representation of, 130f
Aortic area, auscultation of, 21
Aortic clicks, absence of, 127
Aortic ectasia, systolic ejection
        murmur and, 168–169
Aortic regurgitation, 86–88
  acoustic spectrogram of, 197f
  acute, early diastolic murmur in,
        197–198
  clinical features of, 88
  hemodynamics of, 62–64, 87
  M/Q scan of, 88f, 119f
  physical signs in, 88
  S₃ in, 141
Aortic stenosis, 84, 319–321
  acoustic obliteration of S₂ in,
        phonophonic representation of,
        131f

Aortic stenosis *(cont.)*
  chest x-rays in, 85f
  congenital, 175–176
  ECG in, 305
  in elderly, 174
  hemodynamics of, 64–65
  hyperlipidemia presenting as, 84–86
  midsystolic murmur in, 171–174
  mild, 172
  M-mode echocardiogram of, 172f
  moderate, 172
  M/Q scan of, 173f
  pulsus parvus in, 173–174
  severe, 172–173
    aortogram of, 320f
Aortic valve
  bicuspid, 174
    calcified stenotic, 175f
    echocardiogram of, 175f
  prosthetic, 146–149
Aortic valve closure (A$_2$), 130–134
  soft, 130–131
  tissue Doppler imaging of, 311f
Aortopulmonary window, 202
Apex, auscultation of, 19–20
Arterial blood pressure
  Doppler recording of, 266
  measurement of, 264–266
    in children, 266
Arteriovenous fistula, 202–203
  coronary, 202–203
  pulmonary, 203
Arteritis, idiopathic, of Takayasu, 255t,
    263
Arthritis
  cardiovascular abnormalities and, 280
  Jaccoud's, 254t
Ascites, 279
ASD. *See* Atrial septal defect
Ataxia, Friedreich's, 254t
Athletes, auscultation in, 22
Atrial fibrillation, 94–95
  auscultatory findings in, 95
  S$_3$ and, 141
Atrial flutter, 95
Atrial pacing, 37, 44, 96–97
Atrial septal defect, 316–318
  auscultatory findings in, 317
  ECG in, 303–304

hemodynamics of, 68
surgical treatment of, 328–329
treatment and evaluation of, 317–318
Atrioventricular conduction defects,
    95–96
Atrioventricular septal defect, 318–319
  surgical treatment of, 329
Auscultation
  areas of, 19–21
  difficult, 16
  dynamic, 37–44
    physiology of, 38t
    techniques of, 24–25
  history of, 2–3
  less known findings in, 141–146
  of normal heart, 18–19
  routine, 23–25
  special considerations in, 21–23
  vascular, 36
Auscultatory position(s), 25–36
  1 (45 degrees supine), 25–26
  2 (left lateral supine), 26–28
  3 (supine with or without legs
      elevated), 28–29
  4 (sitting up), 30–32
  5 (standing), 32–33
  6 (squatting), 33–34
  7 (knee-chest and knee-elbow), 34–35
  physiology of, 35
  with related maneuvers and
      physiological changes, 41t
Austin Flint murmur, 162t, 195

Balloon valvuloplasty, 328
Bang & Olafsen stethoscope, 14
Barham's sign, 265t
Barium swallow, clinical conditions
    detectable by, 306t
Barlow's syndrome, 254t
Bell, stethoscope, 8–10
Bernheim's syndrome, 254t
Bicuspid aortic valve, 174
  calcified stenotic, 175f
  echocardiogram of, 175f
Bisferiens pulse, 257–259
Blalock-Taussig procedure, 321

Blood pressure, 264–271
  arterial
    Doppler recording of, 266
    measurement of, 264–266
      in children, 266
  venous
    abnormalities of, 267–271
    measurement of, 266–271
Blunt trauma, 235
Bornholm syndrome, chest pain in, 226
Bounding pulse, 257
Broadbent's sign, 265t
Bronchopulmonary collateral vessels, 203–204
Bruits, 207
  abdominal, 278
  in lower limbs, 280
Budd-Chiari syndrome, 254t

C wave, 269
Cabot murmur, 162t
Cannon wave, 268–269
Canter rhythm, 143
Carcinoid syndrome, head/neck abnormalities in, 272t
Cardiac arrest, auscultatory findings in, 229
Cardiac arrhythmias, 94–96
Cardiac axis, deviations of
  clinical conditions associated with, 304t
  ECG representations of, 303f
Cardiac dyspnea, 283
Cardiac examination, 247–298
  general, 253–283
  history in, 248–253
Cardiac failure. See Heart failure
Cardiac impulses, 276–278
Cardiac ischemia
  pretest probability of, factors in, 223t
  silent, 75
Cardiac phases, dynamic, 53–58
Cardiogenic shock, 232
Cardiogenic syncope, 288
Cardiomegaly, on chest x-ray, 101f

Cardiomyopathy, 91–94
  dilated, 92
  hypertrophic obstructive (HOCM), 92–93
    hemodynamics of, 61–63, 93
    midsystolic murmur in, 177–179
    pathology of, 93
    physical findings in, 93
    pressure curves in, 62f, 173f
  restrictive, 93–94
    auscultatory findings in, 93
    physical findings in, 94
  S₃ and S₄ in, 140
Cardiorrhexis, 225f
Cardiovascular structure/function, tests of, 250t–251t. See also specific test
Carey-Coombs murmur, 162t
Carotid arteries
  auscultation over, 36f
  traumatic injury to, 237
Carotid pulse, 262–263
Carotid sinus pressure, 37
Carvallo maneuver, 40–42
Cecil Cole murmur, 162t
Changing murmur, 198–199
Chest
  abnormalities of
    auscultation and, 35–36
    findings associated with, 275t
  examination of, 274–278
  palpation of, 275
  percussion of, 275–276
  visual inspection of, 275
Chest pain, 221–228
  in angina, 281–282
  auscultatory findings in, 222t
  cardiac/vascular sources of, 221–224
  gastrointestinal sources of, 227–228
  musculoskeletal sources of, 228
  pulmonary sources of, 224–227
Cheyne-Stokes respirations, 265t, 284
CHF. See Congestive heart failure
Cine MRI, 306–307. See Magnetic resonance imaging (MRI)
Circumflex coronary artery, anomalous origin of, 205
Click-murmur syndrome, 125
  phonophonic representation of, 126f

Clicks
  absence of, 127
  diastolic, 146
    in mitral valve prolapse, 118f
  nonejection (NECs), 125–127
    absence of, 127
    hemodynamics of, 60–61
    phonophonic representation of, 126f
  presystolic, pulmonary stenosis and,
    128
  pseudoejection, 127
  systolic, in mitral valve prolapse, 118f
Coarctation of the aorta, 176–177, 319
  2-D and Doppler echocardiograms of,
    176f
  surgical treatment of, 330
Collapsing pulse, 257, 258f
Collateral arteries, intercostal, 203
Collateral vessels, 203–205
  bronchopulmonary, 203–204
Commotio cordis, 236
Computed tomography (CT), 305–306
  clinical conditions detectable by, 306t
Congenital heart disease, 316t
  ECG in, 302–303
  electrophysiological abnormalities in,
    328, 332–333
  surgical treatment of, 328–332
    complications of, 329t
Congestive heart failure, 105
  S₃ in, 141
Constrictive pericarditis, 97–99
  hemodynamics of, 68–69
  pulsus paradoxus in, 260f
  triad of signs in, 68f
  venous pulse in, 271f
Continuous murmur, 199–205
  acoustic spectrogram of, 200f
  algorithm for auscultation of, 199f
Cornelia de Lange syndrome, 254t
  head/neck abnormalities in, 272t
Coronary arteriovenous fistula,
    202–203
Coronary artery(ies)
  anomalous, 204–205
  circumflex, anomalous origin of, 205
  left anterior descending, anomalous
    origin of, 205

left main, anomalous origin of,
    204–205
  right, anomalies of, 205
  in sinus of Valsalva, anomalous origin
    of, 205
  traumatic injury to, 237
Coronary spasm, 76
Coronary syndromes, 74–76
  chest pain in, 221–223
Corrigan's sign, 265t
Cough, 289
Critical care, auscultatory findings in,
    219–244
Cruveilhier-Baumgarten murmur, 162t
CT (computed tomography) scan,
    305–306
  clinical conditions detectable by, 306t
Cushing's syndrome, 254t
Cv-y wave, 269–270
  tricuspid regurgitation with, 285f
Cyanosis, 292–293

Damping, 6
de Musset's sign, 265t
Deep venous thrombosis, 240
Dermatologic disorders, 271
Dermatomyositis, head/neck
    abnormalities in, 273t
Diaphragm, stethoscope, 10
Diastolic clicks, 146
  in mitral valve prolapse, 118f
Diastolic heart sounds, 129t, 135–141
Diastolic murmur, 189–198
  algorithm for treatment of, 191f
  early, 195–198
    algorithm for auscultation of, 196f
  flow, 190–191
  mid-, 189–195
    algorithm for auscultation of, 190f
    differential diagnosis of, 195
Diastolic overload, ECG in, 304–305
Diastolic snaps, 146
Dicrotic pulse, 253–256
Dilated cardiomyopathy, 92
Directed echocardiography, 309–310
  clinical conditions and cardiac tissues
    associated with, 311t

Dissecting aneurysm, 238
  auscultatory findings in, phonophonic
    representation of, 224f
  chest pain in, 224
  types of, 238f
Dock's murmur, 162t, 204
Doppler blood pressure recording, 266
Doppler imaging, 307–310
  heart diseases that can be diagnosed
    with, 308t
  tissue, 309, 310f, 311f
Down's syndrome, 254t
  head/neck abnormalities in, 272t
Drugs
  cardiac emergencies related to,
    234–235
  in dynamic auscultation, 37–40
  use/abuse of, in patient history,
    249–252
Duroziez' murmur, 162t, 265t
Dynamic auscultation, 37–44
  physiology of, 38t
Dyspnea, 283–286
  anxiety-induced, 286
  auscultatory findings in, 283–284
  cardiac, 283
  episodic, 284–285
  inspiratory, 286
  paroxysmal nocturnal, 283

Earpieces, stethoscope, 8
Ebstein's anomaly, 323–324
  surgical treatment of, 331
Echocardiography, 307–310
  diagnostic indications for, 308t
  directed, 309–310
    clinical conditions and cardiac
      tissues associated with, 311t
  stress, 312–313
  transesophageal (TEE), 309
Edema, 291–292
Effusion, pericardial, 97
Ehlers-Danlos syndrome, 254t
Eisenmenger complex, 103
Eisenmenger's syndrome, 103, 126,
    254t
Ejection murmur, systolic, 168–180

Ejection sounds (ES), 124–125
  hemodynamics of, 60
  in pregnancy, 22f
  pulmonary, 125
  timing and causes of, 123t
Electrocardiogram (ECG)
  in common clinical situations,
    304–305
  complexes, intervals and segments of,
    302f
  in congenital heart disease, 302–303
  in differential diagnosis, 303–304
  normal complex of, 302t
  with pressure curves, 52f, 54f, 55f,
    56f, 57f, 59f
Electrocardiography, 301–305
Electronic stethoscopes, 12–14
Embolism
  air, chest pain in, 227
  pulmonary, chest pain in, 226
  systemic, 239–240
End systolic heart sounds, 128–135
Endocarditis
  infective, 99–100
    physical findings in, 100
  Libman-Sacks, 255t
Episodic dyspnea, 284–285
Eponymous disorders. *See also specific
    disorder*
  cardiovascular findings in, 254t–255t
Eponymous heart murmurs, 162t. *See
    also specific murmur*
Eponymous signs, 265t. *See also
    specific sign*
Eruptions, skin, 271–274
Esophageal stethoscopes, 12, 13f
Extremities, examination of, 279–281

Facial discoloration, 271
Fallot, tetralogy of, 321–323
  ECG in, 304
  midsystolic murmur in, 180
  physical findings in, 321–323
  surgical procedures for, 322f, 330–331
  treatment of, 323
Family history, 252
Fast cine MRI, 306–307

Fatigue, 289–290
Femoral artery, traumatic injury to, 237
Femoral pulse, 263
First heart sound (S₁), 18–19, 114–124
  absence of, 120
  hemodynamics of, 58–60
  loud, 115–116
    interpretation of, 116f
    in mitral valve prolapse, 118f
  malposition of, 135
  PR interval and, phonophonic representation of, 116f
  soft, 116–120
  split, 122–124
    conditions characterized by, 122t
    differentiation of, 123f
  variations in, 120–122
    conditions causing, 117t
Fist clenching, sustained, in dynamic auscultation, 37
Flow murmur, 190–191
Fontan procedure, 332f
Fourth heart sound (S₄), 135–138
  absent, 138
  auscultation of, 136f
  hemodynamics of, 62
Friction rubs, 96
Friedreich's ataxia, 254t

Gaisbock syndrome, 254t
Gallavardin murmur, 162t
Gallops, 142–144
  phonophonic representation of, 140f
  presystolic, 142
  protodiastolic, 143–144
  summation, 143
Gibson murmur, 162t
Glenn procedure, 332f
Graham Steell murmur, 162t
Great arteries, transposition of. See Transposition of the great arteries (TGA)

Hand, tendon xanthoma of, 87f
Hand grip, in dynamic auscultation, 37

Head/neck, abnormalities of, in syndromes with cardiovascular symptoms, 272t–273t
Headphone stethoscope, 14, 15f
Hearing
  physiology of, 6
  selective, 5
Heart
  rupture of, post-traumatic, 236–237
  traumatic injury to, 235–236
    penetrating, 238–239
Heart block
  complete, Cannon venous waves in, 269f
  congenital, 327
Heart disease
  acquired, echocardiography in, 308–309
  congenital, 316t
    ECG in, 302–303
    electrophysiological abnormalities in, 328, 332–333
    surgical treatment of, 328–332
      complications of, 329t
  in pregnancy, 237–238
  symptoms and signs of, clinical evaluation of, 281–293
  valvular, 73–87
Heart failure, 103–106, 228–229
  congestive, 105
    S₃ in, 141
  emergency treatment of, 229
  high-output, 106
  left, 104
  low-output, 106
  right, 105
    and mitral stenosis, pulmonary hypertension with, signs of, 194t
Heart murmur(s)
  audibility of, 3–4, 5f
  changing, 198–199
  classification of, 163–166
  continuous, 199–205
    acoustic spectrogram of, 200f
    algorithm for auscultation of, 199f
  diastolic, 189–198
    algorithm for treatment of, 191f
    early, 195–198
      algorithm for auscultation of, 196f

flow, 190–191
mid-, 189–195
  algorithm for auscultation of, 190f
  differential diagnosis of, 195
eponymous, 162t. *See also specific*
  murmur
grading of, 166t
mechanics of, 163
phonophonics of, 166t
right ventricular outflow tract,
  167–168
supraclavicular, 168
systolic, 162–189
  early, 184–186
    acoustic spectrogram of, 188f
    algorithm for auscultation of, 185f
  holo-, 181–184
    acoustic spectrogram of, 182f
    algorithm for auscultation of, 181f
  innocent, 23, 166–167
  late, 186–189
    acoustic spectrogram of, 188f
    algorithm for auscultation of, 187f
  mid-, 166–180
    acoustic spectrogram of, 168f
    algorithm for auscultation of, 167f
    stenotic, 171–180
  systolic ejection, 168–180
  timing and associated causes of,
    164t–165t
  to-and-fro, 205–206
    algorithm for auscultation of, 206f
Heart sound(s)
  first (S_1), 18–19, 114–124
    absence of, 120
    hemodynamics of, 58–60
    loud, 115–116
      interpretation of, 116f
      in mitral valve prolapse, 118f
    malposition of, 135
    PR interval and, phonophonic
      representation of, 116f
    soft, 116–120
    split, 122–124
      conditions characterized by, 122t
      differentiation of, 123f
    variations in, 120–122
      conditions causing, 117t

second (S_2), 19, 128–135
  acoustic obliteration of, in aortic
    and pulmonary stenosis,
    phonophonic representation of,
    131f
  hemodynamics of, 61
  loud, 129–130
    sounds and causes of, 130f
  loudness/timing of, variations in, in
    pulmonary and aortic area, 129f
  malposition of, 135
  physiological pseudosplitting of, 133
  and shunts, 135
  single, 134–135
  split, 132–134
    fixed, 133–134
    phonophonic representation of,
      132f
    physiological (A_2P_2), 133
    reversed (P_2A_2), 132–133
    variations of, 136t
    wide, 134
  tissue Doppler imaging of, 11f
  third (S_3), 138–141
    causes of audible, 139f
    hemodynamics of, 61
    physiological, 141
    pseudo-, 141
  fourth (S_4), 135–138
    absent, 138
    auscultation of, 136f
    hemodynamics of, 62
  audibility of, 3–4, 5f
  diastolic, 129t, 135–141
  end systolic, 128–135
  hemodynamics of, 51–69
  normal
    at different locations, 20f
    timing and amplitude of, 115t
  pitches and character of, 114t
  systolic, 114–128
  venous waves and events associated
    with, 268t
Heart valves. *See also specific valve*
  prosthetic, 146–151
    phonophonic representation of, 147f
  traumatic injury to, 237
Hemodynamic diagrams, 52–53
Hemoptysis, 289

Herpes zoster, chest pain in, 228
High-output heart failure, 106
High-output states
  S₃ in, 140
  systolic ejection murmur and,
    169–170
History, 248–253
  family, 252
  past medical, 252
  principles of taking, 248–249
  social, 249
HOCM. *See* Hypertrophic obstructive
    cardiomyopathy (HOCM)
Holosystolic murmur, 181–184
  acoustic spectrogram of, 182f
  algorithm for auscultation of, 181f
Holt-Oram syndrome, 254t
Homan's sign, 265t
Hurler's syndrome, 254t
Hutchinson's syndrome, 254t
Hyperlipidemia, 84–86
Hypertension, 100–103
  forms of, schematic diagrams of, 101f
  pulmonary, 100–103
    auscultatory findings in, 102f
    causes and subtypes of, 104f
    chest x-ray of, 103f
    mechanisms and clinical conditions
      associated with, 102t
    middiastolic murmur in, 194–195
    P₂ in, 104t, 131f
    primary, pulsus paradoxus in, 260f
    with right heart failure and mitral
      stenosis, signs of, 194t
  systemic, 100
  systolic ejection murmur and, 170
Hypertrophic obstructive
    cardiomyopathy (HOCM), 92–93
  hemodynamics of, 67, 89
  midsystolic murmur in, 177–179
  pathology of, 93
  physical findings in, 93
  pressure curves in, 67f, 178f
Hyperventilation, acute, 286
Hypotension. *See also* Shock
  auscultatory findings in, 231t
  orthostatic, 287–288
Hypothyroidism, head/neck
    abnormalities in, 272t
Hypovolemic shock, 230–232

Imaging, 305–310
  modalities of, and associated clinical
    conditions, 306t
Infective endocarditis, 99–100
  physical findings in, 100
Infundibular pulmonary stenosis,
    179–180
Innocent murmurs, 23, 166–167
Inspiratory dyspnea, 286
Intercostal collateral arteries, 203
Intraaortic hematoma, chest pain in,
    224
Ischemia
  pretest probability of, factors in, 223t
  silent, 75
Ischemic cascade, 76f
Isotonic exercise, in dynamic
    auscultation, 37

Jaccoud's arthritis, 254t
Janeway lesions, 265t
Jugular venous hum, 201–202
Jugular venous pressure, measurement
    of, 266–267

Kaposi's sarcoma, 254t
Kawasaki syndrome, 254t
Kearns-Sayre syndrome, head/neck
    abnormalities in, 272t
Klinefelter's syndrome, 255t
Klippel-Feil syndrome, 255t
  head/neck abnormalities in, 272t
Knee-chest position, 34–35
Knee-elbow position, 34–35
Korotkoff sounds, 265t
Kussmaul's sign, 265t

Learman's murmur, 162t
Left heart enlargement, 105f, 106f
Left heart failure, 104
Left ventricle
  tissue Doppler imaging of, 310f
  traumatic injury to, 236
Left ventricular clot, echocardiogram
    of, 150f

Left ventricular dysfunction, on chest x-ray, 101f
Left ventricular impulses, 276–277
Lentige's syndrome, 255t
Levine's sign, 265t
Libman-Sacks endocarditis, 255t
  head/neck abnormalities in, 272t
Liver, enlarged, 278–279
Locke's murmur, 162t
Loeffler's syndrome, 255t
Low-output heart failure, 106
Lupus erythematosus, head/neck abnormalities in, 272t

Magnetic resonance imaging (MRI), 305–307
  fast cine, 306–307
Male genitalia, examination of, 278
Mammary soufflé, 22f, 204
Maneuvers, 40–44. *See also specific maneuver*
Marfan's syndrome, 255t
  head/neck abnormalities in, 272t
Mean's murmur, 162t
Middiastolic murmur, 189–195
  algorithm for auscultation of, 190f
  differential diagnosis of, 195
  flow, 190–191
Midsystolic murmur, 166–180
  acoustic spectrogram of, 168f
  algorithm for auscultation of, 167f
  stenotic, 171–180
Migraine, pulse and, 263
Mitral regurgitation, 80–81
  acute, 81
    early systolic murmur in, 184–185
    hemodynamics of, 65f
  causes of, 182t
  holosystolic murmur in, 181–183
  massive, Doppler imaging of, 183f
  S₃ in, 141
Mitral stenosis, 78–80
  acoustic spectrogram of, 192f
  clinical features of, 79
  differential diagnosis of, 79–80
  hemodynamic changes in, 78–79
  middiastolic murmur in, 191–194

physical findings in, 79
  right heart failure and, pulmonary hypertension with, 194t
  TEE and Doppler imaging of, 193f
Mitral valve
  prosthetic, 149–151
  repair of, 151
  tissue Doppler imaging of, 310f
Mitral valve prolapse, 82–83
  causes of, 82
  clinical features of, 82–83
  flattening of spine in, 83f
  late systolic murmur in, 187–189
  loud S₁, late systolic/diastolic clicks in, 118f
  M-mode echocardiogram of, 188f
  prognosis for, 83
Mitral valve ring, calcification of, 84, 185
  2-D echocardiogram of, 170f
Morton's syndrome, chest pain in, 224
Mouth, abnormalities of, in syndromes with cardiovascular symptoms, 274
MRI (magnetic resonance imaging), 305–307
  fast cine, 306–307
Mulibrey nanism, head/neck abnormalities in, 273t
Müller maneuver, 44
Muscular disorders, cardiovascular abnormalities and, 280–281
Musculoskeletal examination, 280–281
Musset's sign, 265t
Mustard-Senning procedure, 326f
Myocardial infarction (MI), 76
  chest pain in, 221–223
  ECG in, 305
  heart failure with, 228
  phonophonic representation of, 77f
  ruling out, 223
Myocardial rupture, 232–233
Myocarditis, 91
Myocardium, ischemic, 75f
Myotonia dystrophica, head/neck abnormalities in, 273t

Nanism, mulibrey, head/neck abnormalities in, 273t

Neck, abnormalities of, in syndromes with cardiovascular symptoms, 272t–273t
NECs. *See* Nonejection clicks
Neurogenic shock, 234
Nocturnal orthopnea, 283
Nonejection clicks (NECs), 125–127
  absence of, 127
  hemodynamics of, 60–61
  phonophonic representation of, 126f
Noonan's syndrome, 255t
  head/neck abnormalities in, 273t

Obesity, head/neck abnormalities in, 273t
Obstetric stethoscopes, 11
Obstructive shock, 233–234
Opening snaps (OS), 144–145
  hemodynamics of, 62
  phonophonic representation of, 145f
Orthopnea, nocturnal, 283
Orthostatic hypotension, 287–288
Ortner's syndrome, 255t
OS. *See* Opening snaps (OS)
Osler-Rendu-Weber syndrome, 255t
Osler's nodes, 265t
Osteogenesis imperfecta, head/neck abnormalities in, 273t
Ostium primum, ECG in, 303–304

P_2. *See* Pulmonary valve closure (P_2)
Pacemaker sound, 128
Palpation
  chest, 275
  in position 3, 28–29
  pulse. *See* Pulse
Palpitations, 290–291
Papillary muscle dysfunction, 189
Paroxysmal nocturnal dyspnea, 283
Patent ductus arteriosus, 319
  continuous murmur in, 199–201
  Doppler imaging of, 200f
  surgical treatment of, 329–330
PDA. *See* Patent ductus arteriosus
Pediatric cardiology, adult. *See* Adult pediatric cardiology

Pediatric stethoscopes, 11, 12f
Penetrating injuries, to heart, 238–239
Percussion
  chest, 275–276
  in position 3, 28
Pericardial diseases, 96–99
Pericardial effusion, 97
Pericardial friction rubs, 96
Pericardial knock, 144
Pericardial tamponade, 97
  echocardiographic sign of, 61
  hemodynamics of, 59–61
  pressure curves in, 62f
  severe, pressure curves in, 64f
  venous pulse in, 270f
Pericarditis
  chest pain in, 224
  constrictive, 97–99
    hemodynamics of, 68–69
    pulsus paradoxus in, 260f
    triad of signs in, 68f
    venous pulse in, 271f
  schematic diagram of, 98f
PET (positron emission tomography) scan, clinical conditions detectable by, 306t
Pharynx, abnormalities of, in syndromes with cardiovascular symptoms, 274
Pheochromocytoma
  dyspnea in, 285–286
  head/neck abnormalities in, 273t
Phonocardiography, 310
Pigmentation, changes in, 274
Pleurisy, chest pain in, 224–225
Pleurodynia, 226
Pneumomediastinum, acute, chest pain in, 226
Pneumothorax, chest pain in, 225–226
Polychondritis, head/neck abnormalities in, 273t
Polymyositis/dermatomyositis, head/neck abnormalities in, 273t
Positron emission tomography (PET), clinical conditions detectable by, 306t
Postpause, in dynamic auscultation, 44
Potts procedure, 322f, 323

PR interval, phonophonic representation of, 116f
Pregnancy, 333–335
  auscultation in, 21
  ejection sound and mammary soufflé in, 22f
  heart disease in
    auscultatory findings in, 333–334
    management of, 334–335
  normal, auscultatory findings in, 333
Prescription medications, cardiac emergencies related to, 235
Pressure curves
  in aortic regurgitation, 63f
  in aortic stenosis, 64f
  ECG with, 52f, 54f, 55f, 56f, 57f, 59f
  in HOCM, 62f, 178f
  during inspiration and expiration, 58f
  in tamponade, 62f, 69f
Presystolic clicks, pulmonary stenosis and, 128
Presystolic gallop, 142
Prinzmetal's angina, 75–76
Prosthetic valves, 146–151
  phonophonic representation of, 147f
Protodiastolic gallop, 143–144
Pseudoaneurysm, 86f, 233
Pseudoejection clicks, 127
Pseudohypertension, 266
Pseudo-third heart sound (pseudo-S_3), 141
Psychoacoustics, 6
Pulmonary area, auscultation of, 20
Pulmonary arteriovenous fistula, 203
Pulmonary atresia, 180
Pulmonary branch stenosis, 204
Pulmonary clicks, absence of, 127
Pulmonary disease, chronic obstructive, auscultation in, 35
Pulmonary edema, syndrome of early, 283
Pulmonary ejection sounds, 125
Pulmonary embolism, chest pain in, 226
Pulmonary hypertension, 100–103
  auscultatory findings in, 102f
  causes and subtypes of, 104f
  chest x-ray of, 103f
  mechanisms and clinical conditions associated with, 102t
  middiastolic murmur in, 194–195
  P_2 in, 104t, 131f
  primary, pulsus paradoxus in, 260f
  with right heart failure and mitral stenosis, signs of, 194t
Pulmonary regurgitation, 91
  early diastolic murmur in, 198
  organic, middiastolic murmur in, 195
Pulmonary stenosis, 90–91
  acoustic obliteration of S_2 in, phonophonic representation of, 131f
  chest x-rays in, 90f, 179f
  differentiation of, 180t
  ECG in, 305
  infundibular, 179–180
  midsystolic murmur in, 179
  pathology of, 90
  physical findings in, 91
  presystolic click of, 128
  pulsus paradoxus in, 260f
  surgical treatment of, 330
  symptoms of, 91
Pulmonary valve closure (P_2), 130–134
  auscultation of, in pulmonary hypertension, 104t
  loud, 130
  soft, 130–131
Pulse, 253–264
  anacrotic, 256–257
  bounding, 257
  carotid, 262–263
  collapsing, 257, 258f
  dicrotic, 253–256
  femoral, 263
  and migraine, 263
  normal, wave pattern in, 256f
  small volume/thready, 257
  temporal, 263
Pulse volume, 263–264
Pulseless disease, 263
Pulsus alternans, 261–262
Pulsus bisferiens, 257–259
Pulsus paradoxus, 259–261
  hemodynamics of, 65, 66f
  reversed, 261
Pulsus parvus, 173–174

Quadruple rhythm, 143–144
  phonophonic representation of, 143f
Quadruple sounds. *See* Fourth heart
  sound (S₄)
Quincke's sign, 265t

Radiculitis, herpes zoster and, 228
Radiography, 305
Rashes, 271–274
Rashkind septostomy, 322f
Rastelli procedure, 322f
Raynaud's phenomenon, 255t
Reflexes, examination of, 280
Reiter's syndrome, 255t
Renal disorders, head/neck
  abnormalities in, 273t
Restrictive cardiomyopathy, 93–94
  auscultatory findings in, 93
  physical findings in, 94
Retz syndrome, 255t
Review of systems, 252–253
Rheumatic fever
  auscultatory findings in, 78t
  Duckett Jones criteria for, 78t
  valvular sequelae of, 77–78
Right heart failure, 105
  and mitral stenosis, pulmonary
    hypertension with, signs of, 194t
Right ventricle, traumatic injury to,
  236
Right ventricular impulses, 277–278
Right ventricular outflow tract
  murmur, 167–168
Roth spots, 265t

S₁. *See* First heart sound (S₁)
S₂. *See* Second heart sound (S₂)
S₃. *See* Third heart sound (S₃)
S₄. *See* Fourth heart sound (S₄)
Sail sound, 128
Scratches, 127
Second heart sound (S₂), 19, 128–135
  acoustic obliteration of, in aortic and
    pulmonary stenosis, phonophonic
    representation of, 131f
  hemodynamics of, 61

loud, 129–130
  sounds and causes of, 130f
loudness/timing of, variations in, in
    pulmonary and aortic area, 129f
malposition of, 135
physiological pseudosplitting of, 133
and shunts, 135
single, 134–135
split, 132–134
  fixed, 133–134
  phonophonic representation of, 132f
  physiological (A₂P₂), 133
  reversed (P₂A₂), 132–133
  variations of, 136t
  wide, 134
tissue Doppler imaging of, 11f
Septic shock, 234
Shock, 229–234
  cardiogenic, 232
  clinical evaluation of, 230, 231f
  hypovolemic, 230–232
  neurogenic, 234
  obstructive, 233–234
  septic, 234
  types and common causes of, 230t
Shoulder-hand syndrome, 228
Shunts
  hemodynamics of, 67–68
  S₂ and, 135
Signs, eponymous, 265t. *See also*
    specific sign
Silent ischemia, 75
Sinus of Valsalva, anomalous origin of
    coronary arteries in, 205
Sitting position, 30–32
Skin
  examination of, 271–276
  of extremities, 280
  texture/elasticity of, changes in, 274
Snaps
  diastolic, 146
  opening (OS), 144–145
    hemodynamics of, 62
    phonophonic representation of, 145f
Social history, 249
Sound
  absorption of, 6
  physics of, 4

recognition of, 3–4, 5f
training effect of, 6–7
Special populations, auscultation in
    care of, 315–335
Spectrography, acoustic, 14
Spine
  abnormalities of, cardiovascular
      abnormalities and, 280–281
  flattening of, in mitral valve prolapse,
      83f
Squatting position, 33–34
Standing position, 32–33
Stethos, 13, 14f
Stethoscope(s)
  Bang & Olafsen, 14
  comparison of, 15
  electronic, 12–14
  esophageal, 12, 13f
  headphone, 14, 15f
  historical, 2–3
    binaural, 4f
    monaural, 3f
  obstetric, 11
  pediatric, 11, 12f
  placement of, positions for, 23–24
  speciality, 11–12
  standard, 7–11
    comparative features of, 11t
    dimensions of, 7–8
    earpieces of, 8
    examining end of, 8–11
      combination, 11
    recommended attributes for, 8t
    tubes of, 11
  Stethos, 13, 14f
Still's murmur, 23, 162t, 167
Stokes-Adams syncope, 255t, 289
Stress echocardiography, 312–313
Stress testing, 310–313
  forms/auscultatory results of, 313t
Subaortic stenosis, 176
Substance use
  cardiac emergencies related to,
      234–235
  in patient history, 249–252
Summation gallop, 143
Supine position
  45 degrees, 25–26

left lateral, 26–28
with or without legs elevated, 28–29
Supraaortic stenosis, 176
Supraclavicular murmur, 168
Supraventricular tachycardia, 95
Switch procedure, 322f
Syncope, 286–289
  auscultatory findings in, 288
  cardiogenic, 288
  causes of, 287–289
  Stokes-Adams, 255t, 289
  vasomotor, 287
Systemic embolism, 239–240
Systolic clicks, in mitral valve
      prolapse, 118f
Systolic ejection murmur, 168–180
Systolic heart sounds, 114–128
Systolic murmur, 162–189
  early, 184–186
    acoustic spectrogram of, 188f
    algorithm for auscultation of, 185f
  holo-, 181–184
    acoustic spectrogram of, 182f
    algorithm for auscultation of, 181f
  innocent, 23, 166–167
  late, 186–189
    acoustic spectrogram of, 188f
    algorithm for auscultation of, 187f
  mid-, 166–180
    acoustic spectrogram of, 168f
    algorithm for auscultation of, 167f
Systolic overload, ECG in, 304–305

Tachycardia
  supraventricular, 95
  ventricular, 95
Takayasu's syndrome, 255t, 261
Tamponade, 97
  echocardiographic sign of, 65–67
  hemodynamics of, 65
  pressure curves in, 66f
  severe, pressure curves in, 69f
  venous pulse in, 270f
Tangier's disease, 255t
Taussig-Bing syndrome, 255t
TEE (transesophageal
      echocardiography), 309

Temporal pulse, 263
Tendon xanthoma, 87f
Tests, cardiovascular structure and
    function, 250t–251t. *See also*
    specific test
Tetralogy of Fallot, 321–323
  ECG in, 304
  midsystolic murmur in, 180
  physical findings in, 321–323
  surgical procedures for, 322f, 330–331
  treatment of, 323
TGA. *See* Transposition of the great
    arteries (TGA)
Thallium scan, clinical conditions
    detectable by, 306t
Third heart sound (S_3), 138–141
  causes of audible, 139f
  hemodynamics of, 61
  physiological, 141
  pseudo-, 141
Thready pulse, 257
3M stethoscope, 13
Thrills, 144, 276
Thrombosis, deep venous, 240
Thyrotoxicosis, head/neck
    abnormalities in, 273t
Tietze's syndrome, 255t
  chest pain in, 228
Tissue Doppler imaging, 309, 310f,
    311f
To-and-fro murmur, 205–206
  algorithm for auscultation of, 206f
Train wheel sound, 143
Transesophageal echocardiography
    (TEE), 309
Transposition of the great arteries
    (TGA), 324–327
  comparison of normal circulation
    with, 324f
  congenital, 325–327
    treatment of, 327
  corrected, 324–325
    physical findings in, 324–325
    treatment of, 325
    ventricular inversion in, diagram of,
      325f
  surgical procedures for, 322f, 331
Traube's sign, 265t

Trauma
  to chest, blunt, 235
  to heart, 235–236
    penetrating, 238–239
  vascular, 237
Treadmill testing, 310–312
  phonophonic representation of
    auscultatory findings in, 312f
Tricuspid atresia, 327
  ECG in, 304
  surgical treatment of, 331–333
Tricuspid regurgitation, 89–90
  classification of, 89t
  with c-vy wave, 285f
  2-D imaging of, 184f
  early systolic murmur in, 186
  holosystolic murmur in, 184
  physical signs in, 90
  pulsus paradoxus in, 260f
Tricuspid stenosis, 89
  middiastolic murmur in, 195
  pulsus paradoxus in, 260f
  venous pulse in, 268f
Tricuspid valve
  prosthetic, 151
  repair of, 151
Triple ripple, 138
Tubes, stethoscope, 11
Tumor plops, 145–146
Tuning effect, 7
Turner's syndrome, 255t
  head/neck abnormalities in, 273t
"Type A" personality, head/neck
    abnormalities in, 272t

V wave, 270
Valsalva, sinus of, anomalous origin of
    coronary arteries in, 205
Valsalva maneuver, 42–44
Valvular heart disease, 77–91
  systolic ejection murmur and,
    170–171
Vascular auscultation, 36
Vascular emergencies, 239–240
Vascular trauma, 237
Vasomotor syncope, 287
Vein graft, patent, CT scan of, 307f

Venous blood pressure
  abnormalities of, 267–271
  measurement of, 266–271
Venous pulsations, identification of,
    267
Venous thrombosis, deep, 240
Venous waves, 267–271
  events and heart sounds associated
    with, 268t
Ventricular aneurysm, 86f
  ECG in, 305
  S_3 and S_4 in, 140
Ventricular contusion, 236
Ventricular inversion, in corrected
    TGA, diagram of, 325f
Ventricular septal defect, 318
  atypical murmurs of, 185–186
  holosystolic murmur in, 183
  surgical treatment of, 329
Ventricular septum, aneurysms of, 189
Ventricular tachycardia, 95

Vital signs, 253–271
VSD. *See* Ventricular septal defect

Waterston procedure, 322f, 323
Wave descents, venous, 270–271
Wenckebach rhythm, phonophonic
    representation of, 121f
Werner's syndrome, 255t
  head/neck abnormalities in, 273t
Whipple's disease, 255t
Williams' syndrome, 255t
  head/neck abnormalities in, 273t
Windsock sound, 128

X descent, 270
X' descent, 270
Xanthoma, tendon, 87f

Y descent, 270–271

DEMCO